Clinical Cas
Paediatri

A Trainee Handbook

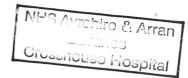

Clinical Cases in Paediatrics

A Trainee Handbook

Ashley Reece MBChB MSc FRCPCH Pg Cert (Med Ed)
Consultant Paediatrician
Department of Paediatrics, Watford General Hospital,
Watford, UK

Anthony Cohn MBBS MRCP FRCPCH
Consultant Paediatrician
Department of Paediatrics, Watford General Hospital,
Watford, UK

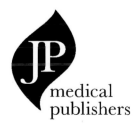

JP
medical
publishers

London • Philadelphia • Panama City • New Delhi

© 2014 JP Medical Ltd.
Published by JP Medical Ltd,
83 Victoria Street, London, SW1H 0HW, UK
Tel: +44 (0)20 3170 8910
Fax: +44 (0)20 3008 6180
Email: info@jpmedpub.com
Web: www.jpmedpub.com

The rights of Ashley Reece and Anthony Cohn to be identified as the editors of this work have been asserted by them in accordance with the Copyright, Designs and Patents Act 1988.

All brand names and product names used in this book are trade names, service marks, trademarks or registered trademarks of their respective owners. The publisher is not associated with any product or vendor mentioned in this book.

Medical knowledge and practice change constantly. This book is designed to provide accurate, authoritative information about the subject matter in question. However readers are advised to check the most current information available on procedures included and check information from the manufacturer of each product to be administered, to verify the recommended dose, formula, method and duration of administration, adverse effects and contraindications. It is the responsibility of the practitioner to take all appropriate safety precautions. Neither the publisher nor the editors assume any liability for any injury and/or damage to persons or property arising from or related to use of material in this book.

This book is sold on the understanding that the publisher is not engaged in providing professional medical services. If such advice or services are required, the services of a competent medical professional should be sought.

Every effort has been made where necessary to contact holders of copyright to obtain permission to reproduce copyright material. If any have been inadvertently overlooked, the publisher will be pleased to make the necessary arrangements at the first opportunity.

ISBN: 978-1-907816-47-5

British Library Cataloguing in Publication Data
A catalogue record for this book is available from the British Library

Library of Congress Cataloging in Publication Data
A catalog record for this book is available from the Library of Congress

JP Medical Ltd is a subsidiary of Jaypee Brothers Medical Publishers (P) Ltd, New Delhi, India

Commissioning Editor: Steffan Clements
Editorial Assistant: Sophie Woolven
Design: Designers Collective Ltd

Copy edited, typeset, printed and bound in India.

Preface

Paediatric trainees in their first years of training rapidly develop the skills and knowledge required to manage acute paediatric problems. But with greater experience comes a new set of challenges which require more reflection than reaction; nowhere are these more evident than in the outpatient setting or paediatric clinic. Changes in paediatric practice over the last few decades mean that many conditions are now managed more or less exclusively in the outpatient setting, where previously they would be managed on the wards. For doctors who have spent their first few years learning on the wards and in emergency departments, this means tackling a new set of problems which require a different set of 'tools'.

Clinical Cases in Paediatrics: A Trainee Handbook has been written in response to these changes, to provide paediatric trainees with the practical guidance they need as they start to manage patients in the outpatient clinic. We also believe that this book will prove extremely useful for those preparing for work-place based assessments, supervised learning events and postgraduate examinations and assessments.

One of the great advantages of editing this book has been that we have also been able to learn from our colleagues' expertise. There have been numerous occasions when, in our own clinics, we have been able to refer to the chapters submitted when we felt we wanted more information.

Whilst we have presented cases in a fairly formal way, we are aware that there are often many ways to manage a problem. Whilst we hope that this book will provide effective strategies for dealing with many of the children seen in paediatric clinics, we do not claim a monopoly on the truth, and encourage people to follow their own teaching and local advice.

Ashley Reece
Anthony Cohn
December 2013

Acknowledgements

We are grateful on a daily basis to be part of the paediatric team at West Hertfordshire Hospitals. Our patients and colleagues make coming to work a true pleasure.

One of the great strengths of our team – in no small measure down to our long serving Clinical Director, Emmanuel Quist-Therson – is that each of us is given the encouragement to develop individually and we feel completely supported in our work.

This is a multi-author work and we would not have been able to complete it without all of our contributors. Their knowledge highlighted gaps in our own and we have learned so much from reading their work. We realise that some of them found the challenge daunting, but we hope they share our pleasure and satisfaction in the completed work. We are delighted to have contributions from other consultants in the Trust with whom we work closely and are especially gratified that some of our former trainees, who are still very much 'part of the family', have been able to contribute as well.

Thanks to everyone at JP Medical, in particular Steffan Clements, who stood by us as deadlines came and went.

Working together has strengthened our great friendship and we are both fortunate to be supported in our endeavours by our families. To Julie, Danielle, Gav, Eitan, Elny, Natasha and Strudel we owe you everything and you make everything worthwhile.

AR, AC

Dedication

For Danielle, Natasha and my dear parents who have always supported me, my education and endeavours; and my dear late grandparents who would have been so proud.

AR

For Julie, Gav, Eitan, Elny, Opa and Oma o'h

AC

Contents

Contributors

Freddie Banks MD FRCS (Urol)
Cases 32, 74
Consultant Urologist
Watford General Hospital,
Watford, UK

Kapila Batta MBChB MRCP MRCGP
Cases 3, 28
Consultant Dermatologist
Watford General Hospital,
Watford, UK

Anthony Cohn MBBS MRCP FRCPCH
Chapters 1, 2, 3, 5; Cases 1, 9, 10, 11, 13, 15, 16, 17, 18, 19, 23, 37, 41, 42, 47, 49, 51, 56, 57, 61, 63, 70, 71, 77
Consultant Paediatrician
Watford General Hospital,
Watford, UK

Carole Anne Colford MBBS MRCPCH
Cases 21, 22
Consultant Community Paediatrican
St Albans Children's Centre,
St Albans, UK

Amanda Equi MBChB MRCP MRCPCH
Case 8
Consultant Paediatrician
Watford General Hospital,
Watford, UK

Neeti Ghali MBChB MRCPCH MD
Case 45
Consultant Clinical Geneticist
Northwick Park & St Marks Hospital,
Harrow, UK

John Heckmatt MBChB MD FRCP FRCPCH
Chapter 6; Cases 14, 20, 53, 75
Consultant Community Paediatrician
Peace Children's Centre,
Watford, UK

Jane Hislop BA MB BChir MRCP FRCPCH
Cases 46, 62, 78
Consultant Community Paediatrician
Pat Lewis Children's Centre,
Hemel Hempstead, UK

Ritika Kapoor MBBS MRCPCH PhD
Case 68
Consultant Paediatric Endocrinologist
Kings College Hospital,
London, UK

Vasanta Nanduri MBChB MRCP MRCGP
Cases 7, 44, 58, 67, 69
Consultant Paediatrician
Watford General Hospital,
Watford, UK

Sankara Narayanan MBBS MD MRCPCH
Cases 43, 66
Consultant Paediatrician,
Watford General Hospital,
Watford, UK

Rohit Pratap MBBS BSc DLO MRCS FRCS (ORL-HNS)
Cases 40, 65
Consultant Otolaryngologist
Watford General Hospital,
Watford, UK

Emmanuel C Quist-Therson MBChB MRCP FRCPCH DCH
Cases 39, 48, 76
Consultant Paediatrician
Watford General Hospital,
Watford, UK

Chaniyil A Ramesh MBBS DCH MRCP FRCPCH
Fellowship Neonatology(Toronto)
Cases 2, 24, 34
Consultant Paediatrician
Watford General Hospital,
Watford, UK

Ashley Reece MBChB MSc FCRPCH Pg Cert (Med Ed)
Chapters 2, 7; Cases 4, 5, 6, 12, 26, 30, 33, 35, 54, 55, 60, 64, 72, 79
Consultant Paediatrician
Watford General Hospital,
Watford, UK

Katharine Riley BSc MBBS MRCPCH
Cases 31, 73
Consultant Paediatrician
Hinchingbrooke Hospital,
Huntingdon, UK

Viji Rudran MBBS DCH MRCP FRCPCH
Case 25
Consultant Community Paediatrician
Peace Children's Centre,
Watford, UK

Pearl Selvadurai MBBS DCH FRCPCH MSc
Case 38
Consultant Community Paediatrician
Peace Children's Centre,
Watford, UK

Pradnya Sheth MBBS DCH MD MRCP MRCPCH
Cases 36, 59
Consultant Paediatrician
Watford General Hospital,
Watford, UK

Zdenek Slavik MD FRCPCH
Case 52
Consultant Cardiologist
Royal Brompton Hospital,
London, UK

Eduardo Szaniecki PgDip DCP MTSP MRCPsych
Chapter 4
Consultant Child and Adolescent Psychiatrist
Hertfordshire Partnership NHS Foundation Trust,
St Albans, UK

Deepshikha Thakur MBBS MD (Paediatrics) MRCPCH
Case 9
Consultant Community Paediatrician
Peace Children's Centre,
Watford, UK

Chee Toh BSc MBBS FRCS(ORL-HNS) FRCS ENT FRCS ENT Ed FRCS
Cases 29, 50
Consultant ENT Surgeon
Watford General Hospital,
Watford, UK

Anthony Vandersteen MA PhD BM MRCP
Case 27
Consultant Clinical Geneticist
Northwick Park & St Marks Hospital,
Harrow, UK

Section 1

Introductory chapters

Chapter 1

How to run the clinic

Basic paediatric training is heavily focussed on providing immediate solutions to acute paediatric problems. The outpatient clinic is quite different from the acute setting. The conditions that present here will be more long term and often more complex with solutions that are not always straightforward, if they exist at all.

Preparing for clinic

It is sensible to check the notes of the patients who are due in clinic. If possible discuss the cases with the consultant before the clinic starts. This can provide a reasonable general approach to the patient but should not be allowed to cloud future judgement because:
- The original symptoms may have resolved and the patient may have other issues
- The symptoms may have changed and a different course of action may be required
- Previous assessments may be wrong
- The referral letter may not address what the patient perceives is the main problem

Preparing the room

There will be a limit to the changes that can be made, but think about the geography of the consultation. There are many obvious things like trying not to place a desk between yourself and the family, so think about the best way of arranging the chairs. If the patients' chairs are near an overhanging cupboard and whenever they stand up they bang their heads then move the chairs or remove the cupboard.

Try sitting in the chairs that the patient will sit in–what does it feel like? If there is a desk, don't leave confidential information, such as the last patient's file, open so that another patient can read it. If there is a computer, think about what is on the screen.

Who should sit on which chair? Generally the patient would be expected to sit next to the doctor. In paediatrics this will be the child or young person. This may mean directing the child to a particular chair 'come on Jennifer, you are the important one, I would like you to sit in this important chair here.'

There are other things that you can't control but may be able to mitigate, as follows.

Noise and disruption

If there are major building works outside, be prepared for a difficult clinic. However, don't make life needlessly hard. For example, most clinic rooms will have a selection of toys: the noisy toys can be relegated to the waiting area.

Siblings can be a further source of disruption, and it is invariably the younger sibling who is jealous of the attention given to an older one, who will do their best to interrupt the clinic and steal the parent's attention. Parents should be encouraged to try to ignore this and focus on the patient. Let the parents know that you have seen this before, and even if it is the worst behaviour you have ever seen, reassure them that it is not.

Light

Make sure that there is adequate light for a good examination. It is always wonderful to have the sun streaming through the windows, but if it is landing directly in the patient's eyes then rearrange the room or close the blinds and switch on the electric lights. Make sure that other people cannot look into the clinic room.

Smell

Bad nappy smells are unpleasant for everyone. If the room seems smelly, imagine what a new patient might feel walking into it. Clearing smells can be difficult. Try opening the windows and doors, using any available air freshener. It is polite to explain to subsequent patients 'excuse us, there has been a bit of a nasty nappy, I have done my best to make it bearable.' It might be desirable or necessary to try and relocate to a different room.

Interruptions

These should be kept to a minimum. In some clinics the team will bring each patient's notes into the consulting room as the patient arrives in clinic. In mid-consultation, the clinic nurse might come in three times, each time bringing a set of notes. This seems rude and intrusive. The nurses are only doing that because that is how other doctors have worked before. You can change things. Ask them to leave the notes outside the room, then after saying goodbye to one patient, pick up the notes of the next one.

Phones and bleeps are more of an issue. Parents may be forgiven for forgetting to turn their phone off, but the doctor should be polite enough to avoid taking any calls which are not clinically urgent. Try to keep these interruptions to a minimum, switching off phones and bleeps wherever possible.

Preparing yourself

A clinic requires a specific type of focus: make sure that you are calm and able to focus, and that any physiological needs have been addressed before meeting a patient.

Making conversations work

The consultation is the heart of medicine, yet it is something that we often get very limited training in. Numerous studies show that as doctors we talk too much and listen too little, giving our patients between 10% and 40% of the consultation time to talk, and using the rest ourselves. This is unfortunate because study after study shows that the more a patient is allowed to talk the higher they rate the consultation experience, and better consultations have been shown to:

- Make patients happier and more content
- Make them more likely to adhere to the treatment plan
- Make them less likely to complain
- Increase doctors' job satisfaction

Doctors tend to believe that if they give patients free reign and let them speak, they will go on for hours. The evidence suggests that if you ask them 'what is the problem?' and then listen attentively without interrupting, the overwhelming majority of patients will speak for < 2 minutes. During this time they will give you essentially all the information you will need.

Unfortunately, it seems that this is beyond most of us, and patients are invariably interrupted after about 22 seconds. This puts them off their track and makes them feel that they are bothering the doctor. Clinic skills are something that we all have to work on.

In paediatrics the issue arises of how the child should be involved. The answer is 'as much as possible'. Even very young children are able to give some history and will want to understand what is going on. Obviously, the parents are essential for corroboration and elucidation as some children may be unable to give a complete history or may decide to play 'opposites' – giving all the wrong answers on purpose.

As regards explanations, it is easy to overestimate the medical knowledge of patients who may be too polite and/or intimidated to admit that they have only a fleeting recollection of the path of the facial nerve. Therefore, directing explanations to the child in a style of language that a child can understand means that the parents are more likely to understand this explanation as well. The message can be reinforced by explaining the same thing to the parents in slightly more sophisticated terms.

Writing and listening

Clearly there is a need to record the consultation. Unfortunately, what normally happens is that the doctor speaks to the patient, and when the patient replies the doctor writes this down. This means that there is only eye contact when the doctor is talking, and the implication is that the doctor is not really focussing on the patient's answers. Solving this is difficult, but can be done, e.g. by only making brief notes and completing them afterwards.

The consultation

The consultation can be divided into four components (Kurtz et al. 2003)
1. Initiating the session
2. Gathering information
3. Explaining and planning
4. Closing the session

An underlying theme of all parts is taking into account the patient's agenda. Old attitudes – that patients' problems primarily provide intellectual interest or that doctors should only have to deal with organic pathology – have no place in modern practice. Actually, what matters most is what the patient thinks and needs. Consider the patient's **ICE**:
- Ideas about what the cause of their problem is
- Concerns about the implications of their problem and
- Expectations about management and outcome

It can be useful to use direct questions in this respect:
- What did you want to happen in clinic today?
- What is it that you are most worried about?
- Does my explanation make sense or are there areas that I need to try to explain better?
- Is the treatment plan manageable (e.g. if mornings at home are chaotic can medications be prescribed for the afternoon)?

During the consultation, it is essential to continuously keep in mind the patient's perspective.

Initiating the session

This starts by meeting and greeting the patient. There are some clinicians who let the clinic nurse or medical students call the new patient, who is ushered in as the doctor finishes off dictating notes on the patient who has just left. Remarkably, this rudeness still continues.

Go out to greet the patient. This means going to the waiting room and calling them. If they are accompanied by their parents there is a dilemma of who to greet first (are you a childrens' paediatrician or an adults' paediatrician?). Remember it is hard to over-involve the child in the consultation. As the child is the patient it seems appropriate to greet them first, and offering your hand in a friendly, 'grown up' manner is often a good ice breaker. Decide how to introduce yourself and what you want to be called, also ascertain this for the child and parents. The dialogue might be:

'Hello, are you Johnny?'

[*Shake hands.*]

'My name is Matilda and I am the doctor that you are going to see today, please come along to my room.'

[*After engaging with the child, greet the parents.*]

'Hi, my name is Dr ..., I am Professor ...'s paediatric registrar.'

It is always good to engage the child during the walk to the room, discussing their clothing, hair or soft toy that they have brought along. Sometimes, the discussion with the child can be so absorbing that the parents get overlooked. As long as they become involved, most parents will happily forgive this oversight.

At the beginning the child is likely to be nervous. Any reassurance now will help, but don't give false reassurance. Most children will be scared that they are going to have to undergo a painful test. If it is clear that this is not going to be necessary, say so from the outset.

Gathering information

Think about how to take a history. In an acute setting, the essence is to make a rapid diagnosis and treatment plan – it is more hierarchical in that the doctor determines and often delivers treatment. In outpatients it is more about establishing a collaborative relationship with the patient to agree a longer term treatment plan which they will administer.

The first goal is to put the patient at ease. This is usually done by 'small talk' but actually this often provides the most important information. It is so much more than just setting the scene, which is why it fits more neatly under the heading of gathering information rather than initiating the session. Rather than starting the consultation by asking 'what is the problem?' you can start by taking the demographic data.

Remember that in all peoples' lives there are factors which are going to impact on their health. For example, if a child is being bullied at school, or has recently been bereaved, this may not only be an underlying cause for physical symptoms but is also likely to impact on management of chronic organic disease.

Consider a child with poorly controlled diabetes; it is easy to think of numerous social and psychological reasons why this may be the case, and simply asking her to take more insulin, without addressing the other issues is unlikely to improve her condition.

Don't forget to give acknowledgement and positive feedback, rather than just nodding or grunting in response to the questions. Many people just say 'OK' when given any answer. This can be misplaced. If a mother explains 'He is a bit upset today because my husband just ran over the dog on the way to his mother's funeral,' have a better response than a nod and saying 'OK.'

Standard opening questions would include:

- How old are you now?.... so you are a really big boy
- Which school do you go to?
- Which year are you in?
- Who is your teacher? .... what is she like?
- What is your school like?
- What do you like best about school?
- Is there anything that you don't like about school?
- How many brothers and sisters have you got?
- What are their names?
- How old are they?
- Who lives at home with you?
- Do you have any pets?

Be prepared for where these questions might lead. Major issues at home or school may come to light; be prepared to address these (most patients do not get upset about seemingly intrusive questions, as long as they are asked sensitively and seem relevant.).

Once a rapport is established, gather information about the 'presenting complaint'. It should go without saying to avoid leading questions and remember that repeating the last few words of somebody's last sentence gives them the impetus to carry on.

Carry on, as mentioned before; try to let the patient speak without interruption and, as much as possible, make the child the patient. From the letter and history begin making a differential diagnosis, using supplemental questions which will allow this to be narrowed, rather than firing off a random checklist of questions. For example, if the differential diagnosis is narrowed down to 2 or 3 most likely causes the questions should focus on these.

Beware of limited thinking. It is easy to presume a diagnosis and cling to this, even in the presence of mounting evidence that it is not the correct one. A favourite aphorism is: 'if you are barking up the wrong tree you have two options. The first, which is most commonly practised, is to simply bark louder, whilst the second more sensible one is to find another tree.'

Be prepared to challenge not just your assumptions, but also the assumptions of others. Everybody gets things wrong sometimes. If another doctor, of whatever grade, has seen a patient and made a diagnosis, but seems to have missed a more likely one, it is essential to discuss this with the doctor concerned – who may be grateful rather than exasperated. Clearly how this is discussed is important and having a blazing row in front of the patient is unlikely to be of benefit to anybody.

For the majority of problems the history alone will suggest the diagnosis or have significantly narrowed the possibilities. Now comes the physical examination. Much has been written about the value of physical examination, with perhaps its greatest value being the 'laying on of hands.' Even if the diagnosis seems certain from the history, patients may feel short changed if they have not had a physical examination.

Whilst the physical examination should be focussed, it should not appear dismissive. Again, think about language. The same examination may be preceded by 'Let's just have a quick look at your tummy' or 'I am interested in your tummy – and I would like to have a good look it.' Which of these sounds most reassuring (the opposite may be more appropriate for sensitive examinations)?

Try to explain exactly what is going to happen. Children expect that a trip to the doctor may be painful, and it is important to be honest with them. If they are just having a physical examination they should be reassured that nothing horrible is going to happen.

There are often issues of consent and invasion of privacy. This may appear at any age, but especially in older children. Remember that it is highly unlikely that the examination will make the difference between life and death. In some cases a suitable colleague may be able to help, e.g. children may prefer to be examined by a doctor of the same sex. In other cases gentle negotiation may generate consent, but if they still refuse and you examine the child then this could constitute an assault.

Explaining and planning

Think about what words to use. If the child is going to be included, use language that they can understand. It is helpful to pause frequently asking if anybody has any questions.

The discussion will involve either a clear diagnosis or a number of possibilities. The absence of an exact diagnosis should not prevent appropriate reassurance. For example, 'I am not entirely sure what is causing your tummy pains, but I am confident that there is nothing about them that makes me think that you have a serious underlying condition.' At this stage further tests might be considered. They can often confirm a diagnosis, exclude a serious differential diagnosis, or identify the appropriate management. But before ordering a test it is worth asking the following:

- Will it change the management? If the diagnosis seems clear how will this test change things?
- What is the 'cost' of the test? Consider:
  - The child: is the test safe (e.g. does it involve radiation exposure), will it hurt, and will school or other activities have to be missed?
  - The family: will they have to see the child being distressed by the test, will they have to miss work and will there be high fees?
  - The organisation: paying for 10 MRI for simple headaches is not a good use of funds
- How will the family get the results?

Most tests are probably unnecessary, and it is worth thinking about each one. Unfortunately, in some clinics there will be a requirement that certain tests are 'routinely' performed. This may be due either to clinical necessity or consultant idiosyncrasy. Whilst ordering the tests, for educational purposes always ask why they are necessary and consider whether or not you would order them if you were in charge.

When ordering a test or investigation, it helps to know exactly what it will entail, including how long any wait will be. So, become familiar with common tests. Some may be carried out in other hospitals and again this should be explained to the family. Have some idea of the wait, and avoid false promises. For example, if the average wait for an MRI is 6 weeks, suggesting it will be performed tomorrow, is unhelpful to the patient and hospital.

As regards radiological examinations, specific guidelines are available from the Royal College of Radiologists: Making the best use of clinical radiology services. This advises which investigations are indicated for specific conditions.

It is a shame how often the expertise of radiologists is overlooked. If a patient does need imaging, rather than just filling out a form, a discussion with the radiologist will help determine the most appropriate test.

If you have arranged any tests, the sooner the patients get the results the better. If they only have a follow-up appointment in 3 months' time this is a long time to wait. More importantly, unless somebody is chasing the test it is liable to get lost. If at the follow-up appointment a result is discovered that should have been acted upon 2 months ago it makes for a very uncomfortable clinic.

There are a number of ways of forwarding results to patients, and this will vary from clinic to clinic. As a trainee, follow local practice, but establish ideals of your own. In general, rather than offering to contact patients with results of tests, ask them to contact you a week or so after the test has occurred. This can be done quite easily by phone or email, but avoid using your personal phone number or email address.

The next part is to discuss management; this can vary from 'masterly inactivity' (temporising, observing and reassuring, but not starting any treatment or organising any tests on this visit) to emergency admission. Explain the diagnosis and its implications. Often, there will be a range of treatment options and you should discuss these with the family. For example, some families with a child with epilepsy will want medication, whilst others will not.

Practise how to approach this and give unbiased information to help the family make a decision. In medicine, we tend to believe in: 'Don't just stand there do something' whilst many people prefer the approach of 'Don't just do something – stand there' As long as patients have appropriate information about treatment options, what they decide is up to them.

If drugs are required, name the drug; explain how it works and common side effects. Try to give some idea of how quickly it will work and how long it will be required for. If providing only a limited supply of the medication from clinic, explain that they can visit their general practitioner for an additional prescription. If a referral is needed for further consideration, such as to a specialist, explain the reasons for this, and who they will be referred to.

Closing the session

At the end of the session, make sure that the family understand the conclusions of the consultation. Ideally this is with a diagnosis, but if not with a plan outlining how a diagnosis is to be reached. They should know what they have to do, e.g. keep a symptom diary.

The family should be clear about management and follow up, including how they will receive results of any tests. Do some 'safety-netting,' advising what the family should do if the situation changes, and relevant contact details.

After this, a follow-up appointment can be arranged if necessary. Again, think about this. Could they be followed up in primary care? Or do they need any follow up at all? If it is for reassurance, is this more for the benefit of the patient or the doctor? Make sure that they know how to book any follow-up appointment.

At the end check that all of their questions have been answered – 'Is there anything that we haven't covered? That's quite a lot to take in; do you want me to go over anything again? Have you got anything at all that you want to ask me?'

Closing the session can be tricky. Formally close the consultation, 'So that seems to be OK, let's see you again in 10 months' time.' Sometimes body language is required such as 'subtly' standing up and making a move towards the door.

Time keeping

For most new patients, the appointments are 20–40 minutes depending on the clinic. Part of the clinic skill is ensuring they run to time. If the clinic is running late, apologise to patients personally, 'I'm sorry that you have been waiting.' After clinic, administrative work should be completed in a timely fashion (see Chapter 2).

If things go wrong?

Occasionally, the consultation does not go to plan. You may need to say, 'Sorry I just need to get things a bit clearer in my mind, do you object if we go back a bit?'

Further reading

Blau JN. Time to let the patient speak. BMJ. 1989; 298(6665):39.

Kurtz SM, Silverman JD, Draper J. Teaching and Learning Communication Skills in Medicine. Oxford: Radcliffe Medical Press, 1998.

Silverman JD, Kurtz SM, Draper J. Skills for Communicating with Patients. Oxford: Radcliffe Medical Press, 1998.

Kurtz S, Silverman J, Benson J, Draper J. Marrying Content and Process in Clinical Method Teaching: Enhancing the Calgary-Cambridge Guides Academic Medicine, 2003; 78(8):802–809. www.gp-training.net

Chapter 2

Clinic letters – writing, dictating and being assessed

Who is the letter for?

Convention dictates that letters are written back to the referrer (usually the general practitioner, but could be a health visitor, school nurse, other health care professional or a doctor from another speciality). However there is no reason why the letter cannot be written to the child – it is about them after all. This can be especially helpful for older children with chronic conditions.

What is the letter for?

The letter can serve a number of purposes including:
- As a (legible) part of the medical record
- Communicating the current medical situation with other professionals
- Identifying what may be expected of the patient, writer and recipients
- As a reminder to the patient of the consultation and significant outcomes arising from it

When composing a letter try to ensure that it fulfils all of its intended purposes. Some doctors will write separate letters to health professionals and the patient, but this can place pressure on the system, and more importantly might lead the patient to suspect that they are being excluded from some medical communication, and therefore worry about what information they are not receiving.

Writing letters

In order to get all of the clinic letters out on time, it is imperative that they are brief. Short letters are easier to dictate, quicker to type and may reach the general practitioner (GP) more quickly. They are more likely to be read too. Research shows that GPs value letters with a clear structure.

When writing letters, think about the following dos and don'ts:

Do

- Be clear, concise and to the point
- Be accurate – patients may complain if the letter says the pain has been present for 6 months when it has been there for 28 weeks
- Ensure the letter is understandable by all of the intended audience – GP, family, other health professionals – so avoid jargon, acronyms and abbreviations as much as possible
- Ensure the letter contains all results available, or indicate if results are outstanding

Don't

- Repeat the history as given in the initial referral letter
- Give excessive details of investigations – 'the full blood count was normal' is fine
- Patronise the GP by giving a medical lecture; if the problem is asthma the GP does not need to know that the child has frequent episodes of cough, wheeze and shortness of breath which are worse at night and on exercise. Describe atypical signs or what has led to an unexpected diagnosis. However, consider fuller explanations when letters are copied to parents

Dictating letters

The most common method for producing clinic letters is for them to be recorded onto a hand held device and then transcribed, by either a real or 'virtual' secretary. As technology advances, handheld digital devices are more affordable and voice-recognition software becomes more user-friendly. Whichever method is used, there are some specific tips for dictation which should be considered:

- Speak slowly and clearly – listen to your own recordings occasionally. If you can't understand what you are saying nobody else will be able to either
- Identify yourself, the date of the clinic and the consultant in charge
- Let the secretaries know how you would like your names spelt
- Leave a number or NHS/hospital e-mail address that you can be contacted on to deal with results and queries
- Identify each patient by name and hospital or NHS number
- At the end of the tape say 'That is the end'
- Place the tape in an envelope with your name and the date of the clinic
- 'Please', 'thank you' and smiles are always welcomed – even on tapes! An example of a structure for a clinic letter back to the GP is shown in **Table 2.1**.

Assessment of written communication

Doctors in training will be assessed on their written communication by their supervising consultant. This may be their clinic notes or more usually the clinic letter. The tool used to make the assessment may change over time but will always be against accepted good practice. One validated and used until recently was the Sheffield Assessment Instrument for Letters (SAIL). The Royal College or Paediatrics and Child Health's assessment and training site will provide useful information and guidance (www.rcpch.ac.uk/assess-exams). Guidance on the required number of such assessments in a training year will be given but aim for quality and not quantity. Ensure you are assessed on different types for clinic letter - letters back to the referee or GP, speciality referrals as well as letters informing parents about test results or management plans.

Table 2.1 Structure of clinic letters

Hospital Headed Paper – NHS Logo
Hospital address
Contacts details for secretary/clinic

Name of clinic/consultant
Reference number (usually hospital number)
Date of clinic
Date of letter

General practitioner address

Dear Dr,

Name, date of birth, hospital or NHS number, and address of patient

Problems/assessment: 1. List problem is order of importance. If there is a diagnosis mention this first.
2. Include all relevant details, not just a list of symptoms.

Management
- Any specific instructions (e.g. changes in lifestyle – eat more fibre, drink more fluid, etc.)
  - Investigations
  - Medications
- Referral to other clinicians, therapists or health care professionals

Follow up: Where and with who, or 'None arranged'

Please can you arrange: A helpful addition to ask the general practitioner or person you are writing to do
something specific for this child.

Rationale
(relevant history and examination)
Include here any pertinent information that is not contained in the focussed summary above.
It is not necessary to go over detail in the referral letter unless there is new or different information.
It is good to include an assessment section which assimilates all the information so far into a coherence synopsis
of, and rationale for, the plan
Yours sincerely,

Dr Dick Tate
ST 5 Paediatric Trainee to Dr Sue Perviza
Copies to:
All relevant health care professionals involved in the care.
Parents/child

Further reading

Crossley JGM, Howe A, et al. Sheffeld Assessment Instrument for Letters (SAIL): performance assessment using outpatient letters. Medical Education, 2001; 35:1115–1124.
Department of Health. Copying letters to Patients. Good practice guidelines. 2003. www.dh.gov.uk

Chapter 3

Managing nonattendance

Missed appointments

People may fail to attend an outpatient appointment for many different reasons including forgetting the appointment, dissatisfaction with the service, moving out of the area or feeling that their problem has resolved. Given that there is an expectation that adults should take responsibility for their health, it is reasonable not to offer a repeat appointment to an adult who fails to attend, unless there has been an error on the hospital's part, such as not informing the patient of the appointment in the first place.

However, children are in a different situation, in that they are dependent on an adult to bring them to an appointment. If they are not brought there may be a concern that their genuine medical needs are not being acknowledged by their carers. Additionally, if a parent/carer does not present a child for medical care this can be a sign of neglect or abuse. Certainly one of the markers of serious child maltreatment is a failure to engage with medical care. However, it is important to put this into perspective in that in the overwhelming majority of children who fail to attend appointments there are no safeguarding issues.

Clearly there are also great pressures to make the outpatient system efficient, and every missed appointment makes this worse. The system does not have sufficient capacity to offer repeat appointments which are unlikely to be kept. On many levels it is inappropriate to offer further routine appointments, in the expectation that they will not be kept, for the main purpose of accumulating evidence of child maltreatment. In a situation where there is a need for the child to receive medical input, or there are safeguarding concerns, the doctor has a responsibility to actively pursue these, by communicating with the family, general practitioner (GP) health visitor (HV) or other professionals.

The guidelines below try to ensure that children who are not brought to clinic will not be deprived of appropriate care. In these children their GP, who has the primary medical duty to the patient, should be informed, and they can ensure that their medical needs are met and consider any safeguarding concern. Where safeguarding issues have already been identified, children should have their nonattendance highlighted to the appropriate professionals.

It is good practice to copy all correspondence to parents/guardians. Local policy will vary; discuss with a senior before sending letters that could possibly be interpreted as inflammatory. The guidelines below offer one option, although there is much scope for variation.

Letter 1: Did not attend first appointment – no medical social concerns

Dear patient/parent

We did not see [Child's name] in clinic today. We hope that this means that your problems have resolved. We are unable to offer you a further appointment at present. If you feel that you do need to be seen, we would recommend that you make an appointment with your general practitioner.

Copy to general practitioner

Letter 2: Did not attend safeguarding concerns

Dear GP

[Child's name] did not attend clinic today. We hope this means that their medical problems have resolved. If you feel that they need a medical review we would be happy to help-on receipt of a further referral.

There have been previous safeguarding concerns raised.

Please could we ask you to ensure that safeguarding issues are being addressed?

Copy – Named Nurse Safeguarding Children, HV/school nurse

Consider copying to social services

Letter 3: Did not attend medical and safeguarding concerns but further appointment not wanted

Dear GP

[Child's name] did not attend clinic today. We have contacted the family who do not want an appointment at this time. Please could you try to ensure that all medical and safeguarding issues are being addressed? We would be happy to send a further appointment at your request.

Copy – Named Nurse Safeguarding Children HV/school nurse

Consider copying to social services

Letter 4: Did not attend medical concerns, no safeguarding concerns, repeat appointment offered

> Dear GP
>
> [Child's name] did not attend clinic today. We have contacted his/her parents/carers and have made a further appointment. If He/She does not attend this we will not send a further appointment unless you make a further referral.
>
> Copy – parents/child

Letter 5: Did not attend for second time

> Dear GP
>
> [Child's name] did not attend his/her clinic appointment today. The appointment was made directly by the parents/carers who expressed concerns about [Child's name]. We are unable to offer a further appointment unless we receive a new referral.
>
> Please could we ask you to ensure that there are no healths or social concerns regarding [Child's name].
>
> Copy: Named Nurse Safeguarding Children
>
> HV/School Nurse
>
> Copy – Parents

Letter 6: Did not attend – medical concerns, family do not want another appointment

> Dear GP
>
> [Child's name] did not attend clinic today. We have contacted the family who do not want an appointment at this time. Please could you try to ensure that all medical issues are being addressed? We would be happy to send a further appointment at your request.
>
> Copy – Parents/child

Chapter 4

Learning and teaching in the outpatient clinic

Overview

The outpatient setting uses all the generic skills of acute paediatrics (history, examination, investigation and treatment) as well as other skills (continuity of care, information-giving and education). Ambulatory services such as day care units and acute assessment units are sometimes considered as an outpatient setting, and many, if not all, of the principles discussed here will apply in these settings as well. Some influences on learning and teaching within a consultation are shown in **Figure 4.1**.

How a clinic is run (see Chapter 1) may affect the ability to teach. With time at a premium, conducting the clinic in an educational way becomes a challenge which requires innovative thinking. Whilst every patient encounter provides learning and teaching opportunities, remember that although some patients will normally try to be helpful, the doctors are there for the patient's benefit rather than vice versa. This chapter will discuss how to use clinics both as a learning experience and as a teaching tool.

Learning in clinic

There is no substitute for running clinics. Most departments will allocate a trainee their own clinic list. A supervising consultant will have overall responsibility for these patients, and should be in clinic themselves. Consultants vary widely in their approach, but the following outline should work in most settings. If there is no obvious system in place, take the initiative and suggest one.

Pre- and post-clinic meeting

A meeting before starting the clinic, reviewing the notes of the expected patients, is invaluable in providing information on how to manage the patients on the list. If the consultant manages patients in a particular way this allows clarification of what is expected or, perhaps, an opportunity to challenge their beliefs. Although many of the referral letters will suggest a course of treatment, new information may present itself which will cause a rethink of the original plan.

After the clinic, discuss the patients and their management. This is a good opportunity to focus on one case in some detail as a 'supervised learning event/case-based discussion'.

How and when to interrupt

For a trainee seeing his or her own list, obtaining an opinion during the consultation can be stressful. Set up the 'rules' before clinic. This helps the clinic flow and relieves any anxiety about interrupting. Hovering outside the consultant's room is distracting, and it may be inappropriate just to walk in during the middle of a consultation. However, waiting around

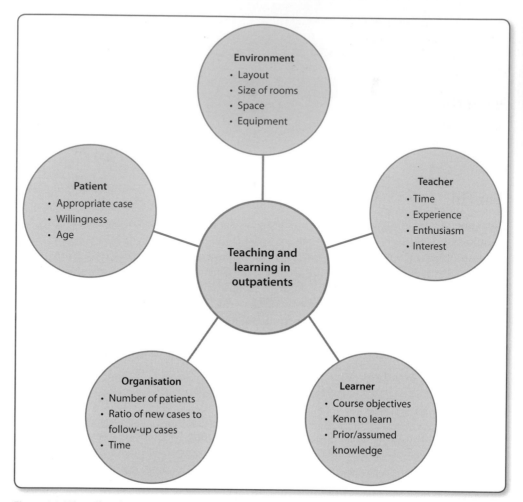

Figure 4.1 What affects learning and teaching in outpatients?

is counterproductive. The clinic nurse will usually advise on the best course of action in uncertain situations.

A good doctor must know the limits of their expertise, and when to ask for help. In a situation where the consultant needs to be consulted think about how to explain this procedure to the parents, e.g. 'I have listened to the problem and examined you, but I think it would be helpful to discuss your case with my consultant, just to make sure that he/she knows about you and can give any further advice.' If leaving a patient alone in the room, think about what else is left behind. This bit can be tricky; taking valuables with you seems like a sensible precaution. It is harder to protect other patients' case notes, although even anecdotally patients do not seem to pick these up and start reading them.

Follow up and chasing up

Most trainees will routinely follow up the children they have seen . However, it is worth checking what the consultant's preferences are. It can be disempowering to general practitioners to have to follow-up trivial conditions endlessly. Chasing up results on patients a trainee has seen is a good way of ensuring case-based learning. Have a system for tracking the results and know whose responsibility it is for chasing results and reporting them back to the family.

Bank the learning

Trainees should be encouraged to log their clinics in their e-portfolio and reflect on cases, presentation, results and diagnoses. Clinic is a good opportunity to do workplace-based assessments.

Teaching in clinic

The general aims of clinic attendance for the undergraduate medical student 'observer' should be to:
- Learn how to diagnose and manage paediatric problems
- Learn about consultation skills by observing different senior doctors – sometimes learning how not to do things.

Learners

It is helpful to consider two types of learners. The novice, such as a medical student or junior trainee who needs to acquire knowledge as much as its application; and the more experienced doctor who will possess more knowledge, but is learning how to apply it. Learners in clinic change the doctor-patient dynamic, and it is probably best to have only one but never more than two in a clinic. They do not need to sit through an entire clinic, but can dip in and out of different clinics that are running simultaneously.

Room layout

The position of learners in the room should be given some thought. The traditional arrangement of having the learner sitting behind the doctor seems to go against an inclusive learning environment. Try to bring the learner into the group and let them feel part of the consultation; make sure that this does not seem intimidating to the patient. Experiment with the seating, e.g. try breaking with convention and create a circle (**Figure 4.2**).

Calling the patient

It is good practice to go to the waiting room to greet the patient and so the consultation begins informally on the walk from the waiting room (See Chapter 1). During this time, inform the patient and parents that there are some learners in clinic (a medical student/ junior doctor/nurse/observer) and check that the parent and/or child are comfortable with that. Because people don't like upsetting the doctor, any suggestion of unease should be taken as not wanting the learner present. A poster in the waiting room informing patients that learners might be present in the consultation, and asking them to opt in or out, can save a lot of blushes all round. Generally children and their parents are happy to contribute to training the next generation; even those with 'embarrassing problems'.

Occasionally, if there is a very sensitive consultation, the learner may be asked to leave and join another clinic. Sometimes this may happen mid-consultation, if it is clear that the learner's presence is hampering communication.

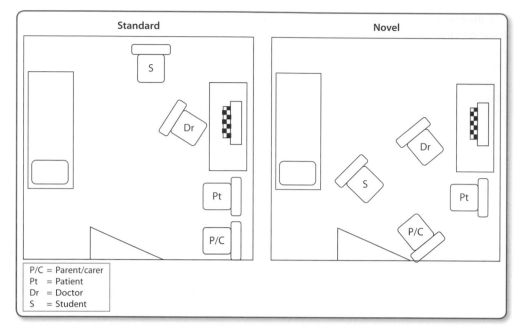

Figure 4.2 Standard versus novel arrangements for room set up, to effect more inclusion of the medical student

Introductions

Introduce the learner by name to the family. 'This is Melissa, she is the medical student I have told you about – Melissa, this is Rory and his parents.'

How to involve learners

Work out with the learner how they can reinforce their learning in this clinic. Before a patient enters they can be shown the clinic letter or given the history and asked to consider a differential diagnosis or management plan.

Two very useful 'tasks' are to ask the student to take a history whilst being observed (apprenticeship model) or ask the student to actively listen to the history being taken (observation). In the first scenario, explain to the family what will happen, and make sure that they are happy with this. Deciding where to sit is important. Behind the student is a good position as it is less undermining and allows eye contact with the family. Staying in the room removes any feeling of the family being 'short changed', by not being seen by the senior doctor. Hearing the history directly from the family, rather than second hand via the learner, means that the family do not need to repeat the history and important messages are less likely to be missed. Try not to interrupt till the student has reached a natural end. Agree at which point the student will finish rather than letting them just fizzle out. Once the student has done their bit, swap seats to assume control. If space allows, the student could act like a member of the team and see the child in a separate room (team-member model). However, the student will miss children seen by the doctor while they complete their consultation, and vice versa.

If the learner is listening to the history, ask if they have any questions at a relevant break in the history taking. This can provide a useful insight into their knowledge and confidence (they may ask something that has not been considered). The interrupting learner can be a challenge, who may need politely reminding at what stages of the consultation their interjections are helpful, and to avoid them at other times. At the end of the history, ask the learner to make a diagnosis or compose a provisional problem list.

Decide when and how cases will be discussed with your learners. There may be a few minutes between patients, and a slightly longer time at the end.

Learning outcomes

Find out how the learner wants to benefit from sitting in the clinic. Try to extract more tangible objectives than just 'to see lots of different cases'. Set some learning outcomes. **Table 4.1** gives other ideas to help stimulate learning in clinic.

Benefits

As doctors we need to be able to teach, be it ourselves, our juniors or our patients. Even more so, we can fulfil the old adage of 'Who is wise? He who learns from everyone'. One of

Table 4.1 Ideas to help stimulate medical students learning in clinic	
Task	**Details**
Get the learner to examine a focussed system	General multisystem examinations are not normally required. Ask the student to examine a system, if the child and/or parent do not mind
Send the learner to watch the nursing aspects of care	For example weighing, measuring height, lung function tests, skin prick tests, dipping urine, taking BP, inhaler technique
Set 'homework'	Give the student a topic or area to research
Guess the child's age	Based on the size and developmental skills displayed on observation, asks the student to guess the child's age. Siblings can be included.
Assess the child's development	Watching the child play and interact during the consultation can allow an assessment as to whether their development is within normal limits
Arrange for the student to sit in with another member of the multidisciplinary team	Dietician, specialist nurse or therapist
The student may play with a younger child – as long as this is not too distracting (peekaboo, turning pages of a book, drawing pictures)	This can be welcome distraction for them, and may allow their parents to discuss issues more thoroughly with the doctor
Observe the interactions	Suggest the learner observes the various inter-relationships and interactions during the interview mother/child, mother/doctor and child/doctor
Frame an evidence-based question	Ask the student to look for published evidence to answer the questions
Do some reading!	Suggest they make notes about the cases and then go and read up about them

the great benefits of having learners in clinic is that they make the doctor think, and a good teacher will gain as much, if not more, from their teaching as their students.

Further reading

Dent, JA. AMEE Guide No. 26: clinical teaching in ambulatory care settings: making the most of learning opportunities with outpatients. Medical Teacher 2005; 27(4):302–315.

Chapter 5

School issues

It is impossible to understand children or childhood without understanding school, and the impact it has on children and their health. Autobiographies demonstrate that school has the potential to make or break people, and the fact that two people can have completely different experiences of the same school suggest that this is as much due to the individual as to the school. Whilst every school is different, there are many recurring themes when it comes to school issues.

Attendance

There is unequivocal evidence that prolonged school nonattendance is linked to life nonattainment. Essentially, children that miss school do not only have poorer academic and career outcomes but also have higher lifelong psychological morbidity than school attenders. So, whilst attending school may be either good or bad for children, not attending is uniformly bad. It is postulated that school itself has some redeeming qualities, and the long term outlook for a particular child can be improved by attending school. This is based on the idea that the home environment is producing and reinforcing negative attitudes which will only be challenged by an external agent – school. Alternatively, it is possible that school nonattendance is merely a surrogate marker for other issues – such as extreme anxiety, and these may not necessarily be modified merely by attending school.

Asking about school should be a routine part of the paediatric encounter. It is remarkable how often prolonged absence is not noted. As a general rule, sick children, not in hospital, go to school. Children with malignancy or juvenile idiopathic arthritis usually have good attendance records. Significant school nonattendance, even for supposed medical reasons, usually has a strong behavioural and/or psychological component.

School nonattenders may be divided into different categories. Probably the most useful distinction is between those that are off school with parental consent and those whose absence is unknown by parents.

Sanctioned absences

There are a number of different scenarios where school absence is maintained with parental knowledge and at least some level of approval. These include:

- **School refusal/phobia:** This will often present as physical symptoms – usually the physical manifestations of anxiety, or conversion disorders. It is easy to fall into the trap of focussing on the physical symptoms, overlooking the fact that the child is not attending school. The challenge is to identify, explain and explore the underlying anxiety. In most children school anxiety is linked to separation anxiety. In separation anxiety the question to ask is who is most worried about separating – the child or adult? A smaller number of children may have school anxiety linked to a specific issue, e.g. bullying, tests, etc.

- **Masquerade syndrome:** Most children that have prolonged medical absence from school do not have a strong medical reason for their absence. They are often presented with frequent minor symptoms or with symptoms that are difficult to corroborate, (there is significant overlap with fabricated or induced illness – previously known as Münchausen syndrome by proxy). A major contributing factor is poor communication between school and doctors. The doctors presume that as the child's symptoms are mild they would be attending school, whilst the parents report back to the school that the child is constantly unwell and has frequent medical appointments, often with significant embellishment. When challenged, the family will say this was due to misunderstanding. The school does not feel in a position to challenge the family. In simple terms this could be perceived as the parent creating a sick role for the child, where the child then learns to play his part and this 'conspiracy' can be very hard to break. Strong multiagency working is required to deal with this.
- **Conversion disorders:** These can be driven by anxiety, but may have no obvious precipitant. In contrast to masquerade syndrome, this could be viewed as the child taking the lead in adopting an inappropriate sick role.
- **Chronic fatigue syndrome:** (see case 13).
- **Sanctioned social absence-parenting issues:** Most pupils need parents to help them get to school. They might need waking in the morning, feeding and being told to go to bed. In families with inadequate supervision, this may not happen, and the children will not attend. This may also occur where a child has become a carer, either to adults who have health, mental health or addiction issues, or in situations where the child is 'needed' to represent the family. For example, in immigrant families the older children may be the best English speakers and be required to act as the family's interpreter.
- **Conflict with school:** Issues often arise with schools and if families feel that their concerns have not been addressed properly, they will not let their children attend school as a result.

Truancy

Children who miss school without their parents' knowledge are a different group. They are likely to have a high level of behavioural and learning issues, and often home issues as well. As a group they are likely to have limited educational achievement and a higher rate of antisocial and criminal behaviour. They are more likely to indulge in high risk activities. Persuading these young people to return to education is a tremendous challenge – which requires a multiagency approach.

Excluded students

These young people have been permanently excluded from school – usually on account of repeated antisocial behaviour. They have significant overlap with the truancy group. Poor behaviour has been their hallmark, and as a result they can have unrecognised educational, physical or psychological problems. For example, a teenager with some learning and behavioural issues with frequent absence seizures may have the former noted and acted upon, whilst the latter is overlooked.

Home educated

Students are home educated for varying reasons, they are a generally vulnerable group, and should be known to, and registered with, the local education/social service authorities.

School's impact on health

There are a number of ways in which schools can impact on health. The following is an indicative rather than exhaustive list.

- **Sleep:** Pupils – especially in secondary schools may need to wake up very early to get to school. By the time they get home, do homework and unwind they may have inadequate time for sleep.
- **Eating and drinking:** Many children – especially in secondary school will skip breakfast, and may not eat and drink till the early afternoon. This is a common cause of headache. Schools have varying eating and drinking policies, but most adults would not accept the restrictions that are imposed on children. A strict 'water only' policy means that most children will not drink adequately during the school day. As well as impacting on school performance, they may drink more in the evenings and this can make treating enuresis more difficult. A longer-term problem is the over-availability of junk food and drinks.
- **Toilets:** At least 60% of children would never open their bowels in a school toilet. 15–20% won't even pass urine. Toilets are always difficult places and children have particular concerns about privacy, hygiene and bullying. In many schools access to toilets is also an issue. As a consequence continence problems can develop or get worse. Minimally, holding on to stool and urine has a deleterious effect on behaviour and learning. Schools that implement a good drinking, eating and toilet policy see benefits in pupil satisfaction and academic performance.
- **Availability to take medication:** Young people do not like to be different. If on medication, they need to be able to take this confidently and often confidentially. Sometimes the technicality can be difficult. For example, some schools insist that all medication is stored centrally. If a child feels the onset of a migraine, by the time they access their medication it may be too late to abort an attack.

Health's impact on school

Health problems can clearly have an impact on school. Repeated absences will not only disrupt learning, but also make it harder for children to remain involved with friends. Children with chronic health needs may also have other limitations that may exclude them from the full curriculum, e.g. unable to do sports, or be involved in activities with friends outside school.

The school will also have to provide suitable facilities for young people's health needs, e.g. be able to store medication safely and provide a suitable environment for treatment.

All state schools in the UK will have a school nurse. Each nurse may be responsible for a number of schools, so will not be on-site all the time. The school nurse should be aware of any significant health or social needs of pupils.

Transition

There are particular times which are challenging for all children, and these are usually around change, a new school year, a new teacher, etc. The biggest of these challenges is changing school, which happens in the UK to most children in the autumn before their 12th birthday. This is known as secondary transfer, and the process and build up to this can start 18 months earlier. For some children this process causes immense stress and is a trigger for school phobia/refusal.

The other major change is in the nature of the school. Primary schools are generally forgiving places, where minor problems are often masked by a caring system. Pupils are surrounded by other children that they have grown up with and accept, generally, any of their weaknesses. The change to secondary school exposes children to new people who, because they do not know them, may be less forgiving of differences. Added to this there is an expectation that pupils will start taking responsibility in organising their lives – being in the right place for the right lesson, with the right book. Children with minor organisational issues, who have coped at primary school, can find this overwhelming.

The discipline in a secondary school is also usually more formal, and sensitive children may feel anxious about getting into trouble. Also the work becomes harder and exams become more serious, a further cause of increasing anxiety.

Bullying

It is impossible to write about school without mentioning bullying. Reported episodes of this are on the increase, which may represent changes in society and/or changes in definition and classification. The suggestion being that a lot of normal conflict is categorised as bullying. Nevertheless about half of all UK schoolchildren report being bullied.

Bullying can be divided into three categories:
- Verbal bullying (teasing)
- Physical bullying
- Social exclusion

Clearly a child may be bullied in more than one way. Children who are 'different' are more likely to be victims, and this includes children with chronic health needs.

Bullying is important, because it lies behind numerous health consultations and affects physical and psychological well being. Bullying involves both bully and victim, with many young people being both simultaneously – the bully/victim. It is hard to identify bullies in clinic because people are usually only prepared to discuss victimhood. This can give the impression that only the victims present, whereas studies show that bullies present with symptoms of stress and anxiety as much as their victims do, perhaps acting out adverse experiences in their own lives. Generally, the bullies are said to 'have fallen in with the wrong crowd' or be 'misunderstood'; rarely do they seem to take responsibility.

Families usually only give one side of the story: happy to discuss the terrible things that are happening to their child at school, but overlooking the terrible things that their child may be doing. Give the family support and information to address the issues themselves, but try to avoid intervening personally. Ideally treatment should involve prevention. However, successful antibullying programmes in school require significant and repeated sessions, so whilst some school have active antibullying strategies, all too often they seem to be one of either 'we don't have bullying here' or 'we don't tolerate bullying here'.

Victims may suffer the same fate in different settings, suggesting that the problem is that they effectively exude vulnerability. Resilience training can help them. Bullies may need some relationship, empathy and anger management training.

Further reading

Jones R, et al. Frequent medical absences in secondary school students: survey and case–control study Arch Dis Child, 2009; 94:763–767.
Thambirajah, et al. Understanding School Refusal. London: Jessica Kingsley Press, 2008.

Patient information

Kidscape
www.kidscpape.org.uk

Chapter 6

Safeguarding issues

Dear Paediatrician,

Thank you for seeing this 6-week-old infant urgently. He has had an upper respiratory tract infection over the last week and has had some bleeding from his nose. There is a small excoriation just in his nostril, and he has a tiny subconjunctival haemorrhage.

I have been worried about the family as his mother is known to me. She has a learning disability having attended a special school. I do not know the father well at all as he is not a patient at this practice. I referred the mother to social care during the pregnancy at about 36 weeks; they have a programme in place with frequent visits to support the parents. The health visitor has told me she saw what may have been a small bruise on the infant's cheek about 2 weeks ago but she was not sure about it and the mother thought it had occurred when the baby was feeding. It is difficult to obtain a clear history, but the mother says that the father dropped the baby a few days ago.

He seems otherwise well and his head circumference is on the 75th centile.

Many thanks,

Dr Simon McClelland

Case analysis

There are a number of warning signs. This is a young baby presenting with seemingly spontaneous bleeding. Babies under 6 months should not do this, so any bruise or bleed in a child of this age must be taken seriously.

There are a number of other factors which are of concern. The mother's learning issues may be so severe that they are impacting on her mothering skills and also make it more likely that she will be in a vulnerable relationship.

The history of trauma needs to be explored, specifically the bruising and reported dropping of the baby.

Clearly if the baby presents with symptoms, such as persisting bleeding, or is in need of urgent medical care this should be attended to immediately.

Differential diagnosis

Suffocation

Bilateral nose bleeds are rare, and are said to be almost pathognomonic of recent suffocation, accidental or nonaccidental. In accidental suffocation there will be a history, whilst in nonaccidental suffocation this is not forthcoming. If this is suspected it needs to be investigated. The nose bleeds are often accompanied by blood from the mouth. Usually, this is blood from haemorrhagic pulmonary oedema. If possible a specimen can be collected in a 'haematocrit' (capillary) tube and spun down. The packed cell volume will be very low. An MRI of the brain can show changes consistent with suffocation. If this is suspected a full child protection investigation will be required including a skeletal survey and ophthalmology review, and involvement of police and social services.

Significant trauma

The baby had a past history of a bruise, the so called herald or precursor bruise. In babies, minor bruising which may appear to require little attention can be followed by significant or life-threatening trauma.

If there has been significant intracranial bleeding there is likely to be an increasing head circumference. It is vital to plot this. Diagnosis can be confirmed by imaging. CT is usually the easiest to arrange and management should be discussed with the neurosurgeons. Again this should trigger further multiagency investigation (see above).

Scratching

Babies do scratch themselves, and usually leave marks. They can draw blood but it is unlikely to be anything more than a superficial scratch around the nose.

Haemorrhagic disease of the newborn

This is rare now. However if the baby did not receive vitamin K and is breastfeeding this can occur. This should be evident from the results of the clotting screen. Treatment is with vitamin K.

Bleeding diathesis

If there is a bleeding tendency it will be identified on the clotting screen.

Infection

This is an unlikely cause. It is unusual for a viral infection to cause bleeding. The child could have impetigo which would bleed, but that would usually be around the nose rather than through the nostril. This would be evident on examination and would be treated with antibiotics.

Birth injury

Coughing, especially pertussis, may cause subconjunctival haemorrhage but this would need to be fairly notable coughing. Subconjunctival haemorrhages can also be present after birth, but by the age of this child they should be resolving rather than appearing.

Consultation essentials

This baby presents with significant symptoms, and needs a diagnosis urgently.

History

It is essential to get as much history as possible, including the birth and neonatal history. Given the mother's learning issues this may be limited. Try to find out about the fall and any other falls or knocks. Ask if the baby is thriving, alert and well (**Figure 6.1**).

More information about the bleeding is helpful, including where the blood was coming from and how much of it there was. In this case the mother said 'blood just poured out of the nose' which suggests something highly significant occurred.

Examination

Obviously look around the areas where the baby has bled. The general examination must include head circumference which should be plotted and compared to previous readings. Check for any other bruises on the baby.

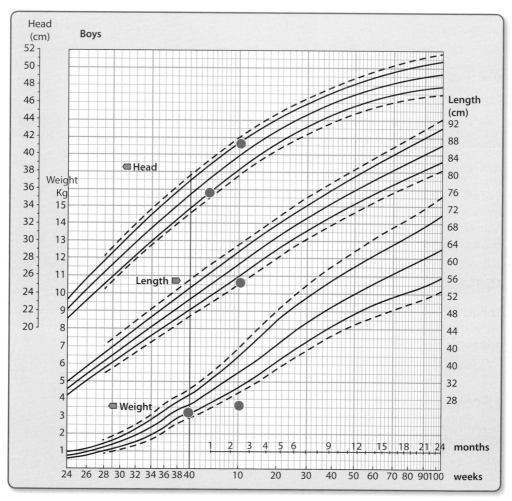

Figure 6.1 Growth chart of infant described in the case.

Tests/investigations

Clotting is a must. If a bleeding diathesis or vitamin K deficiency, haemorrhagic disease of the newborn (HDN) is revealed, this should be treated urgently. Further imaging may be required depending on symptoms and sign; HDN can lead to intracranial bleeds.

If the clotting is normal, then inflicted injury becomes the most likely diagnosis and further investigations including neuroimaging, skeletal survey and ophthalmology assessment will be required.

Diagnosis

In this particular case, the mother fortunately brought the personal child health record. The infant was rather lethargic, with an anxious expression and a full fontanelle. The charts showed the infant had gained weight poorly but the head circumference had increased in size over a 2-week period from the 25th to the 75th centile. There was an excoriation at the base of the left nostril which might have been infected and there was a subconjunctival haemorrhage in the right eye medial to the pupil. The excoriation had been thought to be a source of the bleeding but the maternal history suggested a more serious cause.

Management

Clotting was normal. In view of the head circumference changes and the subconjunctival haemorrhage a CT of the head was arranged which showed large bilateral subdural haemorrhages. There were no retinal haemorrhages but a skeletal survey showed a recent fracture of the left 7th rib. Social services and the police were immediately informed. A strategy meeting was arranged. A police protection order was placed on the child, pending court proceedings for an interim care order. Background searches revealed that the father had children from a previous relationship. As they lived far away it was felt that their safety was not immediately threatened. The baby was immediately admitted and a neurosurgical opinion sought. He had a chronic subdural haemorrhage, which was managed conservatively.

Follow up

The acute paediatrician may not have a need for medical review of the child depending on the extent of the medical issues. In this case neurodevelopmental assessment is important and that could be offered by the community paediatrician. Multiagency liaison is critical, as is collating accurate medicolegal reports to inform the safeguarding process.

Discussion

In retrospect the nose bleed was probably unrelated to the excoriation and was secondary to head trauma, as was the subconjunctival haemorrhage. The problem of a parent not known to primary care is common and impairs assessment of the family but there is no simple solution unless the family is subject to a child protection investigation. The small bruise on the cheek was likely to be significant and ideally should have triggered a medical examination and a further evaluation of the family.

A referral at 36 weeks' gestation was late for notifying concerns prebirth. Where one parent has learning difficulty it is usually the mother and it is the father who constitutes the risk to the child but is not learning disabled.

Safeguarding concerns can present in a number of ways in an outpatient setting.

Situations where the child has an acute medical need, as highlighted in this case are rare and should obviously be discussed with a senior practitioner immediately. The management is to, firstly, attend to the child's urgent medical needs; which will often entail an acute admission to hospital. At this stage, although there may be suspicions of child maltreatment, these are unconfirmed. Therefore, it is reasonable to explain to the family that their child has signs of a serious medical problem, which will need further, urgent investigations and treatment in hospital. If the clinic is in the community, or on a site away from the acute hospital, then the child should be transferred by emergency ambulance.

More common, but still rare, will be the child who displays coincidental signs of injury. For example, a child presenting at the asthma clinic may have multiple bruising in suspicious areas. As with all medical work, everything must be taken in context. Reasonable explanations for the bruising may mean that no urgent treatment is required, although if it is severe, looking for an underlying bleeding disorder may be merited. However, in the absence of an explanation, maltreatment becomes a serious possibility. Again, this should be discussed with a senior, but if there are any concerns a referral should be made to social care immediately. As above, a more detailed investigation may be required. Where this is undertaken should be negotiated with social services.

It is important in these situations to strike a balance. It is often helpful to explain to parents that as a routine, legal requirement, in any child who has unexplained bruising a report is made to social services. This is in no way an accusation of abuse on the part of the doctor, merely a statutory requirement. Explain that the prime concern is that the child's needs are addressed. Further tests and investigations will be undertaken to see if there is a medical problem so that the child can receive any treatment required.

Less rare are the situations where there is some form of disclosure in clinic. This may be of the nature that 'Dad hits me with a stick when I am naughty' or 'my bottom only hurts when Grandpa rubs it.' Often this is met by disbelief or denial from the family. However, if the allegation is significant it needs addressing. Asking for a full explanation is helpful, and may highlight a benign cause. For example, in the latter case, it may be that a child with an anal fissure is looked after by the grandfather, who has to wipe the child's bottom after going to the toilet, and there may be no contact other than this. Obviously, there may be more sinister explanations. In situations of concern, an immediate referral to social services is required. The family can be told that, as an allegation has been made, there is a legal requirement to inform social services. In this setting it is essential to speak to a social worker so that a plan can be made.

The most common need to refer to social services is in situations where the family are clearly struggling, e.g. there may be health or mental health issues in the family, intimate partner violence, drug and alcohol problems, extremely challenging behaviour, etc. Mostly, these are chronic problems, but often remain festering, and often, 'compassion fatigue' means that they do not get appropriate support. Families like these create the bulk of safeguarding work. Explain to the family that they seem in need of help and support and highlight that social services are the team who will co-ordinate this. Unless there is an acute deterioration, this referral can be made nonurgently.

It is important to develop an awareness of other avenues of support, e.g. health visitors, school nurses, general practitioners and other local services.

References

GMC. Protecting children and young people: The responsibilities of all doctors. London, 2012.

Kemp A, Abusive head trauma: recognition and the essential investigation. Arch Dis Child Educ Pract Ed 2011; 96:202–208.

Kemp AM, et al. Patterns of skeletal fractures in child abuse: systematic review. BMJ, 2008; 337:1518a.

Maguire S, Mann MK, Sibert J, Kemp A. Are there patterns of bruising in childhood which are diagnostic or suggestive of abuse? A systematic review. Arch Dis Child 2005; 90:182–186.

Maguire S. Which injuries may indicate child abuse? Arch Dis Child Educ Pract Ed 2010; 95:170–177.

National Institute for Health and Care Excellence. When to Suspect Child Maltreatment Clinical Guidelines 89. London: National Institute for Health and Care Excellence, 2009.

The Royal College of Paediatrics and Child Health, Child Protection Companion. London: The Royal College of Paediatrics and Child Health, 2006.

Chapter 7

Family issues

Dear Paediatrician,

You will remember John who is 9 years old with well-controlled type I diabetes. His mother brought him today to see me because he has been having episodes of abdominal pain. His sugar profile is good and his HbA1C is normal. In addition, he has not been his usual self at home and school, has been isolating himself, more withdrawn and tired, impatient, starting to show poor academic performance and not interacting much with his friends. His mother is also a patient of mine, currently being treated for recurrent depression, having recently separated from John's father.

I would appreciate your assessment and suggestions for further management.

Yours sincerely,

Dr Denise Andrews

GP Registrar

Case analysis

Physical illnesses and chronic adversity impacts on a child's general and emotional development and affects the whole family. This can be understood by considering the situation in a developmental, cognitive and familial context, taking into account the child's current life circumstances.

The impact that an illness or problem has on the family will vary with the number of other stresses and the family's ability to cope with this. The family issues could be causing or exacerbating the problems. John's main carer is going through personal and marital difficulties, and this will impact on John. Considering how he has adjusted to challenges in the past and forming a picture of the family structure and function provide – not only understanding but often suggests strategies for dealing with the present and future.

In considering the psychological impact of illness on the child, there are factors which affect not only the doctor-patient relationship but also the treatment and outcome, including the duration of time taken to reach a definitive diagnosis, the accuracy of the diagnosis and the sensitivity with which it is transmitted to the child and family.

Impact of chronic illness on the child

For varied and context dependent reasons, children with chronic illness have high rates of affective and anxiety disorders. Multiple hospitalisations, especially in the first 2 years of life, may lead to disruption in the formation of a primary, secure attachment, with a possible effect on later relationships and emotional development.

In school-age children, illnesses may restrict and interfere with school life, affecting attendance and participation both in and out of the classroom. This can negatively impact learning, peer group bonding, and destroy any sense of 'belonging'. In adolescence, illness can interfere with becoming independent, and generate anxiety related to being different, cause low self-esteem, and issues of acceptance by peers. Physical deformity or difference will exacerbate this.

Impact of chronic illness on the family

Having a child with chronic illness places stress on marital relationships, which in turn interferes with parenting and can precipitate 'systemic dysfunction'. For example, because the family is focussing on the ill child, a sibling may feel left out and present with behaviour problems.

Parental/family factors

Parental factors play a major role in children's behaviour and these include:
- Parental mental illness, especially when associated with other adverse factors, such as social disadvantage (unemployment, overcrowding, limited space, etc.) is a strong predictor of problematic behaviours in the children.
- Parents with an affective disorder, e.g. depression, are likely to have a low family involvement (low communication, neglect responsibilities), which can generate guilty feelings in the parents; as a result, they may use compensatory behaviours, such as withdrawal and/or over protectiveness.
- Interparental conflict/divorce: children are doubtless sensitive to the strains of family life that occur in conflict; conflict and separation initiate changes, including altered social status, diminished parenting, change of school, new stepparents and stepsiblings.

Adjustment to life events

Adjustment reactions tend to have a better prognosis and be briefer than depression. The adjustment in John's case is to his parents' separation; a range of difficult feelings can arise from this which may be barely acknowledged let alone discussed. These include rejection, fear and anxiety about the future, both in the child and parent, hopes for reconciliation, and impact on the child's internal 'image' or idea of a family. Inconsistent parenting, especially with conflict can exacerbate this.

Somatisation

This is a manifestation of psychological difficulty or distress through somatic symptoms which have no organic basis. The patient presents with the somatic symptoms expecting a medical diagnosis and treatment. In many cases a genuine physical illness or problem may precipitate future somatisations, e.g. children with epilepsy may have nonepileptic seizures. Many children with somatisation have associated anxiety or depression.

Child temperamental features commonly found in somatisation include the conscientious, obsessional, sensitive, insecure, and anxious. Relevant family factors, such as family health problems, preoccupation with illness and high academic expectations also impact.

Common clinical presentations include:
- Aches and pains
- Tiredness
- Dizziness, blackouts faints

- Poor sleep
- Memory 'loss'
- Paralysis
- Nonepileptic seizures
- Palpitations
- Chest pain
- Tachypnoea, dyspnoea
- Paraesthesiae

Emotional disorder (anxiety and/or depression)

Depression in children of John's age is somewhat difficult to define, with symptoms varying according to age, developmental stage, and context. Anxiety is a very common comorbid presentation to depression. Common features are persistent unhappiness and social withdrawal. Younger children may have frequent crying, poor appetite, and nightmares. Worries, 'nervousness' and irritability are others symptoms of emotional disorders. There is a link between parental depression and child mental health disturbance. Nonverbal expressions of affect are helpful diagnostically, e.g. sad facial expression, absence of smiles. Others symptoms include: irritability, worsening school performance or school refusal, diminished socialisation, and somatic complaints.

Other issues

Issues including parenting difficulties (contributed to by parental mental health problem and/or other psychosocial adversities), a significant life event (parental separation), and a temperamentally shy child need to be considered. Parenting is multifactorial and multilayered, it is influenced by a whole range of individual, historical, social, and circumstantial characteristics; and it is very hard. There are different parenting styles: the authoritarian, authoritative, permissive or disengaged which impact on children's future outcomes. In this case, a now single parent has to manage her personal, marital and mental health issues, as well as a child with a chronic condition with significant long term outcomes.

There are models linking early temperamental traits with different outcomes later in life, e.g. features such as high levels of negative affectivity (withdrawal) and low levels of positive affectivity (approach) have been linked with later depression. Another model postulates that temperament may well be a mediator to people's responses to stressful situations.

Consultation essentials

The following should be covered in the consultation:

- Unless specifically asked not to, there is no reason to avoid raising familial issues such as the recent parental separation and mother's depression.
- Previous mental health service contact:

Explore any previous contact with mental health, psychological, special educational needs services, and what have they provided.

Family history

Ask about the family including John's relationship with parents and siblings, and level of contact with his father since the separation. If possible, ask about his mother's mental health history. Identify any other family members with similar problems or long term health needs, and determine important variables that can affect family adjustment such as social support, especially when under stress. Consider siblings who may resent the parents' involvement with a sick child, and/or may become (mini) carers themselves. Often asking the parents who the child 'takes after' is instructive, e.g. if John has his mother's temperament she may be able to identify with him. Finding solutions may not necessarily be easier as this may require his mother to confront some of her own issues. Alternatively, if he has his father's temperament this may generate ambivalent or negative feelings in his mother.

Protective factors

Explore protective factors – these include:
- The level of the child's adjustment to his physical and psychosocial situation
- His temperament and coping styles
- Extended family support
- The security of the child's environment and wider network, including school

Parental buy-in

Try to establish:
- The parents' level of understanding of the condition
- The impact it has on their child and on them, as individuals and as a family
- Their relationship to the medical team. Low commitment or a relationship that is adversarial, confrontational, or non-committal can interfere with engagement and recovery
- The temperament and coping style of the parents
- How the family functions
- How the child and family are adjusting

Guilt or blame

There may be all sorts of reasons parents may feel guilt, or be blamed for, their child's illness or condition, e.g. as a carrier of a genetic condition. Try and sensitively raise this issue as the guilt that a parent may be carrying may be an important maintaining factor that could become a future protective one, if thought about.

Implications

Explore implications of the illness on the future of the child and family, e.g. the actual and perceived degree of disability or limitation involved, and how the condition may affect current and future independence. Acknowledge the stress in bringing up a chronically sick child and its effect on family functioning, remembering that every family is unique and responds in its own way.

Diagnosis in this case is adjustment to life events through somatisation in context of a chronic physical illness.

Management

Children have a range of effective coping strategies to deal with their problems, which are highly influenced by their physical and emotional environments. Resilience, the ability to readjust or recover from personal difficulties, varies greatly between people, with high levels being protective. The combination of adverse and protective factors contributes to how a child sees the illness and shapes their experience of it. These issues need to be explored and worked on, either within the family or with the help of professionals.

It is essential to help the family sustain hope for the future.

Follow up

Having excluded an acute recurrence of the underlying condition, offer reassurance and support. It is good practice to try to gauge the child's views on different aspects of his condition and on the current medical and psychosocial/familial situation, and will make him feel included and listened to. Consider a further appointment in 4–6 weeks to:

- Elicit further information not covered at the initial consultation
- Monitor the situation
- Confirm or refute initial hypotheses
- Have time to gather further information, e.g. from school

If the differentials are clarified, offer another follow up in a few months to monitor how the situation is evolving. It is not unusual for such situations to settle subsequent to reassurance, support, and clarification.

Further help can be obtained from relevant agencies, for example:

- Local agencies that help with separation and impact on family, e.g. Relate
- Liaise with the general practitioner about mother's depression – with her consent
- John himself may benefit from counselling sessions – usually available through school
- Check the nature of contact between John and his father; try inviting father to subsequent appointments
- Consider other 'tier 2' agencies, i.e. those that operate between primary care and specialist services which can provide brief intervention and support
- If the situation deteriorates, discuss the case with the local child and family liaison service or child and adolescent mental health service for specialist mental health input

Discussion

Children of depressed parents have factors and signs that constitute vulnerability to potentially future depression, including impairment in social functioning, poor school performance, and negative self-concept. On the other hand, protective factors that often impact on positive outcomes include:

- Good relationships with parents: affection, 'good enough' supervision, authoritative discipline –which uses explanation, attends to the child's view, grants responsibility but retains veto and fosters independence as well as encouraging assertiveness, creativity, friendliness and warmth
- Perceived support of other adults, e.g. grandparents
- Siblings, close friends, a structured, positive school environment
- Adaptable temperament

Further reading

Barlow J, Ellard D. The psychosocial well-being of children with chronic disease, their parents and siblings: an overview of the research evidence base. Child: Care, Health & Development, 2005; 32(1):19–31.

Belsky J, Vondra, J. Lessons from child abuse: The determinants of parenting. In: D Cicchetti and V Carlson (Eds.), Child maltreatment: Theory and research on the causes and consequences of child abuse and. New York: Cambridge University Press, 1989:153–202.

Briggs-Gowan MJ, Horwitz SM, Schwab-Stone ME, et al. Mental Health in Pediatric Settings: Distribution of Disorders and Factors Related to Service Use. Journal of the American Academy of Child and Adolescent Psychiatry, 2000; 39(7):841–849.

Compas BE, Connor-Smith J, Jaser SS. Temperament, stress-reactivity, and coping: Implications for depression in childhood and adolescence. Journal of Clinical Child and Adolescent Psychology, 2004; 33:21–31.

Hysing M, Elgen I, Gillberg G, et al. Chronic physical illness and mental health in children. Results from a large-scale population study. Journal of Child Psychology and Psychiatry, 2007; 48(8):785–792.

Watson D, Gamez W, Simms LJ. Basic dimensions of temperament and their relation to anxiety and depression: A symptom-based perspective. Journal of Research in Personality, 2005; 39:46–66.

Green H, McGinnity A, Meltzer H, Ford T, Goodman R. Mental Health of children and young people in Great Britain, Office of National Statistics, 2004.
www.dh.gov.uk

NICE guidelines CG28. Depression in children and young people: Identification and management in primary, community and secondary care, 2005. guidance.nice.org.uk

Patient information

Royal College of Psychiatrists
    www.rcpsych.ac.uk
Mind
    www.mind.org.uk
Association of Child and Adolescent Mental Health
    www.acamh.org.uk

Section 2

Cases

Case 1

Abdominal pain

Dear Paediatrician,

Thank you for seeing Melody who is a 12-year-old girl with a 4-month history of intermittent abdominal pain, which can be severe enough to wake her at night and cause her to vomit. She is missing a lot of school.

She seems otherwise well, and has a normal bowel habit. She has not started her periods yet.

Other than reflux as a tiny baby she has had no significant past medical history.

Her father has a history of migraine, but she does not see him anymore.

Yours sincerely

Dr Michelle Morris

Case analysis

The letter, whilst nonspecific, does contain many suggestions as to the cause of Melody's pain. She is 12 years old so has changed schools recently, a common trigger for anxiety. At secondary school her eating and drinking will probably change and reluctance to use the school toilets often precipitates stool withholding. Although her periods have not started she is likely to be experiencing hormonal fluctuations as she enters puberty. Pregnancy, though unlikely, must be considered.

Night time waking and pain can be seen in many conditions and are not specific. The vomiting needs more elucidation but can be due to anxiety. Symptomatic gastro-oesophageal reflux occurs at any age, and the fact that she has had symptoms previously increases the likelihood of having it now.

That her father had migraines means she is more likely to get them, but his departure from her life may be even more significant. Although the family may equate chronicity with gravity, the absence of any worrying features makes it unlikely that she has anything seriously wrong.

Differential diagnosis

There can be more than one cause of pain. For example, she may have abdominal migraine, constipation and functional pain co-existing. The separate aspects will need to be teased out.

Functional abdominal pain/anxiety-related pain

The most likely diagnosis given the absence of alarming symptoms. It should not be a diagnosis of exclusion, as most children, if appropriately asked, will readily identify anxiety. The maxim 'the closer the pain is to the umbilicus, the closer it is to the brain', holds true, but anxiety-generated pain can also be more general.

Management includes identifying stress factors and trying to alter them. For example, if a particular lesson is a struggle, or there is bullying these should be addressed through the school. There are many excellent self-help books which can help with management of anxiety. If more help is required, most secondary schools have counsellors. Higher level psychological help is rarely necessary.

Constipation/stool withholding

A likely cause even when the history seems vague. The standard answer to any question about toileting is that it is 'normal'. At this age, most parents have no idea about their children's bowel habits. Don't forget to ask about school toilets: 'Do you ever go for a poo at school?' as up to 80% of secondary school age children will not and this is a common trigger for withholding.

Asking Melody to keep a stool diary might open her eyes to how abnormal her bowel habit is. X-rays are not indicated to diagnose constipation, but are occasionally useful to convince families that this is the problem. This would need negotiating with the consultant and/or radiologists.

Abdominal migraine/cyclical vomiting

A controversial diagnosis. There is some dispute as to the nature of these diagnoses, from whether they are one and the same thing to whether they exist at all. Classically there are periods of abdominal pain and protracted vomiting which can last a few days. After recovery the symptoms disappear until the next episode. A trial of migraine preventers, e.g. pizotifen, may be useful.

Mesenteric adenitis

This can present with generalised acute or chronic abdominal pain. Ultrasound may show enlarged glands. No treatment, except for analgesia is required.

Irritable bowel syndrome

Many paediatricians are reluctant to diagnose irritable bowel syndrom (IBS) in children, perhaps because it tends to stick, and is seen as a lifelong condition. Usually, a more specific diagnosis can be made:
- Gynaecological pain
- Menstrual cycle, e.g. mittelschmerz
- Pregnancy
- Sexually transmitted disease

The fact that she has not started her periods does not mean that she will not have hormonal cycles. In addition, there is the possibility she may be pregnant. It is important to tread carefully as some children will be less informed in this area than others. Some girls will be open with their parents, others will keep them in the dark. If there are other people in the room, they may be asked to leave. It is essential to establish methods of asking the right questions appropriately, which will be much individualised.

Gastro-oesophageal reflux disease

This is well recognised in babies and adults, but is often overlooked in older children. Given that she had gastro-oesophageal reflux disease before, she is more likely to have it again. The most useful test may be a therapeutic trial of medication, e.g. ranitidine.

Coeliac disease

Classically, coeliac disease should present with diarrhoea, weight loss, bloating and general debilitation. Milder cases are reported to present later with less marked symptoms, without diarrhoea or even with constipation. So, potentially every child with abdominal pain could be tested for coeliac disease. However, there is often a discrepancy between pathological results and clinical presentation. Because gluten sensitivity is common, screening will identify a large number of positive results. How much these children will benefit from a gluten exclusion diet is not clear, and in many their abdominal pain is not linked to their 'gluten enteropathy'.

There is no right answer; it is worth establishing what the local policy is regarding coeliac testing.

Food intolerance/insensitivity/allergy

Belief in food intolerance is more strongly held in the lay community than in the medical one. The most useful way to test for this is with exclusion diets. Dairy foods and wheat are the most popular culprits at present. Because excluding major food groups is a dramatic step, ensure that any clinical improvement is real rather than imagined. Re-challenge by introducing the offending food/s back into the diet after a few months to ensure that it does make a difference. If the family are convinced that exclusion is beneficial, a dietetic referral can help to ensure that the diet is balanced.

Families should be made aware of the debate surrounding the value of allergy tests, and the commercial interest for allergy test providers. Many outlets offer allergy tests which can identify different allergies in the same person on different occasions and some of these tests (York, IgG and Vega) are not evidence based and should be discouraged from forming a diagnostic basis..

Rarer causes

Gallstones – particularly spherocytosis or after prolonged total parenteral nutrition (intravenous feeding)
Pancreatitis
Inflammatory bowel disease
Cystic fibrosis
Intermittent volvulus: Can be linked to adhesions
Other organic causes: Hypercalcaemia/lead poisoning
Other rare causes: Rarely seen outside of exam settings

Consultation essentials

History/examination

Worrying features

If any of these are detected discuss the case with a senior.
- Increasing pain severity
- Weight loss
- Too much stool:

- Diarrhoea – distinguish from overflow. In overflow the stool may be soft and frequent but only small amounts are passed each time
- Malabsorption – classic features include steatorrhoea and a stool that does not easily flush. The stool may be frothy, foul smelling and toxic, causing perianal irritation. The presence of undigested vegetables is not unusual; other foods should not be present
- Blood mixed in with stool – as opposed to blood on the outside of the stool or on wiping the bottom which is common in anal fissures
- Systemic features:
  - Fever
  - Rash
  - Jaundice
  - Clubbing (very rare)
- Organomegaly
- Anal abnormality – especially fistulae or abscesses – suggesting Crohn's disease

Nature/severity/radiation

Describing pain can be difficult. An idea of severity can be obtained by finding out what activities have been missed due to the pain. School can be missed for many reasons – ask 'what things have you really wanted to do which you could not do because of the pain?'

Relieving/exacerbating factors

It is helpful to ask what makes the pain better and what makes it worse, e.g. ibuprofen exacerbating gastritis. If families say they have not tried painkillers this can give some idea of how bad it really is.

Timing/periodicity

Anxiety, even if school related, can be present in the school holidays. If the pain is menstrual cycle related it may be irregular at this age.

Bowel habit

Despite the apparent normal bowel habit, always ask specific questions, including the use of school toilets. It is remarkable how abnormal a 'normal bowel habit' can be. If opening the bowels eases the pain, this is likely to be the cause of it.

Social/school history

Identifying anxiety asking about school and home. As well as identifying specific worries, establish if she is an anxious or relaxed type of person.

Tests/investigations

A careful history and examination will often make investigations unnecessary.

It is easy to fall into the trap of thinking that investigations are good because they are reassuring. This overlooks the fact that they can be painful, require further visits to obtain, have side effects and be costly.

The idea that an investigation will provide an answer that has not already been considered is fallacious. Most investigations merely support or refute a clinical suspicion.

Useful information may include a comprehensive symptom diary. A good toilet history is essential and can be referenced to the ubiquitous Bristol stool chart. Often abdominal pain just resolves if left alone for a few months. Waiting, with appropriate safety netting, can enable investigations to be focussed or even unnecessary.

Blood tests

Blood tests should be performed following reflection rather than as a reflex. Inflammatory bowel disease can present insidiously and coeliac disease has a multifaceted presentation, as discussed above.

- Full blood count: Chronic blood loss, e.g through gastritis or enteropathy can cause anaemia (macrocytic or microcytic), and thrombocytosis
- Erythrocyte sedimentation rate/C-reactive protein: Non-specific but usually raised in active inflammatory bowel disease
- Albumin/protein: Often reduced in inflammatory bowel disease
- Coeliac screen: Hard not to include it

Stool tests

Microbiology – rarely indicated.

Elastase/reducing substances

If the stool is formed there is no point doing this.

Radiology

Plain X-ray

Try to avoid ordering plain films unless there is a clear indication, of which there are none for this patient. Occasionally, helpful in 'confirming' a diagnosis of constipation/stool withholding. Some families can dispute the diagnosis but are convinced when shown an X-ray with massive fecal loading.

Abdominal ultrasound

Not needed routinely, latest scanners can pick up alterations in bowel wall, and might help in the diagnosis of inflammatory bowel disease. Useful for gallstones, mesenteric adenitis and other conditions, but beware of incidental findings.

Further tests

Usually only after discussion with a senior.

Diagnosis

At clinic no formal diagnosis was made.

Management

Melody was asked to keep a diary and consider engaging with the school counsellor.

Follow up

Make this long enough for all the information to be available, often allowing 'therapeutic time'. Waiting at least 3 months seems appropriate, with 'safety-netting' as required.

Discussion

Melody's symptoms settled gradually over the next few months. She did have some concerns at school and benefitted from seeing the school counsellor. Her periods started and were a little heavy initially. The diagnosis, somewhat unsatisfactorily, would be abdominal pain – no cause found-resolved.

Further reading

El Metwally, et al. Predictors of abdominal pain in schoolchildren: a 4-year population-based prospective study. Arch Dis Child 2007; 92:1094–1098.

Case 2

Absence seizures

Dear Paediatrician,

I would be grateful for your advice on Abbie who is 6 years old. She is the only child to her parents. She had been well until about 3 months ago. One day she was singing in the school choir when half way through her mother saw her staring out of the window for a few seconds. Since then the parents and staff have noticed her having several episodes of vacant spells. She stops what she has been doing and will not respond to others calling her name. On some occasions, they have noticed her eyes rolling upwards or flickering of eyelids. She can be a little fidgety or may have odd facial movements. She has occasionally been urine incontinent. Her general health is otherwise excellent and there are no concerns in learning or behaviour.

Dr Bill Murphy

Case analysis

This is a classical description of childhood absence epilepsy (CAE). The episodes are usually noticed by those around the child, either family or school teachers, and a school-aged child's performance in class may have deteriorated as they miss important information during the absence. At home they may have been labelled as 'in a trance' at the time, and the 'day dreaming' may have been attributed to 'not listening' or being engrossed in some other activity.

Differential diagnoses

Childhood absence epilepsy

The usual age of presentation is between 4–12 years with a peak at around 5–7 years. There are reports of CAE in children under 4 years and over 12 years, but only exceptionally. Important features of CAE are: short episode duration, between 4–20 seconds with an average 10 seconds, abrupt onset and abrupt termination, severe impairment of consciousness, high daily frequency – anything up to 100 per day. Absences can be precipitated by emotional or metabolic causes (e.g. hyperventilation). In a typical episode the child exhibits a behavioural arrest, stares into space, with or without facial automatisms such as eye blinking, flickering of eyelids or facial twitching, chewing or lip smacking. Autonomic features like papillary dilatation, tachycardia, sweating, piloerection and urinary incontinence may accompany a typical attack. The attacks can be triggered by hyperventilation. The child will return to normal once the episode is over.

Day dreaming

This is a common behaviour in younger children. They appear 'glued' to the TV, or other activity. They are usually easy to distract and the duration is variable. They may continue in their 'trance' until interrupted. On being disturbed, they are alert. There are none of the features of CAE above. These episodes cannot be triggered by hyperventilation. They may occur when bored or tired. The child's development is normal and general behaviour is otherwise normal also. There is no postictal phase.

Juvenile absence epilepsy

This is often seen in children with disability or learning difficulty. It has a slow onset and slow recovery. There may be collapse and postictal confusion. There are typical electroencephalography (EEG) changes aiding the diagnosis.

Hearing

It would be important to ensure that hearing is checked as important correctable parameters which can present with vacant episodes, and be a reason for failing academic activity at school.

Consultation essentials

History

A good clinical history is important with details of the ictal events along with the pre- and postictal features. A record of school performance can be useful, especially if demonstrating a dip from previous levels. Hyperventilation for 2–3 minutes may be useful in demonstrating a typical absence seizure in outpatient settings, but with caution.

Investigations

Video footage

A video recording is very helpful as this will provide direct details of the events.

Electroencephalography

An EEG will show a rhythmic, 3 Hz, bilateral, synchronous and symmetric spike and wave changes during an absence seizure, usually induced by hyperventilation during the recording.

MRI of the brain

Generally, brain imaging is not routinely recommended in classical childhood absence epilepsy.

Diagnosis

Abbie's story is classic for absence seizures. Her EEG showed 3 per second spike and wave appearances when she blew a windmill for 2 minutes. She had a typical episode and then recovered.

Management

The first line treatment for CAE is either sodium valproate or ethosuximide. Other useful AED's are lamotrigine, leviteracetam, clobazam and clonazepam. Drugs to avoid are carbamazepine, oxcarbazepine, gabapentin, tiagabine, phenytoin and phenobarbitone as they can exacerbate the absences.

Abbie responded to standard doses of ethosuximide. Within 3 weeks of starting the medication her absences stopped and her school work gradually improved. She moved up reading levels.

Follow up

It is important to follow up children with CAE to be sure control continues and to monitor any side effects of medication. After 1–2 years of medication, it can be gradually tailed off to see if the control remains. If any episodes are seen, the dose should be increased back to the level which allowed good control.

Discussion

The CAE has excellent prognosis and 80–90% of children will go into remission with 1–2 years of treatment.

Further reading

Panayiotopoulos CJ. The Epilepsies, Seizures, Syndromes and Management. Oxford: Bladen Medical Publishing; 2005.

Wallace SJ, Farrell K. Epilepsy in Children, 2nd ed. London: Arnold publishers; 2004.

The epilepsies: the diagnosis and management of the epilepsies in adults and children in primary and secondary care. National Institute for Health and Clinical Excellence Clinical guideline 2012:137. http://www.nice.org.uk/CG137

Patient information

Epilepsy action
    www.epilepsy.org.uk
Epilepsy society
    www.epilepsysociety.org.uk
Young epilepsy
    www.ncype.org.uk

Acne

Dear Paediatrician,

Please would you see this 13-year-old girl with acne. This condition has not responded to topical treatment or oral erythromycin. It is affecting her confidence and she is reluctant to go out without make-up. I would appreciate your advice on further treatment.

Dr Adrian Cohen

Case analysis

Most teenagers will develop some acne lesions. Acne can be associated with psychological effects such as lack of confidence and impaired social contact and this may not correlate with disease severity. It is important to know about length of previous treatment. Response to oral antibiotics is slow: a minimum of 3 months and up to 6 months may be required to get maximum benefit.

Differential diagnosis

Acne

It usually starts in adolescence. It develops earlier in girls, probably due to earlier onset of puberty.

Keratosis pilaris

Common hereditary condition associated with follicular plugging. Rough texture with tiny red papules due to keratin plugs in hair follicles. It is most common on the upper arms and thighs but can also occur on the face. It may mimic acne.

Tuberous sclerosis

This is an autosomal dominant multisystem disorder with variable penetrance. Angiofibromas which are red papules on the nose and cheeks usually appear in the teenage years and worsen with age. Look for other cutaneous features including ash leaf macules and periungual fibromas.

Perioral dermatitis

Perioral papules without comedones (blackheads and whiteheads), can be associated with use of topical corticosteroids on the face

Consultation essentials

History/examination

Ask about age of onset, previous topical and systemic treatment including length of treatment, psychological and social effects. It can be associated with polycystic ovarian syndrome with obesity, hirsutism and oligo- or amenorrhoea.

Assess type of lesions present and their extent. These may include:

- Non-inflamed comedones
- Papules and pustules
- Nodules
- Scarring, ice pick scars due to damaged collagen, hypertrophic or keloid scars

Tests/investigations

No tests are required in most cases. A skin swab can be done if bacterial folliculitis is suspected. Consider hormone screen if endocrine disorder such as polycystic ovarian syndrome is suspected.

Diagnosis

In the presence of typical acne lesions, acne was the diagnosis in this case.

Management

The choice of treatment depends on the type of lesion, severity and extent of disease and psychological effects of acne. Response to oral antibiotic treatment is slow and may take 4–6 weeks to achieve a response. Treatment is required for 3–6 months to have a maximal effect. The treatment course may need to be repeated. Avoid tetracycline in children < 12 years because of the risk of permanent staining of the teeth.

Mild acne

Acne is mild if there are predominantly non-inflamed comedones – topical retinoids, e.g. tretinoin 0.01–0.025% gel or adapalene 0.1% gel or cream is a usual treatment.

Comedones with pustules/papules – topical antimicrobials, e.g. benzoyl peroxide, clindamycin, erythromycin.

Combination therapies are available (e.g. Duac gel which contains benzoyl peroxide 5%, clindamycin 1%).

Topical antimicrobials can be combined with topical retinoids. Topical retinoids often cause irritation and benzoyl peroxide may also cause irritation. If this occurs, suggest reducing the frequency of use e.g. to 2–3 times weekly and build up to daily over few weeks if tolerated.

Moderate acne

This is typified by a greater number of lesions and more extensive inflamed lesions. Treatment topically is as above for mild acne, plus systemic antibiotic treatment for 3–6 months, e.g. oxytetracycline 500 mg twice daily, lymecycline once daily, doxycycline

100 mg daily, minocycline 100 mg daily, erythromycin 500 mg twice daily or trimethoprim 200–300 mg twice daily.

Second generation tetracycline (doxycycline, minocycline and lymecycline) can be taken as once daily preparations because of their longer half-life and can be taken with meals whereas tetracycline must be taken an hour before meals. Minocycline is usually only recommended as a second line as it has additional side effects including pigmentation and lupus-like reactions.

Moderate to severe acne

This is typified by papules, pustules and/or nodules with deeper inflammation and scarring **(Figure 3.1)**. Consider additional antiandrogen therapy in girls e.g. Dianette (Ethinyloestradiol/cyproterone acetate). Consider oral isotretinoin, 0.5–1 mg/kg/day for 4 months which is highly effective but has potential side effects which include dose dependent mucocutaneous side effects (chelitis, skin dryness, conjunctivitis, and epistaxis), teratogenicity, abnormal liver function and lipids, myalgia, depression and aggressive behaviour. Monthly pregnancy tests are required for sexually active teenagers.

Follow up

Follow up and review depends on severity. Moderate to severe acne needs follow up at 2–3 months to assess the response to antibiotics. Patients on oral isotretinoin need regular follow up until course of treatment is complete.

Discussion

Infantile acne is a rare presentation of acne. It usually presents after the age of 3 months, appears mainly on the cheeks and is more common in boys. Spontaneous healing usually occurs within 2 years. Lesions range from comedones to more inflammatory papules, pustules and nodules. Scarring may occur. The treatment includes topical retinoids,

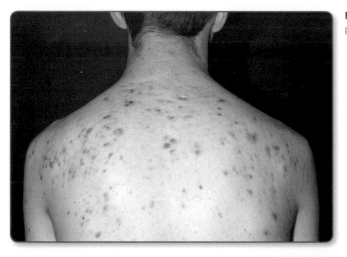

Figure 3.1 Severe acne with pustules, nodules and scarring.

benzoylperoxide or erythromycin. Severe cases will require oral erythromycin or trimethoprim. Rarely oral isotretinoin is required.

Further reading

Thiboutot D, Gollnick H, Bettoli V, et al. New insights into the management of acne; a report from the Global Alliance to improve outcomes in acne. J Am Acad Dermatol 2009; 60:1s–50s.

Layton AM. Disorders of sebaceous glands. In; Rook's Textbook of Dermatology. Breathnach SM, Cox NH, Griffiths CEM, Eds, 8th edn. Oxford: Blackwell Publishing, 2010: 42.1–42.89.

Patient information

The British Association of Dermatologists
     www.bad.org.uk
DermNet NZ
     www.dermnetnz.org
Skin Care Physicians
     www.skincarephysicians.com

Case 4

Allergic reaction to food

Dear Paediatrician,

Thank you for seeing Angie. She is 6 months old. She developed an urticaria rash and lip swelling when given scrambled egg for the first time. Please can you confirm on testing and advise accordingly?

Dr Gordon Winch

Case analysis

The details need to be discussed further but the history of a reaction to a single food product, such as loosely cooked egg, is quite diagnostic. Further information is required as below, but on the basis of the detail in the letter, it seems quite likely that Angie has an allergy to egg.

Differential diagnosis

Egg allergy

This is clearly the diagnosis based on the good, convincing history. The diagnostic challenge to describe the true allergen is more complicated when there is a meal or mixed dish that prompts a more delayed reaction. Egg allergy is an adverse reaction in the immune system caused by egg protein. This is immunoglobulin E (IgE) mediated.

Milk allergy

There could be milk in scrambled egg and clarity on the exact constituents is crucial. Angie is likely to already be having milk and therefore the chance of a true IgE-mediated milk allergy is unlikely.

Consultation essentials

History/examination

A true allergy history will include details of: what was eaten, how much was eaten, timing of any reaction to what was eaten, how long after eating and how long it lasted. Whether the food had previously been eaten, and tolerated, is important, as is any other known allergies to any other foods. What is the exact nature of the reaction? What treatment was given and how it improved the symptoms should also be clarified. Identifying specific symptoms of the reaction including any tongue, throat or laryngeal involvement (which will manifest in a young child as a change in voice, cry or hoarse voice) to clarify the presence of airway involvement or anaphylaxis is important. Any hospital treatment received can also help clarify the type of reaction. Clark and Ewan described a grading system for reactions

Table 4.1 Severity grading of worst reaction before referral		
Grade	Description	Clinical Features
1	Mild	Local skin redness +/- urticarial rash +/- angio-oedema +/- oral itchiness
2	Mild	Generalised red rash +/- urticarial rash +/- angio-oedema
3	Mild	Symptoms of 1 OR 2 above PLUS • gastrointestinal symptoms and/or • nasal mucus discharge or • discharge from eyes
4	Moderate	Change in voice +/- feeling of tightening of the throat +/- mild wheeze
5	Severe	Marked difficulty breathing +/- low blood pressure (collapse +/- loss of consciousness)
Adapted from Clark AT, Ewan PW. Arch Dis Child 2003;88:79–81.		

(Table 4.1). A history of wheeze or eczema should be established as part of the family of atopic conditions.

Tests/investigations

Testing an allergy is tricky. This is because of the phenomenon of sensitisation. The first line test is usually a skin prick test (SPT) dictated by the detail of the history. That should focus the testing towards specific allergens which are likely to the incriminated. In this case, testing the child for eggs is necessary, and milk if there is any suggestion of milk allergy. If not exposed to peanut (and is unlikely to have been at this age), testing for peanut sensitisation would be important.

Skin prick test

A SPT is performed by using glycerated extracts of allergen, specific allergenic proteins from the food or aeroallergen, the placed on the skin. A very fine lance (1 mm) is then used to prick (although it is more of a 'press') the extract into the top dermal layer of skin. A 'positive' control (histamine) and negative control (saline) are included. The former will always react causing an itchy wheal and the latter should not react at all. The test is read after 15 minutes. A positive test is given by a wheal diameter that is 3 mm more

Table 4.2 Skin prick test cut offs for 100% positive predictive values			
Age (years)	Milk	Egg	Peanut
< 2	6 mm	5 mm	4 mm
> 2	> 8 mm	> 7 mm	> 8 mm

Caution: these cut offs are supportive of a diagnosis only in the presence of a convincing history. Without that further evidence, such as IgE and likely an oral challenge is required.

than the negative control, or at the level of the positive control. A negative test is specific to the absence of true allergy, however a positive test is not always very sensitive and it can represent sensitisation, i.e. a reaction on the test without a good clinical history of a reaction to the food. In other words, the positive skin prick test is not a good predictor of a clinically important allergic reaction. That is why testing should not be blanket but directed towards a specific allergen. There is research evidence to support a wheal at various levels to be in the 95% positive predictive range (Table 4.2). In any event, a positive test at any level in combination with a good history is diagnostic.

Specific IgE

If the SPT result is equivocal, further testing is advised. The gold standard test would be a control (double blinded) challenge. However, further evidence can be gathered by testing specific blood IgE levels. Total IgE levels are not very specific but specific IgE levels to an allergen is helpful and can be compared to published cut-offs (Table 4.3).

Challenges

No cut-off can be given for SPT wheal size or serum-specific IgE level which predicts clinical severity. The gold standard test is a blinded challenge to the allergen food which is incriminated. However, in the presence of a positive test with a good history there is no need for a challenge. The most value to be gained from a controlled challenge is when testing suggests tolerance which may have developed on repeat testing or when the history is not very clear.

Diagnosis

Angie had a grade 2 reaction to scrambled egg based on clinical history.

Table 4.3 Predictive value of specific IgE						
	Age	Egg	Milk	Peanut	Fish	Tree nuts
Diagnostic cut off kUa/L	< 2 years	≥ 2.0	≥ 5.0			
	> 2 years	≥ 7.0	≥ 15.0	≥ 14.0	≥ 20.0	≥ 15.0
Challenge value kUa/L		≤ 1.5	≤ 7.0	≤ 5.0	–	< 2.0

This is a guide. Studies on egg vary greatly.

Management

The reaction occurred after a few spoons of a scrambled egg dish containing milk and loosely cooked egg. Angie had been tolerating formula milk without any problem. The reaction self-resolved without any medication. A SPT to egg white showed a wheal of 4 mm, and to raw egg a wheal of 6 mm. These were diagnostic for egg allergy in light of the history. Avoidance of egg was advised and antihistamine prescribed to use as part of a specific allergy plan. Adrenaline pen was not prescribed in the absence of any respiratory effects or signs of anaphylaxis. The SPT to milk and nuts was negative. Nuts could be introduced into Angie's diet.

Follow up

Since egg allergy improves in childhood in the majority of cases (over 50% will outgrow their allergy by 5 years), regular review is recommended. A repeat SPT every 1 or 2 years will give some indication of tolerance. Tolerance to cooked egg develops first, or may be present in the beginning. This means children may tolerate cooked egg products containing egg such as cakes or biscuits. But they are likely to react to rawer forms of egg in meringue, homemade ice cream and loosely cooked forms of egg such as omelette. While anaphylaxis is possible, egg reactions are rarely fatal. Usually safety netting with avoidance and antihistamines in case of a reaction will suffice in the absence of any signs of anaphylaxis in the initial or any subsequent reactions. If testing suggests tolerance, and if initial reactions were mild in a child without asthma, reintroduction can be done at home. Children reacting to hen's eggs will likely react to other avian eggs.

Egg allergy and vaccines

There is a theoretical risk of a reaction to MMR vaccination, since it is cultured on chick embryo, but in reality there is no egg in the vaccine and therefore it should be safe. There is more likely to be a reaction to other constituents of the vaccine. If there is any doubt, or to ensure the child is vaccinated, facilitating this in a controlled/hospital setting could be offered, but is not necessary. Flu vaccine contains ovalbumin but there are versions with low albumin content. Yellow fever vaccine also contains egg proteins. Advice from the local allergy expert or vaccine committee should be sought.

Discussion

The prevalence of egg allergy is 2% in children. It commonly presents in infancy. Severe reactions which involve the airway are rare. As with many allergens, a size of wheal and/or level of specific IgE cannot be used to predict the severity of a reaction. Egg avoidance is important and a dietician involvement is helpful, especially if there are other allergies. Egg allergy in infancy is associated with the development of asthma later in life. The decision to reintroduce (well cooked) egg to children with a mild allergy at a certain time depends on the individual history. Children with a more severe allergy should have cautious reintroduction and may need specialist input.

There is a difference between allergy, intolerance and sensitisation:

True allergy: This describes any adverse reaction to a food, insect sting, and drug or chemical, manifested by a response by the immune system to a substance that would normally be harmless.

Intolerance: This is an adverse response to ingestion of food when the body does not have enough enzymes or chemicals required to facilitate break down, digestion or absorption of the food. This does not involve the immune system.

Sensitivity: This is a response to contact with, often a small amount, of a substance. It is used to describe a positive allergy test, e.g. SPT, where there may not have been a clear clinical reaction to the substance, and therefore the diagnosis of allergy cannot be confirmed without a challenge.

Further reading

Clark AT, Skypala I, Leech SC, et al. British Society for Allergy and Clinical Immunology guidelines for the management of egg allergy. Clinical & Experimental Allergy, 2010; 40(8):1116–1129.

Clark AT, Ewan PW. Food allergy in childhood. Arch Dis Child 2003; 88:79–81.

Clark AT, Skypala I, Leech SC, et al. British society for Allergy and Clinical Immunology. British Society for Allergy and Clinical Immunology guidelines for the management of egg allergy. Clin Exp Allergy 2010; 40(8):1116–1129.

Leung D, Sampson HA, Geha RS, et al. Pediatric Allergy: Principles and Practice, 2nd edn. Philadelphia: Elsevier Saunders, 2010.

Sampson HA. Utility of food-specific IgE concentrations in predicting symptomatic food allergy. Journal of Allergy and Clinical Immunology 2001; 107(5):891–896.

Sporik R, Hill DJ, Hosking CS. Specificity of allergen skin testing in predicting positive open food challenges to milk, egg and peanut in children. Clin Exp Allergy 2000; 30(11):1540–1546.

Patient information

Allergy UK
    http://www.allergyuk.org/egg-allergy/egg-allergy
The Anaphylaxis Campaign
    http://www.anaphylaxis.org.uk/what-is-anaphylaxis/knowledgebase/egg-allergy-factsheet

Case 5

Allergic reaction: nuts

Dear Paediatrician,

Thank you for seeing Peter. He is a 9-year-old boy with mild asthma and eczema. He was at his grandmother's and ate a peanut butter sandwich. After about 5 minutes he developed a red, itchy rash over his face and his lips swelled. He then felt his throat becoming tight and had difficulty breathing. He was brought to the emergency department and given oral antihistamine. This improved the symptoms. He was observed for 4 hours and discharged. I have prescribed an adrenaline pen. Thank you for your assessment.

Dr Jagjit Basharuthulla

Case analysis

This is a convincing history for immunoglobulin E (IgE) mediated peanut allergy. He has atopic conditions (asthma and eczema) which make a food allergy more likely.

Differential diagnosis

Peanut allergy

Peanuts are part of the family of legumes, and are also known as ground nuts (they grow in the ground unlike most other nuts which are tree nuts). Other names include monkey nuts, earthnuts, goober peas, pygmy nuts and pig nuts. The exact reason for the development of peanut allergy is not well known. There may be triggers such as early exposure to soy or peanut oils. The 'hygiene hypothesis' may also be a cause of the increase in prevalence. It is estimated that the prevalence is about 1% in children. Research suggests that delay in introducing peanut into the diet in a child significantly increases the chance of allergy. Similarly there is no need to advise avoidance of peanuts during pregnancy or in breastfeeding mothers. A study comparing rates of peanut allergy in UK children compared to children in Israel showed a lower incidence in Israeli children. Israeli children are given peanuts from a much younger age than children in the UK. Up to 20% of children will outgrow their peanut allergy by the time they are 5 years old. Subsequent reactions are usually more severe but there is no way to predict these. Co-existence of asthma is a risk factor for more severe reactions.

Tree nut allergy

Tree nuts include hazelnut, pecan, walnut, Brazil nut, macadamia, pistachio and cashew. Despite peanut being a legume there is co-reactivity with tree nuts, which, although they are unrelated, is likely to be due to shared homologous epitopes. Management of an allergy is the same, whatever the allergen; strict avoidance.

Consultation essentials

History/examination

The following makes a complete allergy history:

- What is the suspected allergen?
- What was the route of exposure – touch (bird seeds are often 'monkey nuts'), inhalation (relevant for environmental allergens) or ingestion, as in this case?
- What was the timing of the reaction – IgE-mediated reactions occur soon after exposure?
- What was the description of the reaction?
- What treatment was given and how much? Did the child require emergency medication; was an injection given (most likely intramuscular adrenaline)?
- Was this allergen tolerated previously? While this is not usually the case, it can be that some foods become allergenic
- Ask about co-existing conditions of atopy – eczema, asthma (including medications and symptoms to assess control) and hay fever

Assessing for signs of atopy such as allergic 'salute' (transverse line on nose from repeated rubbing in allergic rhinitis), bogginess or swelling under eyes, dry skin.

Tests/investigations

Skin prick test

This test would be a reasonable first step in diagnosis. The published 95% cut-offs can be used as a guide, but in the presence of a convincing history any positive response on the skin prick test (3 mm more than the negative control, or a level at or above the positive control) is considered supportive of the diagnosis.

Specific IgE and component resolved testing

Specific IgE levels in themselves are helpful to describe an IgE-mediated allergy. But a more specific test is becoming more widely available. The 'Ara h' (named after the species of peanut *Arachis hypogaea*) components of the IgE allergenic protein can be tested now and seem a more specific way of assessing peanut allergy. Ara h-2 is the most sensistive marker of significant peanut allergy and if the IgE of this component is raised, the chance of allergy is high and a challenge would therefore be contraindicated. However, if component Ara h-8 is positive, this is a cross reacting protein with birch pollen and lends weight to the possibility of oral allergy syndrome which manifests as hay fever with allergic symptoms of itching or tingling of the mouth, lips or tongue or a scratchy throat when eating certain fresh foods or fruits. This is due to the cross reaction of birch pollen with the skin of the fruit; the symptoms are usually absent when the fruit is cooked.

Challenges

This can be directed by skin prick test (SPT) and IgE (specific or component derived). Usually controlled challenges in hospital are used. Occasionally, a double-blind challenge is required.

Diagnosis

Peter ate one bite of the peanut butter sandwich and had an immediate reaction. An SPT showed a wheal of 6 mm (positive control 5 mm, negative control 0 mm). Despite the positive SPT on usual criteria, it was below the 95% positive predictive value and a specific IgE test was done. This was 25 kUA/L, well above any published cut offs. In light of these results, and the clinical presentation, component testing was not thought necessary at this time.

Management

Avoidance is the key here and strict exclusion is mainstay. Reading labels and ensuring foods are free from any contamination need to become a way of life for Peter. While there is a theoretical chance of resolution (20% by the age of 5 years), this is more common in younger children and by this age the chances are that this will be a lifelong allergy. Peter has always tolerated hazelnut spread and this was advised to continue. He had eaten cashew nuts as part of a Chinese meal and not reacted, so in the absence of any further reactions to tree nuts, his diet was not restricted further. However, skin prick testing to tree nuts would be indicated if there is a concern about any reaction, especially if that nut has not been eaten previously (status unknown). Any positive wheals need further evaluation and in the absence of a clinical reaction, an oral food challenge would be indicated.

The general practitioner prescribed an adrenaline autoinjector (adrenaline pen), which is sensible despite the absence of clear anaphylaxis on the clinical presentation.

Follow up

There is little value in close review but some support to the family in the early stages would be sensible. A 6-month review after introduction of the allergy plan could be followed by annual 2-yearly reviews. Repeat testing could be reserved until Peter is older, and before he reaches an age where he will be discharged from the paediatric clinic. If the testing confirms high responses on either SPT or specific IgE, then continued avoidance or allergy planning should continue. If the testing suggests tolerance with lower skin prick wheals, low IgE, or Ara h components not associated with anaphylaxis (e.g. low levels of Ara h-1, 2 and 3), a formal challenge would be indicated.

Discussion

Indications for injectable adrenaline have been debated. Good summary guidance is available from the Australasian Society of Clinical Immunology and Allergy (see resources). A child diagnosed with a nut allergy should usually be prescribed an adrenaline autoinjector. There are two versions available in the UK: Jext and Epipen. Enforcing carrying the adrenaline pen becomes more of a challenge, as has been shown in studies of teenagers with allergy. Other risky behaviour can contribute to an increased risk of exposure (e.g. kissing). There is also the challenge of schools which do not usually 'pool' the adrenaline pens across children but require individual ones to be available for each student with an allergy plan. Previously it was advised that two pens should be available in case of an anaphylactic reaction, since there is some evidence to suggest two doses of adrenaline are required in a small percentage of children and young people with anaphylaxis. However, from a resource perspective this is untenable and one person one pen ratio is advised, unless there is a clear history of anaphylaxis, uncontrolled asthma or remote location.

Further reading

Du Toit G, Katz Y, Sasieni P, et al. Early consumption of peanuts in infancy is associated with a low prevalence of peanut allergy. The Journal of allergy and clinical immunology 2008; 122(5):984–991.

Scherer SH, Wood R. Advances in diagnosing peanut allergy. J Allergy Clin Immunol: in practice 2013; 1:1–13.

Skripak JM, Wood RA. Peanut and tree nut allergy in childhood. Pediatr Allergy Immunol 2008; 19:368–373.

Australasia Society of Clinical Immunology and Allergy (ASCIA). Guidelines for adrenaline autoinjector prescription. New South Wales: ASCIA, 2012.

Patient information

Allergy UK
   www.allergyuk.org
Kids aware
   http://www.kidsaware.co.uk

Case 6

Allergic reaction: urticaria

Dear Paediatrician,

Thank you for seeing Algie, a 14-year-old boy who has for some months now been getting intermittent hives and urticaria which are causing itching and distress. His mother has changed the washing powder but it has not helped. She has kept a food diary but there does not seem to be an obvious trigger. I have prescribed some antihistamine which has not made any difference either. The frequency is worrying. Am I missing an allergy here and, if so, to what?

Dr Heather Winship

Case analysis

Since urticarial rash is a common manifestation of allergic presentations, there is focus on finding the allergen. However, urticaria has many causes and the main issues here are to try and classify the type of urticaria to make the diagnosis.

Differential diagnosis

Urticaria

This is a group of heterogeneous disorders which manifest with sudden onset of wheals and/or angioedema. The features of urticaria are common to children and adults, and differences in underlying causes are small. Urticaria can be acute or chronic.

The wheal is caused by release (degranulation) of histamine from mast cells which are the primary mediator of the wheal and flare seen. Histamine acts on receptors on epithelial cells of the skin. The effect of histamine on sensory nerves causes the itching. The wheal is oedema of the upper and mid dermis, with dilatation of the venules and lymphatics in that upper third of the dermis consisting of a variably sized central swelling, usually surrounded by reflex erythema. It is associated with itching or a burning sensation and usually resolves to normal appearances within 24 hours.

Angioedema is the result of similar changes but affecting the lower third of the dermis and the subcutis. There is an infiltrate containing many inflammatory cytokines such as neutrophils, eosinophils, macrophages and T-cells. While this describes the pathophysiology, it does not give a clue as to the cause or diagnosis. Sometimes the swelling is painful rather than pruritic, and mucous membranes are often involved. Resolution takes up to 72 hours, being slower than for wheals.

Acute urticaria

A trigger can usually be identified in acute urticaria. The commonest causes are:
- Food reactions – egg, milk, peanut, soya, wheat in younger children and nuts, seafood in older children, scombroid fish poisoning

- Viral infections (mediating urticaria and angioedema via IgE)
- Drugs (by direct histamine release, especially antibiotics such as penicillins)
- Bites, stings, mites
- Mast cell degranulators
  - ingestion/contact – strawberries, polymyxin antibiotics, penetration – nettles, sea life
  - skin contact – latex, chemicals

It is usually generalised. There can be associated joint pain or bleeding into the lesions especially if there is an infective cause. It can be mistaken for erythema multiforme or anaphylaxis. It can be recurrent.

Chronic urticarias

This is characterised as symptoms on most or every day that persist for more than 6 weeks. It is more common in adults. The wheals last 6 hours and fade with total resolution. There may be accompanying angioedema. They may be coexisting atopy. It is caused by functional antibodies against a part of the IgE receptor resulting in degranulation at any time. There is an association with antithyroid antibodies, and reported links with coeliac disease diabetes, arthritis, familial autosomal disease. Investigation is best directed at anything in the clinical history. Inflammatory markers should be checked. Allergy testing will be negative and unless there is a likely allergen identified in the history, testing should be avoided. Serum functional antibodies can be checked if indicated, as can thyroid function and antibodies. Skin biopsy of a lesion may be performed to look for vasculitis. This condition usually remits in the majority after 3 years.

Physical urticarias

Dermatographism causes urticaria on rubbing or scratching the skin. Other physical causes of urticaria include pressure, cold, heat, exercise, sunlight and water. Cholinergic urticaria (often called 'heat rash') features smaller wheals and is caused by heat, exertion or emotion (all thermally provoked). The wheals in exercise-induced urticaria are larger, and it can lead to anaphylaxis. There is an association with sweating.

Mastocystosis

This is a primary disorder of mast cell proliferation. In children this is usually solitary or cutaneous. There are systemic symptoms such as breathlessness, low blood pressure or gastrointestinal upset.

Urticarial vasculitis

This is a rare form of urticaria. It will not respond to antihistamines. In children this is likely to be a Henoch–Schönlein purpura.

Hereditary angioedema

Angioedema without urticaria, which affects nondependent parts of the body, and is not usually itchy, is likely to be hereditary angioedema. The swelling lasts over 72 hours and does not usually occur daily. It may affect the subcutaneous tissues, abdominal organs (causing pain and diarrhoea; it can mimic an acute abdomen) and upper airway which may result in airway obstruction. There are three different types and although this autosomal dominant condition is caused by low levels of the plasma protein C1 esterase inhibitor, there are types with low or normal levels described. The best way to screen for this condition is to measure serum C4 levels which are almost always decreased during attacks and usually low between attacks. It can be treated by giving C1 esterase extract if available, depending on the type of hereditary angioedema. Prophylactic treatments are available for recurrent episodes.

Consultation essentials

A detailed history is going to be the best way to classify the type of urticaria and make a diagnosis. Diagnostic algorithms exist to assist with this purpose (Zuberbier et al. 2009a). When lesions occur, where the child is when they happen, and what associations have the family noticed.

History

Ask about:
- Onset
- Frequency and duration; is it acute or chronic
- Shape, size and distribution of wheals
- Angioedema – swelling of the skin or mucous membranes
- Itching, pain or burning sensations
- Precipitating factors (heat, cold, exercise, emotion, anxiety, food)
- Concurrent illness – such as viral infection
- School and any specific timing of the day
- Medication, including any in the house
- Effect on activity, school attendance and behaviour
- Family history of atopy, urticaria

Examination

A general examination to asses for an underlying connective tissue or endocrine condition is important. An acute viral illness will usually be apparent. Urticaria occurs all over the body, but angioedema is more likely to affect the mucous membranes and the face. It can be helpful, and revealing, to assess for dermatographism by 'drawing' with a blunt point.

Tests/investigations

Test should be directed by the clinical presentation and examination findings. If a known or suspected allergen is reported, then skin prick and serum IgE allergy tests might help rule this in or out. As a minimum, routine blood count, differential and inflammatory markers (C-reactive protein and erythrocyte sedimentation rate) along with urinalysis should be done. A physical urticaria could be brought on in clinic as a 'challenge'. Further evaluation with liver function tests, thyroid function tests and antibodies, anti-IgE antibodies and stool for parasitic infections would be second line.

Diagnosis

Algie was having episodes of recurrent chronic urticaria. A thorough history did not reveal any precipitant causes, although subsequent to the clinic letter he had some episodes at

Christmas and on his birthday. The lesions were small and punctate. This seemed to fit with a cholinergic urticaria. He had noticed he was having similar rash after exercise, although no features of anaphylaxis.

Management

The management depends on the diagnosis. In cholinergic urticaria antihistamines should work since it is histamine and IgE-mediated. Avoiding any situations which may prompt it and dressing appropriately, i.e. not too warmly, will help. For other forms of urticaria, it will depend on the diagnosis.

Follow up

Advice from the immunology or dermatology team may help. There are challenges and more sophisticated diagnostic tests which will be advised by the specialists. Regular follow up 3–6 monthly is required to monitor the condition and to assess the effectiveness of any medication.

Discussion

Management of urticaria generally includes an assessment of disease severity, based on a score (Zuberbier T, et al. 2009). It should be done over a number of days. There are quality of life issues here and school absence may be important. Symptomatic relief using avoidance and medication, usually nonsedating second generation antihistamines. First generation antihistamines may have a longer anticholinergic effect but a shorter antipuritic effect. Oral steroids have been used, as have leukotriene antagonists.

Further reading

Craig T, Pürsün EO, Bork K, et al. WAO Guideline for the Management of Hereditary Angioedema. WAO Journal 2012; 5:182–199.

Leech S. Recurrent urticaria. Paediatrics and Child Health 2012; 22(7): 281–286.

Zuberbier T, Asero R, Bindslev-Jensen C, Canonica GW, Church MK, Gime´nez-Arnau AM, et al. EAACI/GA2LEN/EDF/WAO Guideline: definition, classification and diagnosis of urticaria. Allergy 2009a; 64:1417–1426.

Zuberbier T, Asero R, Bindslev-Jensen C et al. EAACI/GA2LEN/EDF guideline: definition, classification and diagnosis of urticaria. Allergy 2009b; 64:1427–1443.

Patient information

Kids Health
    www.kidshealth.org
Allergy UK
    www.allergyuk.org

Case 7

Anaemia

Dear Paediatrician,

I would be grateful if you could see this 2 year old girl, Anna, who presented to the surgery with a history of pica for months. Blood tests have shown that she has anaemia with haemoglobin of 70 g/L (7 g/dL). Thank you for seeing her urgently.

Yours sincerely,

Dr Abasi Mugwangi

Case analysis

The diagnosis of anaemia can generate anxiety regarding possible causes, including malignancy such as leukaemia. The history of pica (defined as having an appetite for non-nutritive materials such as clay, dirt and sand) points towards a possible nutritional anaemia most probably iron-deficiency. The rest of the full blood count will help to differentiate between most of the common causes of anaemia.

Differential diagnosis

Iron-deficiency

This is the commonest cause for anaemia in toddlers and is usually due to a poor dietary intake of iron. The history is of a child who is a 'fussy eater', likes to drink milk rather than eat and often has a restricted diet with preference for carbohydrates. These children may have other vitamin or micronutrient deficiencies. As well as receiving iron, their diet should be assessed – ideally by a dietician to advice on dietary changes and whether other supplements are required. Pica is a well-recognised feature of iron-deficiency.

Because this is a chronic anaemia, children generally compensate well. It is not unusual for children to present seemingly well with haemoglobin as low as 30 g/L (3 g/dL). The response to iron is excellent and transfusions are rarely indicated, and should only be undertaken with severe caution because of the risk of precipitating cardiac failure.

Congenital anaemias: Diamond–Blackfan anaemia, fanconi anaemia

These are due to red-cell aplasia and are rare conditions. Children may have other dysmorphic features which would suggest a genetic defect, e.g abnormal thumbs, abnormal radius, cleft palate or short stature.

Aplastic anaemia

Acquired aplastic anaemia is very rare and can follow an infection such as parvovirus, cytomegalovirus, Epstein–Barr virus. Certain chemicals can also result in aplasia. Patients usually present with pancytopenia rather than pure red call aplasia.

Spherocytosis

This autosomal dominant condition that can present with jaundice in the newborn period, and episodic anaemia with jaundice during childhood. There is often a family history in one of the parents of anaemia, jaundice, splenectomy or gallstones.

Leukaemia

Leukaemia usually presents acutely with a child who becomes progressively more tired and pale over a few weeks with the additional symptoms and signs of bruising, bleeding, fevers and bone pain. Extremely rarely children will have a prolonged run in time before developing leukaemia, and this period may be marked by general unwellness, and mildly abnormal blood indices with a normal blood film.

Haemoglobinopathies

The newborn universal screening blood spot test should pick up both β-thalassaemia and sickle cell disease.

β-thalassaemia causes severe anaemia and children need to go onto a regular transfusion programme in infancy. β-thalassaemia trait can present with microcytic anaemia, but there is often a family history of anaemia.

α-thalassaemia is less common and tends not to cause significant anaemia unless there are three abnormal alleles, i.e. haemoglobin H disease. Sickle cell disease is seen primarily in the Afro-Caribbean population.

Blood loss

Acute blood loss is usually evident and should not present in outpatients. More chronic blood loss is not common. It may be seen in children who have gastric erosions or severe oesophagitis secondary to prolonged use of nonsteroidal anti-inflammatory drugs. The group most vulnerable to this are those with global developmental delay/spastic quadriplegia, who receive these drugs to treat presumed pain and are unable to vocalise that the drugs are the cause, rather than the cure.

Rare causes

Other causes of anaemia include the anaemia of chronic disease, which is usually mild, and pulmonary haemosiderosis.

Consultation essentials

History/examination

Obtain a history including duration of symptoms, tiredness, pallor, episodes of jaundice, fever, easy bruising,

A dietary history is essential and should include volume of milk intake day and night and the types of food and amounts. A history of pica often is associated with iron-deficiency and may be quite severe with children eating paper, sand, mud, plaster, paint, cloth. The child may be 'thriving' as they get adequate calories from the diet of milk and carbohydrates.

Tests/investigations

A full blood count and film is the most useful investigation in differentiating between the various causes of anaemia.

A hypochromic [low mean corpuscular haemoglobin (MCH), low mean corpuscular haemoglobin concentration(MCHC)], microcytic [low mean corpuscular volume (MCV)] anaemia could be due to iron-deficiency or the thalassaemias. The reticulocyte count may be helpful in differentiating between them as it tends to be low in iron-deficiency and normal or raised in thalassaemia.

Macrocytic (increased MCV) anaemias are very rare in children as isolated folate or B12 deficiencies are not seen.

Normal platelet and white cell counts rule out causes such as aplastic anaemia and leukaemia.

Other useful investigations are – bilirubin (raised in haemolytic anaemias), ferritin (low in iron-deficiency and normal/raised in thalassaemias).

Diagnosis

Her full blood count showed a haemoglobin (Hb) of 70 g/L with an MCV of 49.2 fL, MCHC 24.6 g/dL and Ferritin of 1 mcg/L.

This toddler has the classical presenting features of iron deficiency with chronic anaemia in a young child with a history of pica. A microcytic, hypochromic picture with low ferritin levels confirms the diagnosis.

Management

She was prescribed a daily oral iron supplement for 6 months and given dietary advice suggesting reduction of her milk intake and increase in the intake of red meat, pulses and vegetables. The addition of vitamin C containing products, such as orange juice, with meals and iron supplements increases the absorption of iron. Check compliance of medication and inform parents of the side effects of iron medication – dark coloured stools and constipation – which may need treatment itself.

Follow up

Children with severe anaemia – Hb < 60 g/L should have a repeat full blood count in 5–7 days to assess the reticulocyte response and increase in Hb which is often seen within a few days. If this is adequate a repeat full blood count, reticulocyte count and ferritin should be arranged in 6 months. There is little point testing before then, unless there is a change of symptoms or concerns regarding adherence to treatment.

Discussion

Whilst the diagnosis of anaemia is common, identifying the cause may be more complex. A full blood count with indices and a film should provide clues as to the likely diagnosis. Any child who does not respond to iron supplements may need further investigation and referral to a paediatric haematologist for consideration of other rare causes of anaemia.

It has long been known that iron-deficiency anaemia is associated with negative long-term developmental outcomes, with children being particularly vulnerable in the first few years of life. Periodically there are suggestions to implement universal screening for iron-deficiency anaemia, with a major limiting factor being the availability of a reliable test.

Further reading

Beard JL. Why iron deficiency is important in infant development. J Nutr 2008; 138(12):2534–2536.

Patient information

Centers for Disease Control and Prevention
   www.cdc.gov

Asthma

Dear Paediatrician,

Please could you see this 11-year-old girl whose asthma has become more difficult to control recently. She has required four courses of steroids over the winter and the mother is insisting on a referral to a paediatrician.

Her current treatment is clenil and ventolin inhalers.

Her family have recently moved to the area and as yet we do not yet have any previous notes.

Please see and advise.

Dr Francois Abel

Case analysis

It is likely that this child has had asthma for a while but it has become difficult to control recently. Although no previous history is given, the consultation should elicit that the diagnosis of asthma is correct. During the consultation, identify what has changed to make the child's symptoms worse, and ask about adherence to medication and inhaler technique.

Differential diagnosis

Asthma

The most important question to ask yourself: 'is this really asthma?'. Does she have the classic pattern of recurring episodic symptoms of wheeze, cough, difficulty breathing and chest tightness or does she have symptoms suggesting an alternative diagnosis (Tables 8.1 and 8.2)?

Dysfunctional breathing, habit cough, vocal cord dysfunction

It is important to think of these diagnoses particularly in view of the child's age. A habit cough usually starts with a simple viral upper respiratory infection which then continues as a habit cough despite resolution of the virus. The habit cough will disappear when the child is asleep but can be present on waking and is often disruptive to school classes. The cough is classically harsh in nature. Dysfunctional breathing can have complex causes and can coexist with a diagnosis of asthma. If present, it could be a reason for the failure of the asthma to respond to conventional asthma medication.

Table 8.1 Clinical features that increase the possibility of asthma
More than one of the following symptoms: wheeze, cough, difficulty breathing, chest tightness, particularly if these symptoms:
•   Are frequent and recurrent
•   Are worse at night and in the early morning
•   Occur in response to, or are worse after, exercise or other triggers, such as exposure to pets, cold or damp air, or with emotions or laughter
•   Occur at times other than when the child has 'colds'
Personal history of atopic disorder
Family history of atopic disorder and/or asthma
Widespread wheeze heard on auscultation
History of improvement in symptoms or lung function in response to adequate therapy

Table 8.2 Clinical features that lower the probability of asthma
Symptoms with colds only, with no interval symptoms
Isolated cough in the absence of wheeze or difficulty breathing
History of moist cough
Prominent dizziness, light-headedness, peripheral tingling
Repeatedly normal physical examination of chest when symptomatic
Normal peak expiratory flow (PEF) or spirometry when symptomatic
No response to a trial of asthma therapy
Clinical features pointing to alternative diagnosis

Nonadherence

The importance of addressing psychosocial issues and nonadherence in the management of difficult asthma in children is becoming increasing recognised. Prescription pick up rate can be obtained from the general practitioner as a marker of adherence to prescribed asthma medication. This girl has recently moved house and is at the age of secondary school transfer, both of which can be stressful times for children and their families and can have deleterious effect on asthma control.

Atopy

A history of atopy such as eczema, seasonal rhinitis and food allergies increases the probability of developing asthma through childhood (the 'allergic march'). A positive family history of asthma in the nuclear family, i.e. mother, father and siblings, is an important factor for childhood onset of asthma and persistence throughout childhood. The strongest association is with maternal atopy. It is important to recognise that non atopic wheezing is as frequent as atopic wheezing in school age children.

Upper airway problems

Upper airway issues may manifest as inspiratory noise (stridor) or hoarse voice. Recurrent croup can be confused with asthma. It can be distinguished by a barking cough and the classic features of asthma are not present.

Other respiratory diseases

A persisting wet cough requires investigations as this is not a classic feature of asthma. Finger clubbing is never present in asthma and must be investigated further to look for suppurative diseases such as cystic fibrosis. A history of travel to an area of high tuberculosis prevalence or high prevalence areas within the child's own country might increase suspicion of a diagnosis of tuberculosis. Other diagnoses to consider are ciliary dyskinesia and bronchiectasis.

Gastro-oesophageal reflux and swallowing problems

By 11 years of age most children with appropriate questioning can describe gastro-oesophageal symptoms and an abnormal swallow. Children younger than this may find it difficult to describe such symptoms. A significant neurological problem might suggest an unsafe swallow.

Consultation essentials

Identify any recent changes such as secondary school transfer, move of house, or change in family circumstances that may cause stress or interrupt the routine of being given or remembering to take regular asthma medication.

History/examination

The cardinal symptoms of asthma are intermittent, and repeated, wheeze or cough. Exacerbating factors include exercise, exposure to pets, cold or damp air, or emotions such as laughter (**Table 8.1**). Take a respiratory-focused history to consider all the above differential diagnoses.

It is important to ask about neonatal history and exclude upper airway issues.

Examination and spirometry may be completely normal especially in a child who is currently asymptomatic.

Tests/investigations

Observation of inhaler technique is essential. Most children do not use their inhaler properly and repeated checking of inhaler technique is essential.

In cases of 'difficult asthma', it is important to check that repeat prescriptions are being requested and picked up from the general practitioner. Often poor adherence to medication is a factor and this will need to be discussed openly and sensitively with the family.

Consider testing for atopic status with skin prick tests or levels of specific immunoglobulin E to allergens in the blood. A chest X-ray should only be reserved for children with severe disease, or clinical clues suggesting other conditions.

Spirometry

This may be available to use in clinic. Baseline spirometry is often normal in the outpatient setting especially if the child is asymptomatic. Look for evidence of obstruction with reduced forced expiratory volume in 1 second (FEV1) and evidence of small airways disease with reduced maximal expiratory flow (MEF) 25–75 (25-75% of the forced vital capacity has been exhaled). Look for the bronchodilator response to 10 puffs of Salbutamol (100 μg per puff) given via a large volume spacer device. This can be can be very helpful in assessing reversibility. If baseline lung function is normal then it is unlikely that there will be a significant bronchodilator response. A significant bronchodilator response is > 12% improvement.

Diagnosis

The diagnosis of asthma was confirmed in this girl, based on her past history of suggestive respiratory symptoms. The likely cause of the deterioration is poor adherence, secondary school transfer and inappropriate inhaler technique and device.

Management

It is important to fully explain to parents and the child the different medications and how they work. If possible give children a choice of an appropriate inhaler, e.g dry powder device (such as a turbohaler or accualler) or a metered-dose inhaler (MDI) with spacer. No child should have an MDI without a spacer as very little of the drug will be deposited in the appropriate airways. Older children may take their inhaler without telling their parents but it is important that there is some attempt to observe some of the medications being self-administered, e.g. the twice daily steroid inhaler doses.

It is important to address stresses in the child's life; asking the child directly may yield more important answers than asking the parents who will likely only have a perception of what the stresses are. Secondary school transfer can be a very stressful time. If breathing dysfunction is a component then the child and parent should be taught breathing control exercises by an appropriately trained professional, often a physiotherapist. In some instances a referral to a clinical psychologist will cure their asthmatic symptoms.

Follow up

It is important to have some follow up and also to remember that girls are less likely to grow out of asthma in adolescence than boys. Follow up could be in an asthma clinic setting in secondary care where inhaler technique should be checked at each visit.

Many general practitioner (GP) surgeries have appropriately trained doctors or nurses running asthma clinics. It can be entirely appropriate to ask the GP to continue monitoring of interval symptoms and inhaler technique rather than continue follow up at the hospital.

Discussion

Asthma is one cause of cough and breathing problems in children. Many parents and children will describe all respiratory noises as wheeze including croup and habit cough.

Asking the family to record or video the sound can be helpful. It is important to take a full history including a detailed social history to look for any of the issues raised above. Inhaler technique must be assessed, and an attempt to look for adherence to medication can be very revealing.

Further reading

Bush A Seglani S, Management of severe asthma in children. Lancet 2010; 376(9743):814–825.
Kurukulaartachy RJ, Fenn M, Matthews S, Arshad SH. Characterisation of atopic and non-atopic wheeze in 10 years old children. Thorax 2004; 59(7):563–568.
British Thoracic Society/SIGN- British Guideline on the Management of Asthma. www.sign.ac.uk

Patient information

Asthma UK
www.asthma.org.uk
The Scottish Intercollegiate Guidelines Network
www.sign.ac.uk

Autism

Dear Paediatrician,

Please could you assist in evaluating this 3-year and 2-month-old boy whose parents are concerned about his lack of speech? He has been attending playgroups from 2 years of age but is not showing any interest in socialisation yet. He is good at climbing. His maternal uncle has autistic spectrum disorder.

Dr Kevin Albert

Case analysis

A normally developing 3-year-old will have 2–3 word sentences and a vocabulary of over 300 words, so the absence of speech at this age is abnormal. His social communication appears to be slightly deviant too. A normally developing 2-year-old will parallel play while children between the ages of 3–4 years and will start to show friendship formation.

There is an increasing need to find labels for any behaviour which is abnormal or undesirable. Most of these 'conditions' are spectral in that there is normal variation in these behaviours and at some, essentially arbitrary level, they are differentiated from being normal or pathological. A developmental or social communication disorder should be pervasive, i.e. it would manifest in every setting. A child who is 'a devil at home and an angel at school' will not have a developmental disorder, but the family will probably benefit from parenting support.

Differential diagnosis

Austistic spectrum disorder

This is classified by having problems in social communication and interaction, and unusually restricted, repetitive behaviours and interests. Although the problem should be recognised from early childhood, often this is only possible in hindsight. Later, complex situations unmask difficulties that have been able to be ignored in less challenging surroundings. Language disorders are common with austistic spectrum disorder (ASD) but are not an essential part of the diagnosis. ASD is often an associated condition in children with other neurodevelopmental problems.

The challenge for paediatricians is trying to distinguish the normal from the abnormal. This is particularly difficult when the child's behaviour is seen through a single lens. Most children referred for an assessment for ASD will not have it. They are more likely to have social or educational issues, which although these need attending to in their own right, do not make a diagnosis of ASD. Many families will present having checked their child's behaviour against an internet tool, which can frequently be misleading. Because of the implications of the diagnosis, this should only be made by a developmental paediatrician.

Hearing impairment

This can present with delayed speech because the child has not learnt sounds. A knock-on effect would be isolation which could be perceived as poor socialisation. Children with sensory deficits may display seemingly strange behaviours which they find stimulating.

Selective mutism

Some children will elect not to speak. For the majority this may be situation specific, in that they will talk to close relatives, but not if somebody else is present, or in groups. Children usually grow out of this by school age, although they may remain shy and need help becoming resilient.

Global developmental delay

This should present with delay in all areas. In this case, it seems that his motor skills are fine, which makes global developmental delay unlikely.

Attachment disorders

These could explain this boy's symptoms. Attachment disorder classically arises as a result of a chronic unmet need. For example, a child who is severely neglected, may not have been fed nor had their nappies changed for days. They will have sparse social interaction, and may have been physically hurt. They will not only have failed to learn social skills, but may also display understandable wariness. The features can closely mimic ASD with a child that 'does not connect' – distinguishing between the two diagnoses is not always easy. A history of prolonged abuse might favour an attachment disorder, with the proviso that children with ASD are at a higher risk of abuse. Attachment disorder symptoms can improve somewhat with sympathetic, patient behavioural treatment.

Child abuse

In severe emotional abuse and neglect, a child may display these symptoms. Similarly, in chronic physical or sexual abuse they may display 'frozen watchfulness'. Much of this will overlap with attachment disorders.

Consultation essentials

Ensure that the following are addressed:

Main parental concerns and their duration

Ask about what the parents are worried about. Elucidate speech development, other developmental milestones, social communication and interaction and other coexistent behaviour as described in detail below. Enquire about behaviour in other settings such as nursery. In autistic spectrum disorder, difficulties are observed in more than one setting and present from childhood – although symptoms may be masked in early life by compensatory mechanisms.

Pregnancy and birth history

Autistic spectrum disorder (ASD) has been associated with: prematurity (children born at <35 weeks' gestation), twin or multiple births, use of maternal valproate during pregnancy, increased paternal age and adverse incidents during early neonatal period. A history of difficulty or lack of secure attachment in infancy should be explored as attachment disorder closely mimics ASD.

Development

It is important to establish that the child's developmental profile, including motor (gross and fine), speech and social persona, before considering a diagnosis of social communication disorder. A delay in two or more areas of development may indicate global developmental delay and one must be cautious in interpreting these. A diagnosis of global developmental delay does not exclude autistic spectrum disorder, as the two quite often coexist.

Speech and communication:

Ask about initial speech development, especially if there was delay or regression. Probe about child's communication in the absence of speech; using eye contact or pointing to indicate his need is not in favour of ASD, whilst using somebody else's hand as a tool to point is in favour of autistic spectrum disorder. It is extremely important to rule out any hearing problems which can cause speech delay. Children from a bilingual background may have speech delay.

Social interaction

Ask how the child responds to being approached from familiar or unfamiliar people. Some 'stranger danger' is expected but if he fails to differentiate familiar from unfamiliar people consider child abuse and or attachment disorder. Specifically ask about his interaction with his own age group such as turn taking and play behaviour – children with ASD display difficulty in turn taking and sharing. Look out for parent/carer-child interaction. Social background must be explored to evaluate the possibility of child abuse.

Routines, rituals and sensory behaviour

A history of being bound by routine which, if not followed, will lead to emotional outburst which is 'out of proportion' supports a diagnosis of ASD. Routine or ritualistic behaviour may exhibit itself during bed time or eating. For example, children with ASD may have a very limited food repertoire, and food may need to be placed on a plate in a particular way and then eaten in a specific order.

Hand or finger mannerisms or repetitive behaviours such as toe walking, hand flapping, jumping, running around in circles are also seen in children with ASD.

Sensory behaviour such as insensitivity to pain, apparent lack of temperature regulation wearing coats in summers and minimal clothing in extreme winter climate, or excessive sensitivity to textures, sound, light or taste are often seen in children with ASD. These children may therefore find a school atmosphere particularly challenging. As mentioned above they may have significant food aversion, eating only a very limited repertoire of foods and being very resistant to expanding this. This can pose a serious challenge if they refuse essential medication.

Other

A limited ability to play with toys in a conventional manner, such as being obsessed with the mechanism of a toy or preferring to order cars or crayons rather than play with them, is suggestive of ASD; as are obsessions with a specific toy, DVD or book, i.e. watching the same DVD many times a day and not wanting to watch anything else.

Medical history

Children with Fragile X, tuberous sclerosis, neurofibromatosis, muscular dystrophy, CNS disorders and other chromosomal disorders are at increased risk of developing ASD. A family history of ASD raises the possibility of autistic spectrum disorder in the child.

Look for dysmorphism or neurocutaneous markers as would be found in a diagnosis for tuberous sclerosis. Note the head circumference (can be large initially but normalised later). Observe parent/child interaction and focus on joint referencing, showing and joint attention. Assess for ritualised behaviour and evidence of sensory behaviour. Obtain feedback from other settings such as the educational setting.

Ensure that the other differentials have been ruled out. Hearing impairment as a cause should be excluded. Co-morbidities should be evaluated. A formal assessment process using structured questionnaires, or standardised diagnostic assessment can help in diagnostic process.

The diagnosis of ASD should only be made by a senior developmental paediatrician. Many children may present in a general clinic either by mistake or with behaviour as a secondary complaint. In this instance the general paediatrician may be able to identify an alternative cause, often preventing an inappropriate referral to the developmental team, or suggest that the referral takes place.

Often the diagnosis is hard to confirm, and children should not be 'labelled' unless there is a high degree of certainty.

Management

The management of ASD is needs-dependent. The most important aspect of management is parental understanding of the diagnosis. The role of information leaflets, websites, and voluntary support groups is vital in this aspect.

Most children on the autistic spectrum benefit from speech and language therapy. In addition support from other services such as early years advisory services, autism advisory services, occupational therapy and child psychology can be pivotal. Additionally, the child may need support from child and adolescent mental health team, education psychologist, art and music therapist and challenging behaviour psychology service.

The parents may need parenting support, as parenting a child on the autistic spectrum can be a challenge. In some area, specific groups are available. The National Autistic Society is a source of invaluable help.

Investigate appropriate to clinical needs. Microarray and Fragile X (especially if concomitant global delay) analysis, may help identify the cause of the child's presentation. EEG or MRI is not routinely indicated.

Follow up

For children seen in a general paediatric clinic, a referral should be made to the developmental team. Follow up in the general clinic is not necessary unless there are specific medical needs.

In the community setting, a follow-up within 6 weeks after the initial diagnosis is advisable to address questions that may have arisen. Thereafter, it should be dependent on clinical needs. Children on the autistic spectrum disorder often have coexistent conditions such as sleep problems, dyspraxia, attention deficit hyperactivity disorder and mental health disorders, which will need addressing.

Discussion

ASD is a condition whose diagnosis seems to change as does our understanding of the problems associated with it. The 2013 Diagnostic and Statistical Manual of Mental Disorders (DSM-V) has revised the diagnosis of ASD by attributing different levels: 1, 2 and 3 and removing 'Asperger's syndrome' and 'pervasive developmental disorder – not otherwise specified'. It is possible that a tightening of diagnostic criteria will mean that some people previously diagnosed with ASD may no longer fulfil the diagnostic criteria. Other changes include the requirement that symptoms should be present from early childhood, although they may only become obvious later on, when social challenges increase.

A diagnosis of ASD should be the start of the management process. Children will have widely varying presentations and needs, and these usually vary over time. There is no 'one size fits all' solution. There is no room for a discussion about MMR and autism because there is no link between MMR and autism.

Further reading

Dover CJ, Le Couteur A. How to diagnose autism. Arch Dis Child 2007; 92(6): 540–545, doi:10.1136/adc.2005.086280.
Lai MC, Lombardo MV, Chakrabarti B, Baron-Cohen S. Subgrouping the autism 'spectrum': reflections on DSM-5. PLoS Biol 2013; 11(4): e1001544. doi:10.1371/journal.pbio.1001544.
DSM-V. American psychiatric Association 2013.
    www.dsm5.org

Patient information

Helpguide
    www.helpguide.org
National Autistic Society
    www.autism.org.uk

Case 10

Breath holding

Dear Paediatrician,

Thank you for seeing Ronald, who is now two and a half years old. Over the last 9 months he has had a number of episodes of collapse and loss of consciousness. These usually occur with little or no warning. He cries before each episode.

Last week he had a very severe episode, where he cried, went very pale and dropped to the floor. His mother noticed all of his limbs were shaking. He took a few minutes to come round.

He was born at 32 weeks' gestation and was on a special care baby unit for 6 weeks, but has otherwise been well.

Mum's brother has severe epilepsy.

Today when I examined him he looked quite pale but otherwise had a normal examination.

I would appreciate your further advice.

Dr Chia-Yee Low

Case analysis

The letter gives a good description of breath holding spells. As they have been present for such a long time, there must be a reason as to why the referral has only just occurred. This could be because the latest episode was more dramatic than previous ones, or that the family or general practitioners have doubts about the diagnosis. Obvious concerns would be the possibility of epilepsy and the late effects of prematurity. They may think that premature babies are at higher risk of particular problems, or may remember events on the neonatal unit, such as apnoeas or bradycardias, and wonder if these are related to the current presentation. Ensure that these concerns are explored and addressed.

Differential diagnosis

Breath holding spells/reflex anoxic seizures

This case sounds typical of breath holding spells (BHS), also known as reflex anoxic seizures (RAS). The child is the right age and the history of spontaneous episodes after minor stimulation is a classic sign. As in vasovagal faints, the presence of some twitching after falling is not unusual and does not make this diagnosis less likely.

Some authors differentiate between blue (cyanotic) and white (pallid) breath holding spells or attacks. Although as the colour of the child appears to vary, they are probably the same thing.

In the UK, all of these episodes are more usually referred to as BHS and in the US to RAS. Some people refer to pallid BHS only as RAS. From a parent's point of view, an RAS is more likely to generate anxiety than a BHS.

Episodes usually occur after minor trauma or upset. The child will often let out a long cry and then seem to stop breathing. There is an increase in vagal tone which causes a profound bradycardia and collapse, which can be followed by twitching or jerking. Some children can even have prolonged asystole. Sometimes the spell can be aborted by blowing on the child's face or splashing them with water.

The age range for these episodes is from about 6 months to 6 years with a peak incidence at about 2 years of age. They can vary in frequency from once every few months to many in one day. Boys are three times more likely to have episodes than girls. Although terrifying to observe, particularly if the child collapses, they are remarkably benign. Most children will grow out of them.

Families should try not to let the fear of an episode restrict activity. Similarly, the child should not learn to use BHS to manipulate a situation. There is some evidence that a course of iron therapy, given for 3 months or so, will significantly reduce the number of BHS even in children without iron-deficiency. The mechanism for this is unclear.

Cardiac arrhythmia

Fatal cardiac arrhythmias kill. But they tend to do it early. As he has already had numerous episodes the risk of a serious arrhythmia is miniscule.

Epilepsy

This is highly unlikely. Certainly, these seizures would be quite atypical.

Fallot's spells/congenital heart disease

It is unusual for Fallot's tetralogy to present this late, as this should have been identified antenatally or in the early neonatal period. A child with Fallot's tetralogy would be expected to be cyanosed. Other lesions causing collapse, including aortic stenosis, are unlikely because there has been no murmur detected and the episodes are happening with minimal stimulation. In cardiac lesions there might be an expectation of exertion before a collapse. He is too young to have symptomatic hypertrophic obstructive cardiomyopathy.

Consultation essentials

History/examination

Identifying the presence of a precipitant, however minor, more or less wraps up the diagnosis. If these spells are happening with no precipitant at all, then further thought will be necessary. A family history of sudden death increases the likelihood of arrhythmias – especially long QT syndrome. The presence of neurodevelopmental problems increases the likelihood of a diagnosis of epilepsy.

A normal cardiac examination and the absence of a significant murmur effectively exclude a structural cardiac lesion.

Tests/investigations

Blood tests

These are rarely of use. In some cases BHS (or RAS) are associated with iron-deficiency. However, as many respond to iron treatment even in the absence of iron-deficiency, blood tests rarely alter management.

Electrocardiography

There is some debate about whether all children with BHS (or RAS) need an ECG, with good arguments on each side. A 12-lead ECG is a reasonable screening tool. In the presence of a strong family history of arrhythmias a 24-hour tape may be indicated.

Electroencephalography

No real indication for this, unless there is more information obtained from the consultation. Beware the false positive EEG.

Diagnosis

Ronald has BHS (or RAS).

Management

The family were reassured about the benign nature of the condition and that it was not linked to epilepsy. He was given a 6-week course of iron, following which his episodes of BHS reduced significantly in frequency.

Follow up

Follow up is not strictly required. If there is significant anxiety and appointment after the end of any therapy may be reasonable, i.e. in 4 months' time.

Discussion

Breath holding spells are frightening but benign. Probably the biggest challenge in the consultation is reducing rather than increasing anxiety. The diagnosis is essentially made on the history. It is important to consider the language used in the consultation to ensure that appropriate reassurance has been offered.

Further reading

Stephenson JB. Reflex anoxic seizures ('white breath-holding'): nonepileptic vagal attacks. Arch Dis Child 1978; 53:193–200.
Boon R. Does iron have a place in the management of breath holding spells? Arch Dis Child 2002; 87:77–78.

Patient information

The Syncope Trust and Reflux anoxic Seizures group
www.stars.org.uk

Change in behaviour

Dear Paediatrician,

Thank you for seeing George who is 10 years old and has had a change in personality and behaviour. He becomes quite aggressive and unreasonable, shouting and throwing things about. He is also getting into a lot of trouble at school.

He used to be quite placid, but his parents have noted a marked change over the last 6 months.

His past history is unremarkable, but the family is concerned as one of his uncles has bipolar disorder.

Many thanks,

Dr Miriam Austin

Case analysis

George may simply be displaying normal behaviour – especially given his age, which the parents are interpreting as worrying. Before proceeding it is essential to understand what the worrying behaviour is and what has changed. The most likely explanation is a response to changed circumstances. At this age George should be going through puberty, and the way that he himself, his family and school respond to this will impact on his behaviour. Equally, changes in his life, such as family discord can also affect him.

Organic brain disease will not alter dramatically with a change of environment. If the behaviour is different in different settings, it is more likely to be reactive. A school report can be invaluable. If George is angelic at school, the issue is likely to be based on George's relationship with his parents. Other situational clues may link to toxic causes which could be environmental, e.g. carbon monoxide at home, or may be drug induced.

The difference is if the described behaviour is changing in nature or not. In some rare conditions such as partial seizures, migraines and metabolic disturbances such as porphyria, as well as repeated ingestion of drugs including alcohol, there may be fairly formulaic episodes, interspersed with more or less normal behaviour. The family may be concerned about the inheritability of his uncle's bipolar illness, but may not have considered the possibility of their son having access to and taking his uncle's medication.

A more holistic deterioration in behaviour, especially with deterioration in other neurological functions, increases the likelihood of a progressive cause such as a space occupying lesion or Wilson's disease.

In practice it should be possible to narrow down the differential by a careful history and examination, and this should prevent over-investigation. If the behaviour is improving, then a wait-and-see approach can be adopted.

Differential diagnosis

Normal behaviour

Parents may not appreciate what constitutes normal behaviour, especially as their children enter teenage years. Most children's centres, based in the community, offer courses and support for parents of teenagers.

'Behavioural' – reactive/anxiety/depression

This is usually as a result of a change in the child's life. The family may not be aware of what the cause is but it is also not unusual that the family underplay what, to the child, is significant. Obvious triggers would be family separation, abuse, bullying and relationship issues. In some of these, particularly sexual abuse, disclosure may not be forthcoming. A young person should be given the opportunity to disclose abuse, but unfortunately very few do. Often professionals may have suspicions, but in the absence of a disclosure there is little that can be done.

The history should identify if the behaviour is situational, i.e. worse either at school or home. Depending on the severity of the behaviour, help may be available through:

- Parenting courses
- School – a counsellor may help the child, and some schools organise parenting groups
- Youth clubs and activities
- Counselling services
- Child and adolescent mental health services (CAMHS)
- Social services
- Police/youth offending teams.

The behavioural response to a stress will be exacerbated in the presence of:

- Drug and alcohol issues
- Mental health issues – see below

The possibility of these being contributing factors needs active exploration.

Anxiety and, to a lesser degree, depression are usually bound up with the above issues. Ideally the management should be holistic, involving the child, family and school.

Change in presentation of behavioural problems (e.g. attention deficit and hyperactivity disorder, autism, pervasive demand avoidance)

Usually, by the age of 10 years, the family will know which behaviours are linked to any underlying condition. However, sometimes when the stimulus changes, the response may change as well. Occasionally, the belated change in behaviour will 'unmask' a more pervasive diagnosis. Most of these conditions can be excluded by simple questioning about sociability, friendships and behaviour. If there is serious doubt, then a referral to Child and Adolescent Mental Health Services (CAMHS) or community paediatrics is appropriate.

Remember, children with these conditions may also have other pathologies. For example, a child whose behaviour may have started out troublesome, but has deteriorated further should be assessed and a new diagnosis considered.

Early onset psychosis

This is extremely rare. Social withdrawal is the usual presentation. The presence of hallucinations is not pathognomonic of psychosis in children, and is more commonly due to anxiety. In psychosis there has to be evidence of thought disorder. Whilst many general symptoms may be present as precursors to psychosis, initially they lack specificity.

Medication/drug/alcohol

Intermittent behaviour change may be linked to drugs and alcohol. If the behaviour were a side effect of a drug prescribed for the child, the family would be expected to make the causal link. As the behaviour is intermittent, the ingestion could be happening 'accidentally', e.g. by George taking his uncle's lithium, or by poisoning (accidentally ingesting 'hash brownies'). Similarly alcohol may be taken openly or surreptitiously. Identify when the behaviour occurs, and what toxins may be around at the time.

Toxic (e.g. carbon monoxide or lead)

These would be expected to cause more stupor and sluggishness, but needs to be considered. Other family members would expect to have symptoms as well. Blood tests should be diagnostic.

Epilepsy

The textbooks always mention partial epilepsies so this one should as well. This kind of behaviour is rare in any form of epilepsy. The behaviour should be similar in each episode, fairly short lasting and have no obvious trigger. Unfortunately, an electroencephalography will not diagnose, or completely exclude, epilepsy and will often be inconclusive. Children may have a trial of antiepileptic drugs which seem beneficial, but are more likely to work because of their sedating properties.

Migraine

This is another very rare cause. Sometimes migraine can present in this way, in the absence of more classical features. There should be absolutely no features between attacks, and the behaviour should be formulaic and 'untriggered'.

Tumour

The prospect of a tumour will cause anxiety in doctors and patients. In the absence of any other symptoms or signs this is exceedingly rare. Sometimes neuroimaging is required for reassurance rather than anything else.

Endocrine/metabolic

Under this category, it is possible to construct an almost endless list including:
- Thyrotoxicosis
- Hypoglycaemia
- Wilson's disease
- Porphyrias

Unless there are clear features, they would not be considered in the first round of diagnosis.

Post-infectious

Behaviour change – such as behaviour associated with post streptococcal disease, or Lyme disease would be expected to be more pervasive.

Consultation essentials

History/examination

Clearly, the history will provide the most useful information and can help narrow the diagnosis. Essentially, consider whether the behaviour is:

- Situational – what are the triggers, and when does it happen?
- Static – is the behaviour always the same?
- Specific – are there any other changes in the child's life?

When symptoms are more likely due to organic pathology, the triggers are likely to be absent or highly variable, the behaviour may change in nature over time and there will often be other symptoms such as headache or deteriorating academic performance.

Any third party information, especially from the school can be invaluable. This will require the parent's consent.

Examination can be focussed after taking the history.

Tests/investigations

Because the differential is vast, investigations need to be tailored. If there are clear indications of organic disease then it is best to discuss this with an appropriate specialist prior to organising investigations.

Diagnosis

On discussion, George disclosed that he had been bullied at school. His parents said that they had reported it and believed that everything was sorted, but George said that nothing had changed. There was also a suggestion that there may be some parental violence at home, but his parents were reluctant to discuss this.

Management

The parents were going to approach the school to address the bullying issue, and arrange counselling in school for George. They were given information about relationship advice, and the advice sheet contained contact details for victims of domestic abuse.

Follow up

This depends on the certainty of the diagnosis. If tests are performed then the family need a mechanism to obtain the results. If there is any change in the behaviour then further review is required. A review may also be necessary to collate information from other sources, or provide a safety net. In most cases this would occur after 2–4 months.

If considering a complex diagnosis, liaison with a tertiary centre is likely to be needed.

If there is a confident diagnosis and management plan, then no follow up may be required.

Discussion

Organic causes of behavioural change will usually present with pervasive and persistent changes, sometimes these can be of insidious onset. A useful discriminating question is 'on one of his good days, if a family friend who had not seen your son for a year saw him at a social gathering, would the friend think that there was anything wrong with him?' If the answer is no, then an organic cause is highly improbable. If the answer is yes, then it is imperative to look for an organic cause.

Despite its relative importance, many doctors find it difficult to discuss parenting issues with their patients' parents. A reassuring phrase is 'as parents, although we are not necessarily the cause of our children's problems, we are undoubtedly the main source of their solutions.'

Further reading

Bergese R. Understanding Your 10–11 Year Old (Understanding Your Child series). London: Jessica Kingsley Publishers; 2008.

Patient information

Family Lives
www.familylives.org.uk

Chest pain

Dear Paediatrician,

Thank you for seeing this 13-year-old boy who has a 5-month history of chest pain. It seems to come on at any time, and is not obviously associated with exercise. He has been seen in the emergency department and had an ECG which was reported as looking normal. He has had a month's course of omeprazole without benefit. His parents are concerned as it has been going on for a while now. I have advised him to avoid sports until he has seen you. He had a murmur diagnosed on his 6-week check and a subsequent review by a paediatrician who reassured the family that it was innocent. He has an uncle who had a heart bypass operation last year.

Yours sincerely,

Dr Michael Beattie

Case analysis

This presentation is common in school-aged children and teenagers. Studies suggest that only about 1% of children that present with chest pain will have a cardiac cause for their pain. A considerable proportion of children presenting with chest pain will have significant symptoms of anxiety or depression.

The possibility of there being something wrong with the child's heart is probably causing most anxiety, which in itself may contribute to the pain. A study reporting 10 years' experience of chest pain presenting to an outpatient clinic in the US, including nearly 18 000 patient years, showed three deaths in total – two from suicide and one from a retroperitoneal haemorrhage.

Differential diagnosis

Cardiac causes

The commonest cardiac conditions contributing to morbidity and mortality are cardiomyopathy, arrhythmias and abnormalities of the coronary arteries. On careful evaluation, symptoms which may suggest a cardiac cause of pain include chest pain on exertion, a positive family history, abnormalities on examination and/or abnormal ECG findings. This should prompt further cardiac evaluation. In an unwell child, pericarditis can cause chest pain.

If a child is known to have a disorder with possible cardiac manifestations (e.g. Marfan's syndrome and dissection of the aorta) or an underlying cardiac abnormality (such as mitral valve prolapse), chest pain must be taken seriously and requires prompt attention. Cardiac chest pain is usually retrosternal.

Respiratory causes

The airways, pleura, chest wall or diaphragm can be the site of chest pain, which is usually exacerbated by coughing. Pneumonia or pleurisy, while painful, are usually acute problems and do not have the intermittent chronicity of this presentation.

Exercise-induced asthma is often described as painful. The pain is usually around the chest or may be 'under the heart' on the left side of the chest. Patients may mention associated 'rapid heart rate' which is the normal response to exercise. A trial of β2-agonists prior to exercise is indicated.

Gastrointestinal causes

Oesophagitis, secondary to gastro-oesophageal reflux, may cause severe acute retrosternal pain. There is often a history of previous symptoms if, for example, the child was unsettled as a baby. An oesophageal spasm my cause chest pain in a dysmotility disorder. If patients are receiving nonsteroidal anti-inflammatory drugs this may make oesophagitis (and rarely asthma) worse.

Musculoskeletal causes (Table 12.1)

This is the commonest cause of chest pain. The pain is sharp and well localised with specific point tenderness in one area. There may be a history of trauma, straining or repetitive arm activity such as swimming, tennis or throwing, causing disruption of intercostals or the thoracic muscles. There are a number of possible conditions. As these are all self-limiting, whether these are separate entities – or entities at all – could be a matter of some debate.

Table 12.1 Summary of the clinical features of musculoskeletal causes of chest pain		
Diagnosis	**Presumed aetiology**	**Classic features**
Costochondritis (Tietze's syndrome)	Costochondritis with some swelling of the costochondral joint, often at the 2nd or 3rd ribs	Stabbing central, chest pain aggravated by deep inspiration and lasts from a few seconds to a number of minutes.
Precordial catch syndrome (Texidor's twinge)	Trapping of the pleura within the costochondral 'joint'	Sharp, severe pain occurring usually on the left side of the chest, worse when taking breaths in. Slow, deep, breaths can help improve. Usually lasts 3–30 seconds. It does not usually occur during exercise. The pain resolves quickly and completely in all cases. The cause is unknown but theories include nerve pinching or spasm of intercostal muscle fibres
Slipping rib syndrome	The 8th, 9th and 10th ribs are attached to each other via a fibrous band which means they are mobile. They are also at risk of injury with rupture of the fibrous connections. Rib movement, particularly during lifting, may impinge one of the intercostal nerves	Pain in a dermatomal distribution at the lower part of the thorax, especially after specific movements – such as 'throwing a left hook'
'Stitch' – intercostal muscle strain	Diaphragmatic muscle spasm, or ischaemia of the diaphragm due to diversion of blood to the limbs	Sharp pain in left lower side of the chest or under the ribs, difficult to take a deep breath, usually during exercise. Relieved by rest

Often episodes of pain, though severe, are too short lived to require analgaesia, but if the pain is longer lasting, simple analgesics may help.

Psychological

The pain may be a somatising response, and this will reflect the premorbid character of the child and their exposure to conflict and 'life events' at home and school. It is important to ask about this, and to make a positive diagnosis. Self help books and school or community support are usually all that is required, but more serious problems might need child and adolescent mental health services input.

There may be some organic chest disease in a family member which the child could be mimicking.

Miscellaneous causes

A rash, particularly in a dermatome, should raise the suspicion of herpes infection which can be associated with pain in that area. Less common causes include malignancy (mediastinal), breast tissue development in puberty as well as breast tissue pathology – or the cause may remain unexplained and idiopathic.

Consultation essentials

History

The classic description of myocardial infarction pain would be worrying in the acute setting, but is fortunately rare. Chest pain in children and young people is commonly left sided, but without radiation. There is often a 'stitch' quality to it which can cause the young person to have difficulty with their breathing or catching their breath. This needs to be differentiated from pleuritic chest pain occurring with inspiration.

Timing is important: if the pain started after trauma then think about rib fractures – which are easily missed on an acute X-ray. If the pain occurs after vigorous activity involving the upper limbs this makes a musculoskeletal problem more likely. Ask about what reproduces the pain, especially any movements which may contract muscle or tendon.

A history of dyspepsia, excessive coffee intake or unhealthy and erratic eating habits may suggest peptic ulcer disease of oesophagogastritis. Ask specifically about a personal or family history of asthma.

Asking about psychosocial issues can help put symptoms into context. For example, a sibling of a child with relapsed cancer complained of nonspecific chest pain and after assessment, no obvious cause was apparent. This was put down to it being their time to need some attention and was managed symptomatically.

Examination

The heart sounds are usually normal but a routine cardiac examination is wise, checking for any murmurs. Check the character and volume of peripheral pulses. Pressing on the precordium to try and mimic the pain can be a good clue towards the presence of costochondritis. Movements of the upper limbs should be checked to be sure there is no aggravation of the symptoms by pectoralis muscle contraction. The intercostal muscles could still be causing the symptoms if these manoeuvres prove fruitless.

Look for features of Marfan's syndrome; aortic root dilatation would be an important cardiac cause of chest pain.

Investigations

Usually there are no specific tests which are required. In theory inflammatory markers could be raised in costochondritis, but they rarely are. In a nonacute setting troponin I is not indicated (unless there is a real feature or possibility of a cardiac cause). An ECG would be a reasonable step to exclude an underlying abnormality and may be reassuring for the family. A chest X-ray will help identify focal lung or bony pathology. However, a reasonable approach would be to avoid investigations if the examination is normal.

Diagnosis

In this case the most likely diagnosis was musculoskeletal. On closer questioning the symptom started after some exertions involving upper limb exercises during a fitness test. He had been playing basketball and other racket sports requiring upper limb exertion. Anti-inflammatory medications and rest were advised.

Management

As indicated above the chances of a cardiac cause for the chest pain are very unlikely. If the symptoms suggest a treatable problem such as oesophagitis, asthma or anxiety, this should be treated. Otherwise watchful waiting is required.

Follow up

Offering to review may be supportive, but if the diagnosis is clear and there is no underlying organic condition based on thorough assessment, there may be no need for this.

Discussion

Rather than saying that chest pain generates anxiety it is arguably more accurate to say that anxiety generates chest pain. Many families get fixated on the tests and diagnosis rather than understanding the likely cause and management. It is important to consider all causes. In the rare likelihood of a serious cause this needs appropriate investigation and management, otherwise prompt and emphatic reassurance is required. Underlying psychological issues should be discussed and addressed appropriately.

Further reading

Ives A, Daubeney PEF, Balfour-Lynn IM. Recurrent chest pain in the well child. Archives of Disease in Childhood 2010; 95:649–654.

Lipsitz JD, Hsu DT, Apfel HD, et al. Psychiatric disorders in youth with medically unexplained chest pain versus innocent heart murmur. J Pediatr 2012; 160(2):320–324. doi: 10.1016/j.jpeds.2011.07.011. Epub 2011 Aug 24.

Reynolds JL. Precordial Catch Syndrome in Children. Southern Medical Journal 1989; (10):1228–1230.

Susan F. Saleeb, Wing Yi V. Li, Shira Z. Warren and James E. Lock. Effectiveness of Screening for Life-Threatening Chest Pain in Children. Pediatrics 2011; 128:e1062.

Patient information

The Cincinnati Children's Hospital
    www.cincinnatichildrens.org
KidsHealth
    www.kidshealth.org

Chronic fatigue syndrome

Dear Paediatrician,

Thank you for seeing Caroline, who is 13 years old now. For the last year she has been struggling with increasing lethargy and tiredness. Her symptoms started with a febrile illness, following which she has had tiredness and fatigue. At the time I performed a number of blood tests, including a glandular fever screen. These were all normal.

Over the past year, her symptoms of lethargy have become increasingly severe. She has now not been unable to go to school for the last 4 months. She remains in good spirits, and certainly has retained her humour. Due to the severity of symptoms, I repeated a number of blood tests including a full blood count, liver function tests, thyroid function, erythrocyte sedimentation rate and rheumatoid factor, and these were all normal.

She describes some nausea, and has increasing difficulties sleeping. She tends to get to sleep at about 4 AM and get out of bed at 1 PM. Examination was essentially normal.

I would appreciate your advice.

Dr Felicity Bolam

Case analysis

This is a description of a young woman who has all of the features of chronic fatigue syndrome (CFS)/myalgic encephalomyelitis (ME). The chronicity of the problem, coupled with the normal blood tests which have remained so for a long period of time, makes any other diagnosis very unlikely. Occasionally, the description in the referral letter may be incomplete, and the investigations are always a little lacking. Complacency must be avoided before making a diagnosis.

Differential diagnosis

Chronic fatigue syndrome/myalgic encephalomyelitis

All of Caroline's symptoms are in keeping with the diagnosis of CFS/ME. In many instances, the family will be expecting to receive this diagnosis. There are no specific tests to confirm this condition, and it becomes a diagnosis of exclusion. There are, however, a number of tests that are necessary and these have largely been performed by her general practitioner. The possibility of carbon monoxide poisoning, autoimmune diseases such as systemic lupus erythematosus and other rare conditions may mean that further blood tests are needed.

The glandular fever screening test is not foolproof in detecting glandular fever, and a chronic course may be possible, but effectively the management is the same for glandular fever and CFS/ME. In some families, giving the diagnostic label of prolonged viral illness is more acceptable than CFS.

The criteria for diagnosing CFS/ME in young people require symptoms to be present for at least 3 months. Classic features include fatigue, poor sleep and nausea. There are other varieties, where lymphadenopathy and/or mild fever may predominate. CFS/ME is the paradigm biopsychosocial condition.

The simplest approach is to consider that a physical illness has caused debility which has become prolonged. This has led to a 'de-toning' of the muscles, which makes them seem weak. Added to this, often excessive periods of lying down lead to symptoms of postural hypotension. An inadequate amount of activity disrupts the sleep wake cycle contributing to the feeling of tiredness and fatigue.

In more complicated cases, other factors begin to set in. For example, increasing school absence makes return more difficult, and school phobia or separation anxiety can be increased. In addition, there is often a change in family structure and relationships, and although these may be undesired, they can soon become well established. Any change becomes difficult, even that which is desired such as a return to normal function. This means that turning things around, becomes challenging.

Although there is heated controversy about treatment, the only treatments shown to be of benefit are graded exercises, with or without cognitive behavioural therapy. Some families may feel that the problem is being 'under medicalised'. It is always hard to deal with this issue, and there are no easy solutions. It is essential that well-intentioned medical intervention does not become a potentiating factor for this condition.

In a similar vein, these families may say that once a young person feels better, they will be able to increase their activity. In reality, it seems that it is increasing the activity that makes them feel better. The objective is to turn the vicious cycle into a virtuous one. This usually involves a multidisciplinary approach involving physiotherapy, psychology and school.

Simple advice about sleep hygiene and energy management is helpful. Medication to aid sleep can be of assistance. Melatonin seems to be more successful in the paediatric age group, although adults tend to use Amitiptyline.

As a number of medical conditions can mimic CFS/ME, it is necessary to revisit the diagnosis every 3–6 months, repeating investigations as necessary.

School phobia

One of the possible differentials is a phobia of being at school.

Narcolepsy

This is uncommon, but unfortunately there is often a significant lag between onset of symptoms and diagnosis. In narcolepsy, sleepiness is often situational, at times of reduced activity. This may include falling asleep in lessons or on car journeys but after a restorative sleep normal vigour seems to return.

The formal diagnosis should be made with a proper sleep study, but the Epworth Sleepiness Scale can give a useful guide.

Treatment is with understanding, which requires mediation with the school, and medication. Currently, methylphenidate (as used in attention deficit hyperactivity disorder) is the treatment of choice.

Carbon monoxide poisoning

Presents with features similar to chronic fatigue syndrome. Classically symptoms would improve with prolonged periods away from the offending source of carbon monoxide. Many families have carbon monoxide monitors, or it is easy to ask the gas supplier to check carbon monoxide levels in the house.

Treatment is with removal of the offending carbon monoxide producer – usually an old boiler. Occasionally, patients may need hyperbaric oxygen.

Hypothyroidism

Hypothyroidism can present insidiously. Again, many of the features can mimic CFS/ME. Essentially the only way of establishing whether this is present or not is to check the thyroid function tests. As Caroline has had this repeated twice, the diagnosis in this case seems unlikely.

Depression

Depression in children is often poorly appreciated. Certainly its manifestations include lethargy and withdrawal. In this case, Caroline has kept her sense of humour, which does make depression considerably less likely.

Lyme's disease

This is a condition that presents in a myriad of ways. It does seem rather far-fetched in this scenario. However, if there is a history of travel to an area with deer, then checking serology may be useful.

Autoimmune disease

An autoimmune disease would be expected to produce more systemic symptoms, including fever, rash and muscle and joint pains. It can be difficult to exclude. Rheumatoid factor is a very limited value in this age group. Anti-nuclear antibody (ANA) may be more useful, but also throws up a number of false positives.

Consultation essentials

History/examination

It is easy to fall into the trap of making the diagnosis before the patient enters the room. Reconstructing the patient's day takes a little time but provides most of the rewards. Useful factors include:
- Bed time
- Time to onset of sleep

- Length of sleep
- How she feels upon waking in the morning
- Time to get out of bed
- Daytime activity
- Daytime naps
- Eating and drinking during the day
- Communication with others
- School attendance.
- Social activities
- Changes in the family to accommodate the condition

Symptoms which challenge this diagnosis of CFS/ME, such as fever, weight loss, change in bowel habit and rashes should be asked for. If present the diagnosis will need reconsidering.

A thorough physical investigation will hopefully reassure all parties that there is nothing more sinister going on.

Often, the family come already having made the diagnosis themselves. The greater challenge can be trying to convince them of the proposed management plan.

Tests/investigations

Most, if not all of the investigations have already been performed. Whether it is worth further blood tests at this stage is debatable. A more complete opening set of blood tests would include:

- Full blood count/erythrocyte sedimentation rate
- Urea and electrolytes
- Liver function tests (Ca)
- C-reactive protein
- Glucose
- Thyroid function
- Anti-nuclear antibody
- Coeliac
- Creatine kinase
- Ferritin
- Urinalysis
- Others as indicated – e.g. toxicology screens, Lyme serology, etc.

Diagnosis

Caroline has CFS/ME, and some associated school anxiety.

Management

She was referred to the physiotherapists who introduced a graded exercise program. She was referred to the psychologist, but unfortunately did not engage with them. She did, however, work with the school team. Initially, work was sent home, but she managed to attend school for some lessons and this built up over time.

Follow up

The most important follow up is normally with other members of the multidisciplinary team. However, medical follow up every 3–6 months may be useful, particularly if any medications have been prescribed. Also, if there has been no improvement it is worth revisiting the diagnosis, with investigations where necessary.

Discussion

Simple CFS/ME tends to improve over 6 months or so. If it persists it is worth looking at other factors, including whether the family are fuelling or fighting the problem. Often secondary gains and entrenched behaviour can hamper recovery. Many people with CFS/ME seem to have associated school phobia and/or separation anxiety. It is best to confront this at the time of diagnosis, so that all of the issues can be addressed. Evading this area might seem comfortable, but is not of benefit.

Further reading

Fernández AA, Martín AP, Martínez MI, et al. Chronic fatigue syndrome: aetiology, diagnosis and treatment. BMC Psychiatry. 2009; 9.
National Institute for Health and Care Excellence (NICE). Chronic fatigue syndrome/Myalgic encephalomyelitis (CG53), Clinical Guidance 53. London: NICE, 2007.
http://guidance.nice.org.uk/CG53
www.narcolepsynetwork.org

Patient information

Association of Young people with ME
www.ayme.org.uk

Case 14

Clumsy child

Dear Paediatrician,

Could you please see Edward, age 4 years, who tends to trip over things and is prone to falling over. He is a bright little boy but his nursery says he is clumsy, and he has hurt himself a few times.

Dr Alex Breen

Case analysis

Although some degree of clumsiness is normal as children first master the skill of walking, by this age he should be walking confidently. Distinguish between isolated and more general problems. Edward is quite young to be diagnosed with dyspraxia and this diagnosis is often best made after a multidisciplinary assessment.

Differential diagnosis

Normal development

Even at this age the occasional trip or fall is not unusual. If the symptoms are improving, this makes normal development likely.

Dyspraxia (developmental coordination disorder)

This is a rather ill-defined condition. It is not just clumsiness but includes difficulties with executive functioning such as personal organisation, locomotors and fine movement problems including poor ball skills, immature art work, untidy dressing, indistinct speech and difficulty making friends.

Approximately 25% of children with developmental coordination disorder will be referred before starting school. The remaining 75% will be referred during the first few years in primary school. These children are often poor at organising themselves and may be rather untidy. They tend to have slow, immature and laborious handwriting and difficulties in copying from the blackboard. Some may have been irritable or exhibit difficult behavioural issues. Management is with occupational therapy and school support.

Neuromuscular

Duchenne muscular dystrophy presents at this age with reluctance to walk distances, a tendency to fall suddenly without warning, some difficulty getting up again, more difficulty going upstairs than coming down and inability to jump or run properly. Occasionally mild forms of cerebral palsy may present this late. Other neuromuscular disorders are rarer and include mild forms of spinal muscular atrophy and hereditary peripheral neuropathy.

Mechanical

Hypermobility, or lax ligaments, is a common normal variant and the more extreme forms are variants of Ehlers–Danlos syndrome. They are usually associated with pain, but may rarely present with falls. Treatment is with physiotherapy. Leg length discrepancy alone, unless marked is unlikely to produce these symptoms. Occasionally very severe in-toeing may cause tripping, which may respond to orthotics.

Other causes

Although the history is of tripping up and falling, consider whether the fall is secondary to other causes, such as fits (especially drop attacks, vasovagal episodes, though rare in this age group), or other arrhythmias. Some migraine equivalents can also cause sudden falls.

Consultation essentials

History

There are a number of facts which are needed to help establish a diagnosis:
- Establish if he can run. Inability to run suggests weakness, and a tendency to fall when running suggests difficulty with coordination
- A history of falling, especially whether he trips over objects or seems to fall over 'air'. A child with foot drop may trip; a child with Duchenne may fall without apparent reason
- A child with weakness would have difficulty getting up again and would also tire excessively
- Using stairs: children with coordination difficulties have more difficulty descending than ascending stairs
- If there is global developmental delay then this presents with difficulties in both gross and fine movements
- Establish the 'history': children with neuromuscular disorders, even Duchenne muscular dystrophy, would not show deterioration at this time. Deterioration suggests something else entirely, either a tumour, the early stage of Friedreich's ataxia or a leukodystrophy
- Neuromuscular disorders are often hereditary. Ask if any family members have similar difficulties, foot deformities or muscle weakness
- The presence of incontinence would suggest either global delay or a spinal lesion

Examination

Gross movements give great information, if anything has been revealed by the history. Try to observe this, e.g. time the speed and method of rising up to standing from a sitting position. Children with normal strength and coordination will do this in < 2 seconds, children over 3 years should not pivot (balance on hands and feet) while rising. It is important to observe the gait, walking and running, and observe for any falls. It is useful to have a specific length of corridor and to time a number of children running up and down to get an idea of what is normal. Check for a waddling gait, and consider if he can run or simply just walk fast. See if there is anything odd or bizarre about the way he moves. A 4-year-old should be able to run normally and jump but probably not hop. A child with Duchenne would only be able to walk fast and would tend to waddle.

A general neurological examination should pay particular attention to head size, coordination, eye movements, fundi (although these can be hard to visualise in young children because they may not cooperate) and cranial nerves generally. Check for muscle wasting or hypertrophy, tendon jerks, muscle contracture and joint hypermobility. Examine the back for signs of spinal dysraphism, a tuft of hair or a midline lipoma.

Investigations

Neuroimaging

If there is anything of obvious concern on examination such as a big head, papilloedema or other cranial nerve or long track or cerebellar signs then urgent brain imaging is required. Consider brain imaging (MRI if possible) if there is any suggestion of deterioration or simply that there seems to be an impairment which is extremely static (i.e. a child with significant difficulty which has not improved) or if the gait is odd or unusual in any way. Brain tumours are often diagnosed rather late in children and sometimes first present as coordination difficulties.

Nerve conduction studies

Absent jerks would suggest a possible peripheral neuropathy (if the child has absent jerks, test the parents' jerks as one parent could also be affected without realising it). Arrange nerve conduction studies or make a specialist referral.

Creatinine kinase

Large calf muscles and a waddling gait as described above suggest a muscular dystrophy and a raised serum creatinine kinase would be expected (at least ten times the normal range).

Diagnosis

Edward's lower legs were covered in bruises from frequent falls and he had absent tendon jerks. He did not have overt weakness and his gait was good but there was a hint of foot drop. He could run quite well. He was a cooperative boy, and his general development was normal. His mother also had absent tendon jerks.

Management

Edward was referred for nerve conduction studies which showed slow nerve conductions in him and his mother. The presumptive diagnosis was a hereditary sensory and motor neuropathy which was confirmed on DNA analysis showing a duplication of chromosome 17p12.

Follow up

His gait was helped by the provision of light-weight ankle foot orthoses and he continues to see the physiotherapists and has an annual medical review.

Discussion

Most children referred with coordination difficulties are healthy but it is important to examine these children to exclude any possible underlying medical disorder, as outlined above (see Gibbs et al below for a full list).

Generally only those children with neurologic signs need referral to physiotherapy and occupational therapy. A substantial number of these children also need a detailed educational assessment.

Further reading

Gibbs J, Appleton J, Appleton R. Dyspraxia or developmental coordination disorder? Unravelling the enigma. Arch Dis Child 2007; 92:534–539.

Patient information

Dyspraxia Foundation
http://www.dyspraxiafoundation.org.uk

Case 15

Constipation/stool withholding

Dear Paediatrician,

Please can you help this family who are struggling with Joel who is 6 years old. He has a long history of bowel problems and has always had a tendency to being constipated. However, since starting school things have got significantly worse. He has episodes of soiling, up to 10 times a day, and the stool is very loose. He says that he has no control over it. He is missing lots of school because of his diarrhoea. He is also in a lot of pain.

He found it quite difficult starting school, so his parents think that some of this pain may be caused by anxiety.

Many thanks,

Dr David Carlson

Case analysis

The most likely cause of Joel's diarrhoea is overflow soiling secondary to constipation/ stool withholding (CSW), but it is essential to distinguish this from genuine diarrhoea. In overflow there is often a frequent passage of small quantities of foul smelling soft stool, as opposed to diarrhoea where the quantity passed is large. Undigested food, other than corn, peas and carrots would suggest diarrhoea.

Often the diagnosis of CSW has already been made, and the referral is essentially concerned with management. Sometimes, as in this case, the diagnosis seems obvious, but has been overlooked. But in other scenarios the diagnosis is much less obvious.

For example, CSW can present in a myriad of ways including:

- Abdominal pain
- Soiling
- Backache
- Leg pain
- Lethargy
- Colic
- Seizures

Therefore, a good bowel history is essential. Unfortunately, many guidelines emphasize frequency of defecation, when it is more important to determine how a child goes, rather than how often. For example, some children who go daily might have significant symptomatic withholding, whilst others may be comfortable going once a week.

The reason that CSW is important is because of the effect that it has on children and their families. These children are often overcome by increasing spasms of pain having held on to their stool for a considerable length of time; it affects their mood, behaviour, learning ability, and almost every aspect of their lives – until they have opened their bowels. It is not unusual for families not to want to leave the house because of the severity of the symptoms and their unpredictability.

Families often feel isolated, as professionals fail to acknowledge the severity of the symptoms. With all families, but especially those with children with CSW, it is eye opening to ask how the condition is impacting on their child's and their own lives.

Using the toilets at school is avoided by the majority, 60–80% of children report not opening their bowels at school.

The constipation mantra is 'you should be producing a soft easy regular stool, using an appropriate combination of fluid, fibre and laxatives – the right dose is the one that works.'

It is often hard to know how much a psychological component is at play in these situations. Most children respond to simple treatment, and unless there are other factors it is sensible to treat the CSW from a more physical perspective and then see what, if any, issues remain.

Differential diagnosis

Constipation/stool withholding and overflow

The CSW affects up to 30% of children, but can be downplayed. Direct questioning often reveals that the problems were evident for much longer than they have been acknowledged.

Essentially, at some stage passing stool becomes painful or scary and the child then tries to avoid subsequent discomfort by holding on to their stool. The more they hold on the bigger and harder it becomes so that when they can't hold, it comes out and hurts even more. This reinforces the desire to hold on which can very quickly become a habit.

As the stool builds up, there can be episodes of 'leakage' which are usually either small bits of hard stool, or some liquid stool which has trickled down around the backlogged stool. This can happen numerous times a day, until the backlog is passed, and then the soiling will usually stop for a day or so, until the cycle repeats itself.

Parents' concerns can usually be addressed by emphasising:

- His bowels are almost certainly working normally; it is just the bottom that is holding on
- If there was something wrong with him anatomically it would have been evident earlier
- If there was a 'twist' blockage or hernia these would present in a very different way
- If there was serious underlying illness, you would expect this to have worsened

Consultation essentials

History and examination

It should be possible to make a diagnosis of CSW by the history. Tests are rarely, if ever, indicated. Children from a very young age, sometimes as young as 2 years old, can say if they are holding on to their stool. Good questions to ask are:

- How often do you go for a poo?
- Are your poos nice or not nice?
- When you feel a poo coming do you let it come out, or do you try to keep it in?
- Do you ever look at your poos – what do they look like? (compare with the Bristol stool chart)

If they do not know the answers to the above questions then the 'horrible' questions are:

- Do you wipe your bottom after going for a poo?
- If you wipe, do you look at the paper, and is there poo on the paper when you start wiping? A clean wipe suggests hard, constipated stool

'Red flag' symptoms and signs are important, but rare. Most will present in other ways. Anatomical problems will present at birth or soon after.

- Weight loss/faltering growth
- Blood or mucous mixed in with stool, as opposed to blood on the outside of the stool or on wiping as is often seen in anal fissures
- Undigested food in the stool
- Abnormally placed anus
- Delay in passing meconium greater than 48 hours after birth
- Evidence of neuromuscular problems
- Mouth ulcers/ulcerated anus/anal fistulae

Rectal examination is rarely if ever indicated, and its performance may constitute assault. Even inspection is often unnecessary if it will distress the child. If the parents have seen the anus and say it is normal, this should be sufficient.

Investigations

These are rarely, if ever indicated. A plain X-ray should not normally be used to diagnose constipation, but can occasionally be helpful, if there is doubt or disbelief.

CSW signs or symptoms cannot be used to diagnose child mistreatment. There are some abused children who may have such symptoms, but invariably the abuse diagnosis is made first.

Diagnosis

Joel gave a clear history of CSW, made worse by not using the school toilets. He responded well to laxatives. He had a purging dose initially, over a weekend so that he did not miss school. The fact that he was no longer soiling did boost his confidence, but he was still reluctant to use the school toilet. The laxative dose and timing was altered, and his parents ensured that he had some toilet time before school every morning. This was largely successful. He still had some school issues which were dealt with by the school, with the help of the school counsellor. He remained on laxatives for 2 years.

Management

The essentials of treatment are to get the child to pass a soft, easy regular stool using an appropriate combination of fluid, fibre and laxatives. The right dose being the one that works. 'Regular' is usually once a day, but it is more important that the passing is easy rather than worrying about the frequency.

Once this is achieved, treatment needs to continue until the withholding habit has been overcome. This can take a long time, months or often years, however, as soon as the child is going normally, the symptoms will disappear, with the prolonged treatment being necessary to change bowel habits.

Although excessive fibre is not likely to be effective, boosting fluid and fibre intake to appropriate levels can often help. Written information about fibre content of foods is very useful, as are fluid guidelines.

If families want to try using dietary means, this is fine. There is uncertainty about the role of milk and dairy products in CSW. Certainly, if there is a link between introducing dairy and the onset of symptoms, a trial of a dairy–free diet for a few weeks may be helpful.

If laxatives are required, Macrogols have become the treatment of choice for most children. The National Institute for Health and Clinical Excellence recommends them for children over 1 year, but there is growing experience with using them in even younger children.

For children that do not like Macrogol, choose laxatives that will be tolerated and easy to give. Common favourites would be:

- Lactulose
- Senna
- Sodium picosulphate

The dose of laxatives needs to be titrated to achieve the desired result.

Families are often wary of laxatives, fearing that:

- They will make the bowels lazy; and
- Cause dependence

Neither is true, but stopping them too soon will cause the symptoms to recur.

Follow up

It can take a while to find the correct dose of laxatives, often with setbacks on the way. If families can be offered ready access to help, this will accelerate the time to resolution. This could be offered by a nursing team, or by offering phone or email rapid consults.

As far as follow-up appointments are concerned, an appointment in a few months is useful. Beyond that, the amount of on-going support depends on the child, family and primary care help. Some families will want to manage by themselves and find the appointments an inconvenience, whilst others will want appointments, if only to offer reassurance.

Further reading

Cohn A. Constipation, Withholding and Your Child: A Family Guide to Soiling and Wetting. London: Jessica Kingsley Publishers Ltd; 2006.

National Institute for Health and Clinical Excellence Clinical Guidelines 99. Constipation in children and young people: quick reference guide 2010.
http://guidance.nice.org.uk/CG99

Patient information

Education and Resources for Improving Childhood Continence
www.eric.org.uk

Conversion disorder

Dear Paediatrician,

I would be grateful for your help with this young 12-year-old boy, Leonard, who presents with a number of baffling symptoms. For the last few months, he has been unable to walk. He has difficulty getting out of bed. He manoeuvres himself around the house by crawling, and when he needs to leave the house uses a wheelchair that the family have borrowed from the Red Cross. He is unable to stand up by himself, and needs his parents to take him to the bathroom and toilet. He says that he has no sensation in his legs, from his feet up to his knees.

More recently, he has been unable to speak. He has also developed a cough, which is particularly troublesome during the day.

Many thanks,

Dr Shelagh Chilton

Case analysis

Leonard clearly has physical symptoms, which are anatomically, physiologically and pathologically inconsistent. This would be fully in keeping with a conversion disorder, otherwise known as somatisation or hysteria.

In reality, the situation is often not clear cut. In many conversion disorders, there is some underlying medical pathology, and the conversion disorder may be considered a form of embellishment – many children who have nonepileptic seizures (pseudoseizures) also have underlying epilepsy. Alternatively, there are some situations where there is clear fabrication. For example, in situations where a child is said to be unable to walk, he may, when he thinks no one is looking, get up and play basketball. If challenged, he would usually deny that this had happened, and try to find an excuse for the tracks that he had left.

Making a diagnosis requires a good understanding of neuroanatomy, to make sure that no serious pathology is being overlooked. Sometimes tests and investigations are necessary to convince everybody, not least the patient and family, that there is no significant underlying cause. Any investigations should be fully completed as soon as possible. This is because until an organic cause has been emphatically excluded, the young person and family will usually have difficulty engaging with the appropriate psychological support.

Differential diagnosis

Conversion disorder

A conversion disorder is defined as a mental health condition where symptoms manifest neurologically and they cannot be fully explained by a medical condition, substance abuse, or other mental disorder. It is considered that these symptoms result from the subconscious somatisation of psychological suffering, or that the patient is – subconsciously – converting psychological distress into physical handicap. That is, that the patient is not in control of the symptoms.

Common symptoms include:

- Paralysis
- Aphonia
- Muscle disorders
- Fit like episodes
- Pain/paraesthesiae
- Vomiting/nausea

The symptoms are sometimes inconsistent, and may become progressive. Patients often exhibit certain nonchalance about their symptoms.

The challenge is not only to confirm the diagnosis, but also to explain it so that the young person and their family can understand, and engage in therapy. To this end, various tests may be required. Often the only way to convince the family is to find out what conditions they feel need to be considered in the diagnosis, so that these can be properly excluded. Sometimes this will involve a specialist team, and it is essential that this team are aware of the presumed diagnosis at the time of referral, to avoid setting off a chain of further opinions.

It is usually helpful at the first meeting, to define the limits of any investigation. Often, the family are convinced there is a physical cause, and may find it hard to accept there is an alternative cause.

Appropriate treatment can involve physiotherapy and should involve child and adolescent mental health services (CAMHS).

Embellishment

There is often an underlying physical cause to the child's symptoms and this needs to be investigated, and treated appropriately. Embellishment can occur for a number of reasons. In this situation a significant CAMHS input is likely to be necessary.

Fabrication/malingering

Conscious fabrication of symptoms suggests that the patient or carer is manipulating the situation, and people around them. This is a complex situation which requires joint all the involved professionals to work together. If the parents are driving the fabrication then social services need to be involved.

Consultation essentials

History

Identify precipitants and obtain a very accurate description of the symptoms. This will usually be sufficient to confirm the diagnosis. Trying to understand the patient and family's belief about the symptoms is essential, and sometimes this can best be achieved by speaking to them separately.

It is vital to identify any stresses such as school or family. Although these are sometimes readily disclosed, more often, this does not occur at the first meeting.

Examination

A thorough examination is required. This will allow inconsistencies to be revealed. For example, manoeuvres requested during an examination may require using muscle groups that the patient claims no longer work.

Tests/investigations

Do the minimum amount of tests required to enable everybody to sign up to the diagnosis. Often it is difficult not to perform, blood tests, brain imaging and an EEG. If there is a history of exposure to toxic substances such as carbon monoxide or infections, test for these. All investigations should be completed rapidly.

Diagnosis

Leonard has all the features of a conversion disorder. There is an inconsistency in the pathology of the symptoms: being unable to walk, but crawling around the house, a 'stocking' distribution of pain, and being able to cough but not speak.

Management

Because the family worried that he may have multiple sclerosis, an MRI was performed, which was normal. Sensitive discussion about the symptoms helped them understand the diagnosis of conversion disorder. Superficially, there seemed to be no obvious trigger. He was referred to CAMHS who identified issues within the family. His recovery was also aided by some physiotherapy.

Follow up

No medical follow up is really required, although the family may feel that it gives their predicament some medical respectability. This presents a dilemma, as the family may prefer to see the paediatrician rather than the psychiatrist. It is important to explain that management is multidisciplinary, and medical follow up by itself is likely to fail. It may be necessary to make repeat appointments with the GP in case letters are needed for school, etc.

Discussion

Making a diagnosis of a conversion disorder should be done with some trepidation. Usually, new symptoms reinforce rather than challenge the diagnosis, and they should be assessed in case they suggest an evolving neurological disease. Similarly, there may be organic disease with embellishment, each of which needs its own treatment.

Sometimes there can be pithy explanations for the conversion. In Leonard's case this included, 'You wanted to scream but didn't think anybody would hear you,' and 'you literally didn't feel that you could stand (it) any longer.'

Further reading

Silber TJ. Somatization disorders: diagnosis, treatment, and prognosis. Pediatr Rev 2011; 32(2):56–63.

Case 17

Cough

Dear Paediatrician,

Please could you see Jared, who is 5 years old. He has presented numerous times over the past 3 months with a persisting cough. I have given him amoxil on two occasions to little effect.

A few weeks ago I gave him some bronchodilators, but Mum is not convinced that these have made much of a difference.

There is no atopy in the family.

Dr Ayid Ibrahim

Case analysis

There are numerous causes of chronic cough; whilst most of these are 'benign', occasionally there is a more serious underlying diagnosis. Unless there is overwhelming evidence of a benign diagnosis it is usually appropriate to request a chest X-ray.

Differential diagnosis

Normal child

On average, normal young children without respiratory illnesses will cough 11 times a day. It is rare for this mild intermittent coughing to present unless there is significant parental anxiety.

Recurrent upper respiratory infections/post viral cough

Coughing associated with an upper respiratory infection may persist for a few weeks. Jared may have 'one infection after another' which would not be unusual for a child of this age. This should be evident from the history. Similarly, some infections may take many months to clear. Pertussis cough can persist for months (see below), as may post respiratory syncitial virus (RSV) cough, although this is more likely in much younger children. Exposure to environmental irritants such as cigarette smoke may make this worse. A post viral cough should show signs of improvement over time. If there is an increased number of infections, consider IgA deficiency, which if present justifies a more liberal use of antibiotics, perhaps even given prophylactically.

Asthma

Although asthma is an uncommon cause of non-specific cough, the only practical way of excluding it is with a proper trial of antiasthma therapy which would usually be an inhaled corticosteroid taken for 8–12 weeks, making sure that efficient inhaler technique is employed. In asthma there are usually interval symptoms between exacerbations, so that the child is rarely symptom free. In older children spirometry may help with the diagnosis, but Jared is probably too young to be able to perform this. The seemingly negative history of atopy should be explored. It is remarkable how often this is only revealed on direct questioning. It is only of relevance in first degree relatives.

Rhinitis

Whilst rhinitis is frequently overlooked as a cause of chronic cough in younger children, by this age Jared would be expected to have typical symptoms. In general, treatment with oral antihistamines is usually good enough. It can be difficult to administer intranasal steroids safely and adequately in children of this age.

Pertussis (parapertussis)

Pertussis never goes away. This is true in both individual and societal terms. Even immunised individuals may get some form of pertussis, and pertussis-like infections are common. Pertussis is said to be called in China 'the cough of 100 days'. In the initial period there is usually a specific illness, but even though the child recovers, the coughing persists. It is spasmodic, and although most spasms seem prolonged, the child may be completely well in between spasms. Although there may be a classic whoop noise, or vomiting at the end of each spasm this is by no means universal. The diagnosis is often made clinically. A nasopharyngeal swab taken in the first 2 weeks of the illness can be used for confirmation; polymerase chain reaction of a swab may be useful for up to 4 weeks; and serology for 12 weeks. Lymphocytosis is variable and non-specific. In the first few weeks macrolide antibiotics may be helpful. In younger children apnoeas may be present and this should precipitate admission to hospital.

Protracted bacterial bronchitis/chronic suppurative lung disease/bronchiectasis

These conditions present with a chronic wet cough. The X-ray will suggest the diagnosis and further investigation and treatment would usually involve a tertiary centre.

Inhaled foreign body

A history of choking suggests an inhaled foreign body. An X-ray may show changes of collapse and/or unilateral hyperinflation. If there is any suspicion of this, the child should be referred urgently for definitive treatment with rigid bronchoscopy. Sometimes the diagnosis is only made as a 'coincidental' finding when the child is having a bronchoscopy for a lung problem that fails to improve.

Habit coughs (tic/tourettes)

Habit coughs can sound extremely dramatic, and are often present more or less continuously when the child is awake and aware. The more frequent the cough, the more likely it is to be a habit cough. Habit coughs will disappear when the child is asleep. It is important to ask carefully about this, as the coughing may delay sleep onset but should disappear when the child is actually asleep. In some children the cough may be a feature of a wider tic syndrome. The cough is usually so disruptive that it is hard to remain in school. The first challenge is to convince everybody of the diagnosis. In some children the symptoms, like with many tics, reduce over time. Others may need some psychological support. Sometimes this can be provided in clinic as a brief intervention.

Cystic fibrosis, primary ciliary dyskinaesia, immunodeficiency

It is rare for these to present as an isolated cough, without associated symptoms. Although cystic fibrosis (CF) testing is routine in the UK, it only picks up the commonest mutations. This means about 2% of cases will not be detected on routine screening. If in doubt a sweat test should be organised. In primary ciliary dyskinesia there is often a history of nasal discharge from birth. Diagnosis is by electron microscopy of nasal cilia, and this is usually performed at a tertiary centre. Sometimes even quite severe immune deficiencies can present quite late with seemingly mild symptoms. It is unusual for them to present only with cough. If there are other features, classically faltering growth and diarrhoea, then immune testing may be helpful – this is best discussed with the immunology lab.

Tuberculosis

This rarely presents as a cough without other symptoms and a contact history. An X-ray will usually suggest the diagnosis which can be confirmed by specific tests. Most hospitals have a tuberculosis team who can advise about diagnosis, treatment and contact tracing.

Thoracic mass (lymphoma/neuroblastoma)

An intrathoracic mass is likely to be noticed first as a shadow on the X-ray. Urgent further assessment in a specialised respiratory or oncology centre is indicated.

Anatomical cause: Aspiration, achalsasia/H-type tracheo-oesophageal fistula/neuromuscular, e.g. bulbar palsy

A history of cough in relation to feeding should raise the possibility of aspiration. Obviously, congenital lesions should have been present since birth. Diagnosis can usually be made radiologically, often with videofluoroscopy. As always a discussion with the radiologist is the best way of choosing the right investigation.

Reflux oesophagitis

There is continuing debate about the role of reflux in cough, including which one is more likely to cause the other. Given a history of reflux it may be worth a trial of medication. The area is complicated by the seemingly poor results of treatment, and the suggestion that it may be non-acid reflux that is the problem.

Interstitial lung disease

This is another rare cause, which should be identified on X-ray and treated by experts.

Cardiac failure

Whilst cough may be a feature of cardiac failure, it should not be the presenting feature.

Consultation essentials

History

The general features of a cough to elucidate are:
- Age of onset
- Nature – dry/wet
- Quality – the noise produced
- Timing during the day and night
- Triggers
- Exacerbating and relieving factors
- Associated symptoms

'Red flag' features include:
- Neonatal onset
- Sudden onset
- Cough with feeds
- Chronic moist/wet cough with phlegm production (swallowed in young children)
- Continuous unremitting or worsening cough
- Associated night sweats/weight loss/change in bowel habit
- Signs of chronic lung disease

A general cough history should include how and when the cough started; an acute onset increases the likelihood of an inhaled foreign body. It is essential to understand the quality and nature of the cough. Very young children will swallow excess mucus or blood rather than expectorate, but in this scenario the cough will usually be described as wet or productive. In older children the colour and nature of any sputum produced should be ascertained. Crucially, a cough which is not present when the child is asleep is most likely to be a habit cough.

In some cases there may be obvious triggers to the cough which might suggest an allergic cause, e.g. asthma or rhinitis or an anatomical or physical cause, e.g. aspiration of feeds. Ask about exposure to cigarette smoke, indirectly in younger children, directly in older children. Reports that smoking only occurs "outside" should be met with some degree of scepticism, and even if it is true, a lot of the offending agents linger on the smoker's body and clothes. Similarly, many people give a very conservative estimate of their cigarette consumption. Establish whether the cough is isolated or related to other respiratory symptoms, e.g. wheeze, dyspnoea, tachypnoea or systemic symptoms such as fever, weight loss, diarrhoea, headaches, etc.

Find out what treatments, if any, have been tried, and if they have been effective. If the child has been prescribed inhalers make sure that their inhaler technique is effective. Ask about the family history and whether any people that the child has been in contact with have similar symptoms.

Examination

This should include checking for clubbing, observing the rate and work of breathing, and an ear, nose and throat examination. Auscultation can be misleading in young children and should not be relied upon. The child should be measured, weighed and plotted.

Investigations

Measuring oxygen saturations should be straightforward. In children with chronic cough, spirometry can be helpful but may not be routinely available. In most children with chronic cough, a chest X-ray will be indicated. Further investigations will usually be indicated from the history and chest X-ray. Remember that current CF screening will miss some cases of CF, especially in the non-white population.

Diagnosis

On history, Jared had a dry cough which waxed and waned. He was otherwise well. He had been started on bronchodilators but screamed when his mother tried to give them. A putative diagnosis of asthma was made.

Management

Jared's mother was trained in good inhaler technique. He was commenced on an inhaled steroid for 8 weeks and showed marked improvement, followed by deterioration when this was stopped. He was, therefore, diagnosed with presumed asthma.

Follow up

Most follow up of asthma is done best in primary care, and Jared was referred to the nurse-led asthma clinic at the general practitioners.

Discussion

Chronic cough can be divided into two categories. In the first there is significant concern about underlying disease and fairly urgent action is required. These children will usually exhibit some of the red flag features mentioned above. Specifically, they will be producing mucous/phlegm which will give the cough a wet nature. In the presence of any of these features, further investigation to identify the cause and initiate prompt appropriate therapy is indicated.

In children with a history of a dry cough and in the absence of any worrying features, a trial of antiasthma therapy is worthwhile, even in the absence of a specific asthma history. This should have clear limits including an assessment of efficacy. There may be some value in trials of antireflux and antirhinitis therapy.

Further reading

Shields MD, Bush A, Everard ML, et al. Recommendations for the assessment and management of cough in children. Thorax 2008; 63:1–15.

Lokshin B, Lindgren S, Weinberger M, Koviach J. Outcome of habit cough in children treated with a brief session of suggestion therapy. Ann Allergy 1991; 67(6):579–582.

Patient information

Asthma UK
    www.asthma.org.uk
Kids Health
    www.kidshealth.org

Crying baby

Dear Paediatrician,

Please can you urgently see Matilda, who is 6 weeks old. She is increasingly unsettled, crying all the time. I prescribed some Gaviscon which did help initially, but now seems to have become less effective. It may have made her a bit constipated.

Her mother wanted to breast feed, but was advised against this because she was on a selective serotonin reuptake inhibitor (SSRI) during pregnancy. She has tried a number of different milks but none seems to settle her.

Many thanks,

Dr Ian Connolly

Case analysis

Do not underestimate the impact a crying baby has on the family. Exhaustion and frustration can develop to such a degree that unless you have experienced it yourself, it may be possible to sympathise but almost impossible to empathise.

Unsettled behaviour, often referred to as 'cry-fuss' behaviour, is very subjective, as different parents have different expectations and tolerance levels. In some cases, it is the parental issues that need addressing.

It is vital to offer understanding and support to these families, as it improves outcomes for everybody. There are some medical causes for crying, which must be explored, although treatment is not always effective. It is often realistic to say 'we might not be able to settle her, but we are at least going to try'. Telling parents 'all babies cry' is unhelpful.
In Matilda's case there are a number of factors which may be contributing:
- Maternal issues – Matilda's mother is on an SSRI so is likely to have anxiety and/or depression
- Gastro-oesophageal reflux disease – there was some benefit from Gaviscon
- Constipation/stool withholding – needs to be assessed
- Drug withdrawal – SSRI withdrawal is increasingly recognised

Differential diagnosis

Normal behaviour

It is hard to know whether cry-fuss behaviour is excessive or merely interpreted as such. Try to explore parental expectations and see if any support is available. It is crucial that parents get adequate rest, and giving them permission to let somebody babysit whilst they go to sleep can be helpful. Health visitors offer support and can advise about local parenting groups.

Gastro-oesophageal reflux disease

This is common. The classic symptoms are:

- Crying dependent on position: This is frequently misinterpreted. For example, parents will say, 'she likes being held' when in reality being upright reduces reflux. Similarly 'she hates having her nappy changed' is likely to be because lying flat and lifting her legs exacerbates reflux
- Poor feeding: This is likely to be secondary to the pain of oesophagitis
- Putting hands in mouth: This generates saliva which being alkaline helps neutralise the acid in the stomach and oesophagus
- Posturing: Wriggling, arching, turning the head (Sandifer's syndrome) are all attempts by the baby to deal with the pain

Treatment of gastro-oesophageal reflux disease (GORD) is controversial. Numerous reviews have failed to show that treatments offer significant symptomatic benefit (it is possible that this is because there are other or additional issues). Certainly, the widespread prescription of therapies suggests that the literature is unread and/or disbelieved.

There are many different approaches to reflux management; it is best to follow local guidelines.

Treatment options include:

- Watchful waiting
- Physical measures – raising the bed, keeping upright, winding
- Feed thickeners – these can make the milk difficult for the baby to suck through the teat.
- Anti-reflux milks – note that some anti reflux milks require stomach acid to thicken in the stomach so will not work with acid suppressing drugs
- Medications:
  - Alginates, e.g. Gaviscon
  - Acid suppression, e.g. Ranitidine, proton pump inhibitors
  - Motility agents, e.g. Domperidone
- Surgery – very rarely indicated, usually only if severe/failing to thrive

Reflux generally improves over 9–18 months; it can persist and has probably been under-recognised in older children. As the child grows, the drug doses may need increasing accordingly. After 9 months of age, it is worth trying to wean the drugs to see if they are still necessary.

Stool withholding

This can start at any age. The symptoms are often unrecognised because if the withholding is successful, the only evidence is the struggle. The classic features are:

- Frequent crying – can have a reflux like history. Because feeding stimulates the gastrocolic reflex, stool withholding babies may have feeding difficulties. Because the pain can be at any time, they may also sleep poorly
- Straining– behaviour that can mimic seizures
- Change in behaviour after bowel opening, i.e. calmer, better and less upset
- Passing lots of flatus
- Often infrequent passage of stools – but how a child goes is more important than how often. Babies will on average open their bowels a few times a day, with significant variation. So, a baby going once a day may be stool withholding whilst a baby going

once a week may be normal. Babies stool is usually very soft, first time parents may misinterpret a formed stool (which would be hard for a young baby) as normal. The diagnosis is supported if the symptoms vary with time, especially if they improve after a bowel opening. Treatment involves getting the baby to go easily and comfortably, using an appropriate combination of fluid, fibre and laxatives.

Cow's milk protein allergy

There is a broad spectrum of this condition from the essentially asymptomatic to frank colitis, and debate as to whether this is an intolerance or allergy. Babies with cow's milk protein allergy may be more prone to GORD and stool withholding. If this is a possibility, then a dairy-free diet should be trialled for 2–6 weeks. Breastfeeding mothers should go dairy-free, as cow's milk protein can cross into human milk. If the babies are on formula, they may try 'prescribed' or 'medical' milk. These come in three types:

1. Partially hydrolysed feeds – 'comfort milks' are available over the counter. Often parents will have tried using these already, but if they have not, it is worth trying them.
2. Hydrolysed feeds – whilst effectively the same, different types can vary hugely in price. The dietician can usually advise on this.
3. Elemental feeds – could be reserved for babies with colitis, but it is often hard to refuse them to parents who claim that hydrolysed feeds have helped, but not totally. Also some parents may quote papers that these milks are 'better' in cow's milk protein allergy. They are very expensive. The general practitioner will want reassurance of regular review and of on-going benefit before agreeing to prescribe.

In any child that has started one of these milks they should be challenged with normal milk after 2–6 weeks. If they do need the special milk, they can be challenged again at about 1 year of age, and every 6 months or so thereafter. Children, or mothers, on a dairy free diet may benefit from dietetic input to ensure calcium needs are being met. Soya feeds can be used for children over 6 months of age but are not recommended for younger children. There is some crossover with cow's milk protein and soya allergy so it may be worth advising breast feeding mothers to avoid soya as well as milk initially.

Colic

There are some babies that just cry. There does seem to be an entity whereby babies cry for a few hours a day, usually at the same time, but are completely settled otherwise. This may be the elusive '3-month colic'. Colic has been said to be an acronym for cause obscure lengthy infant crying. Most children with a diagnosis of colic will, on simple questioning, be shown to have a more definitive diagnosis.

Pain – broken bones, muscular contractions, e.g. cerebral palsy

Occasionally, these can be the cause of a crying baby. This should be evident on examination.

Over stimulation

Some babies seem to be over-stimulated. They just need to be left alone. The only way to diagnose this is by putting the baby down to rest. Sometimes this requires a short admission.

Medication/withdrawal

Irritability can be associated with medication, either taking it or withdrawing. A full drug history is essential. Withdrawal may be attenuated by breastfeeding which might be happening against medical advice. Treatment is usually symptomatic. Severe withdrawal may need medication.

Consultation essentials

History

Consider crying to be an expression of pain. The history should therefore mimic a pain history:
- Onset
- Duration – constant or intermittent
- Change in severity – getting better or worse
- Exacerbating/relieving factors
- Associated behaviour

Because there is often a gastrointestinal link the following are essential parts of the history:
- The milk that the baby is taking now, and which others may have been tried. If there has been a change of milks, ask about the reason for the change, and whether it had the desired effect
- The amount of milk taken per feed and number of feeds per day- overfeeding can exacerbate GORD – normal intake is 120–150 mL/kg/day (2 ½ fl oz/lb/day)
- Whether the baby feeds well or not – 'is she easy to feed?' and 'does she seem content and settled after a feed?'
- A bowel history – especially whether opening the bowels causes general improvement in symptoms

Examination

The examination should identify if there are any physical issues. Do not discount the reassurance of a normal exam. The weight and head circumference must be plotted. If there is any faltering growth, then further action is required.

Tests/investigations

These are rarely necessary. Often a trial of treatment is the most useful investigation.

Diagnosis

Matilda had symptoms of GORD.

Management

The diagnosis was discussed with the parents, along with treatment options. She was started on ranitidine. She also had some mild constipation and Gaviscon was stopped but she received extra water. Her mother seemed to be depressed and she was recommended to go and discuss this with her general practitioner.

Follow up

It is important that these families are offered supportive follow up. Often the first measure is only of limited success and further interventions might be necessary (alternatively beware of discarding treatments before giving them time to work). The general practitioner or health visitor may be the best people to follow up, but further clinic appointments may help. Do not underestimate the value of a sympathetic doctor in helping parents manage a challenging child.

Discussion

The most important variable in child development is the nature of the parenting that a child receives. Parents of crying children often have their resilience worn away, which affects their parenting ability. They also tend to believe that there must be something wrong with their baby and feel helpless that they cannot comfort her. There is an obvious circular link with postnatal depression. Furthermore, crying babies are at an increased risk of being abused.

Further reading

Douglas P. Managing infants who cry excessively in the first few months of life. *BMJ* 2011a; 343 doi: 10.1136/bmj.d7772.

Douglas P et al. The unsettled baby: how complexity science helps. Arch Dis Child 2011b; 96:793–797 doi:10.1136/adc. 2010:199 190.

Van der Pol RJ, et al. Efficacy of proton-pump inhibitors in children with gastroesophageal reflux disease: a systematic review. Pediatrics 2011; 127(50):925–935.

Vandenplas Y, et al. North American Society for Pediatric Gastroenterology Hepatology and Nutrition, European Society for Pediatric Gastroenterology Hepatology and Nutrition. Pediatric gastroesophageal reflux clinical practice guidelines: joint recommendations of the North American Society for Pediatric Gastroenterology, Hepatology, and Nutrition (NASPGHAN) and the European Society for Pediatric Gastroenterology Hepatology, and Nutrition (ESPGHAN). J Pediatr Gastroenterol Nutr 2009; 49(4):498–547.

Patient information

Family lives
    www.familylives.org.uk
Cry-sis
    www.cry-sis.org.uk

Case 19

Daytime wetting

Dear Paediatrician,

Please could you see Jemima, who is 5 years old. She has never really been dry by day and has frequent accidents. Mum is very understanding, but is beginning to find things difficult. She keeps being sent home wet from school, and Mum thinks that her friends are beginning to notice the smell. She wears pull ups at night, which are always soaked through in the morning.

Many thanks,

Dr David Coulter

Case analysis

Occasional daytime wetting, due to 'misjudgement' is common in 5 year olds, but Jemima's wetting is happening too often. The challenge is to try and ascertain whether Jemima's problem is anatomical, physiological, and behavioural or even if it is a problem at all. In order to understand the issue, further information is required including when, where and how often the wetting occurs, and how much urine is passed.

Never having been dry might suggest an anatomical cause, but this would normally be associated with a continuous leak. The ability to have been dry for the best part of a day or night – even if this is an infrequent occurrence – makes an anatomical cause highly unlikely. Occasionally, in girls with fused labia, urine can collect behind the fusion and then leak out afterwards.

Physiologically, it is vital to understand whether she has a small overactive bladder or a large 'holding on' one. A history of urgency can apply to both types.

Constipation/stool withholding is a common causal or exacerbating factor in urinary problems.

Concern about urinary symptoms and safeguarding is misplaced. Suspecting abuse because of urinary symptoms alone is misguided.

Bedwetting is not unusual at this age. Focus on the daytime wetting first. In some situations, e.g. over active bladder (OAB) or anatomical causes, the day and night wetting may be linked. Children, who wet, for whatever reason, will often become ambivalent about the wetting, losing the 'yuk' factor, which limits their motivation to be dry. In order to divert their parents' frustration they will often say 'I didn't feel it coming' or 'I didn't know it was there'.

To disabuse families of this notion, ask if the child has ever gone and passed urine by themselves without being asked and remained dry throughout the process. When they answer 'yes' point out that the sensation of needing to pass urine is not one that comes and goes, so if they have been once they know when it is there.

Similarly, if they cannot feel wet knickers this would suggest a total loss of sensation in that area. If that was the case, they would develop bed/pressure sores at night. If they do not have bed sores, they know when they are wet. When they say 'I didn't know it was there' they mean 'I wish it wasn't there and I don't want to get into trouble'.

Differential diagnoses

Unrealistic expectations

Although parents may expect complete dryness, at this age the occasional misjudgement is to be expected. Conversely, there are some parents whose expectations are unduly low.

Over active bladder/detrusor instability/twitchy bladder

The under recognised, OAB is a source of much distress. It presents with frequency and urgency. The child passes small volumes of urine, and has urgency such that they may not have time to get to the toilet. Although frequency is said to be a feature of OAB, many children control this by significantly limiting their fluid intake.

Bladder function is dynamic, and in most people anxiety causes frequency. Quite a few children seem to have a transient period of OAB when starting school, which often settles spontaneously. In some children the bladder seems quite 'twitchy' more or less all of the time.

In adults OAB can be treated with pelvic floor type exercises, but these are not particularly effective in children. Usually children respond well to antimuscarinics such as oxybutynin, which should be given for about 3 months initially. This is all that is required for many children, whereas others may need treatment for longer or continuously. The drug should be weaned every 3–4 months to ensure that it is still needed.

Postponement

If children try holding on to their urine, there is a limit as to how long they can hold before urine starts leaking. Classically, these children are jumping up and down and fidgety, desperate not to go to the toilet. They pass large volumes of urine infrequently. The soiling analogy is that this is like playing football by the windows, and having been told numerous times to play elsewhere, the advice is ignored and a window gets smashed. The wetting is not intentional, but it is predictable and avoidable. It is important to ensure that acceptable toilets are readily available. Children may wet at school because the toilets are unpleasant or they have restricted access to them. What is required in this situation is increased motivation. Whilst being positive is important, often a change only occurs when there is a reasonable consequence to wetting, e.g. Barbie does not want to play with girls that wet their knickers.

Constipation

It is essential that constipation is actively excluded or treated.

Vaginal reflux (abnormal micturition)

Urine can collect in the vagina after micturition. After finishing micturition there will be some leakage. The history is usually of wetting after going to the toilet. Useful management includes double micturition (count to 10 and try again), sitting 'backwards' on the toilet facing the cistern and ensuring proper wiping afterwards.

Urinary tract infection/cystitis

It is unlikely that urinary tract infection this would cause a long-standing problem. Dysuria may lead to wetting because micturition is painful, and this precipitates postponement. More rarely, cystitis may mimic OAB. Infection is unlikely in the absence of dysuria.

Anatomical abnormality

It is very unlikely that there is an abnormality of the anatomy unless the child has spina bifida. Classically there would be a continuous dribble. Fused labia may give symptoms similar to vaginal reflux and can be treated with a short course of topical oestrogen.

Diabetes

Diabetes mellitus is unlikely to present chronically. Diabetes insipidus is very rare and would have accompanying polydipsia.

Poor wiping/shaking/phimosis (in boys)

Boys may wet after passing urine, because they do not complete micturition, usually being impatient to return to playing, or because urine gets trapped behind a bulging foreskin and then drips out later.

Consultation essentials

History

Establish a urinary history asking about volume, urgency and frequency in relation to drinking and try to establish if there is any constipation/stool withholding. Find out when the wetting occurs, especially if it happens before or after passing the bulk of urine, i.e. are your knickers wet before you get to the toilet? In most cases the wetting will be a herald of further urine to come. Understanding the situations in which wetting occurs and the consequences of wetting usually provides avenues for intervention.

Examination

Physical examination should check for any obvious abnormalities including spinal abnormalities, and local soreness.

Investigations

The most useful test is to measure urine volumes over a few days. The family should try to measure this as often as they can, but do not need to stop the rest of their lives to do so.

Bladder volume can be estimated by the following formula:
(Age of child + 1) x 30 = average bladder capacity in mLs
So, when a 5-year-old girl passes urine, she should pass around 180 mL or 6 fl oz each time.

It can also be helpful to measure urinary frequency, but as said above, often children will 'manage' OAB by limiting fluid intake.

Radiological investigations are rarely indicated. Occasionally, a bladder ultrasound may be helpful, and this can also indirectly assess emptying effectiveness by measuring bladder volumes. Even more rarely urodynamic studies or contrast radiology may be helpful.

Diagnosis

Jemima measured her urine volumes which were around 50 mL giving her a diagnosis of OAB.

Management

She started oxybutynin and within a week her symptoms improved and she was dry by day. A few months later she was also dry at night. After 3 months the oxybutynin was weaned but her symptoms recurred. The oxybutinin was re-started with the understanding that weaning would be tried every 3–4 months.

Follow up

The follow up depends on the family and primary care. This can be negotiated with the parents.

Discussion

Soiling can be behavioural, physiological or anatomical. It is essential to establish which is the cause as the treatments are clearly very different for each case.

Further reading

Von Gontard A, Neveus T. Management of Disorders of Bladder and Bowel Control in Childhood. Cambridge: Cambridge University Press; 2006.

Patient information

Education and Resources for Improving Childhood Continence
    www.eric.org.uk
Cohn A. Constipation, Withholding and Your Child: A Family Guide to Soiling and Wetting. London: Jessica Kingsley Publishers Ltd; 2006.

Case 20

Delayed walking

Dear Paediatrician,

Please see Simon who is now 18 months old and is still not walking. He has not shown much inclination to stand either. He does however sit reasonably well and is beginning to get about shuffling sideways on his bottom. He sat at about 9 months old. He was born at term, weighing 3 kg, by a normal delivery. He was well as a newborn infant. He was admitted for bronchiolitis at about 3 months old while away on holiday and was said to have been quite ill. His parents are healthy. He has a sister who did not walk until about 15 months. His language development seems also a bit borderline: he is now saying two words 'mum' and 'ta' for thank you.

Dr Mahmood Gupta

GP Registrar

Case analysis

The letter excludes major birth trauma as an obvious cause. The late walking affecting his sister suggests other family members might have walked late. The bronchiolitis illness needs further enquiry as does his possible late language development. As with all developmental conditions, an artificial cut off point is used to determine when investigation is required. Even at this stage, the majority of children who are not walking will be normal.

Differential diagnosis

Normal development

There is more variability over locomotor development than any other aspect of development. At 18 months many children will still not be walking, and most toddlers who walk late are healthy.

Global developmental delay

Late walking could be a manifestation of overall slow development. This is hinted at by seemingly slow language development.

Cerebral palsy

Spastic diplegia is unlikely because of his term delivery but not impossible. A spastic diplegia is a lesion of prematurity but a complication of pregnancy could have arisen at about 32 weeks which did not lead to delivery. Other possibilities include hypotonic/ataxic cerebral palsy or a hemiplegia where the early signs may not be evident to the uninitiated and the birth history may well be normal. Road traffic accident during pregnancy has been associated with cerebral palsy although usually the severe forms. The bronchiolitis, if associated with severe desaturations or apnoea, could have caused brain injury.

Brain tumour

The general practitioner would have been very likely to have mentioned a big head. A brain tumour would be a rare cause but one that has to be borne in mind.

Progressive conditions

These are highly unusual and there would normally be a history of developmental regression. This group would include neurodegenerative conditions such as leukomalacia, and progressive brain anatomical lesions such as hydrocephalus or a chronic subdural haemorrhage.

Neuromuscular disorder

Duchenne muscular dystrophy (DMD) is the most likely of these, a mild form of spinal muscular atrophy or a hereditary peripheral neuropathy. A child with congenital myotonic dystrophy might occasionally present with delayed walking.

Developmental dysplasia of the hip

Although this should normally be detected at birth, some cases do slip through the net. Also, the pathogenesis of the condition is better understood so that features may not always be present at birth – which is why it is no longer called congenital dislocation of the hip. Developmental dysplasia of the hip (DDH) has to be managed by a specialist orthopaedic team.

Rickets

There is a resurgence of rickets in the UK, sometimes with symptoms sufficient to cause delayed walking. There would likely be other features such as a rachitic rosary and wrist swelling. Although it is most common in dark skinned children, children on restrictive and unusual diets are also at risk, especially if they spend most of their lives indoors. A wrist X-ray will confirm rickets, and the treatment involves vitamin D supplementation and dietary advice.

Hypothyroidism

This can be insidious. Often the only way to exclude it is to test thyroid function.

Inborn errors of metabolism

There may be episodes of acute deterioration, especially at times of illness. If there is any concern this should be investigated, and this is best done either at a time of illness or in a hospital setting during a controlled fast.

Consultation essentials

History

Events in pregnancy, which may seem trivial, could cause non-progressive brain injury. These would include infections and any trauma, especially abdominal trauma. Similarly, if he required resuscitation and/or neonatal care, these could be the cause or consequence of brain injury. Late quickening and polyhydramnios are features of congenital myotonic dystrophy.

Establish when the parents first walked, and if either was a bottom shuffler with late walking. Determine any history of foot deformities, hand weakness, stiffness of the mother's hands, presenile cataract, or uncles with muscle weakness, particularly on the maternal side – all of these are features of congenital myotonic dystrophy.

Enquire about, and clarify the trajectory of the child's development, 'is he getting better, worse or staying the same'. Any regression should raise the possibility of serious disease. Alternatively, the situation may have improved since the general practitioner's letter. Ask about feeding, a child on long-standing doorstep milk and no solids would suggest rickets.

Determine the severity of his previous illnesses. Children with inborn errors of metabolism may decompensate during viral illnesses causing a prolonged or atypical course. Bronchiolitis may cause symptoms ranging from the subclinical to respiratory failure, with obviously varying consequences.

Examination

On examination look for any evidence of a genetic syndrome – if suspicious, a referral to a geneticist is the best next step. Measure and plot head circumference, either macro- or microcephaly might suggest possible underlying causes.

Assess social skills – at 18 months he should have some sense of 'stranger danger'. This is good, although it can make the examination more challenging. He should have several consonant sounds, one or two words, good vocal turn taking, pointing and early imaginative play by 18 months.

Check his sitting skill and assess his righting reflexes: hold him around the pelvis and sit him upright, then tilt him gently from side to side, he should have good body righting reflexes, absence suggests either significant weakness or impairment of motor control. Look for signs of a hemiplegia. Observe for facial weakness. Both mother and child will have some facial weakness in congenital myotonic dystrophy.

Features of advanced language development, fine hand tremor and floppy legs suggest spinal muscular atrophy. Slow general development and enlarged firm calves suggests DMD.

Ask him to try and walk, and check his gross movement. His gait may suggest a particular diagnosis such as DDH.

Investigations

Any tests are determined by the clinical picture.

Creatinine kinase

A major concern is identifying muscular dystrophy. A very important factor is whether the parents are contemplating having further children, indeed one of the reasons for choosing 18 months as the cut off point for not walking is because this is the time when parents are often considering having more children. It is vital not to miss muscular dystrophy at this stage as it would inform choices in relation to a future pregnancy and possible preimplantation genetic diagnosis. So, unless it is clear that he is close to walking and seems otherwise well, performing a creatinine kinase seems sensible.

Hip X-ray

The DDH is easy to miss and hard to diagnose. Discuss with the radiologist beforehand to ensure the correct views are taken. Many radiologists like a 'frog view'.

Neurological imaging

A matter of debate: whilst a scan will provide information, it rarely changes the treatment or outcome. Nevertheless, if there is an identifiable neurological cause, most paediatricians would want to see the MRI.

Metabolic investigations

If there is evidence of regression, or other features of a metabolic condition – discuss with the metabolic team.

Diagnosis

In this case, the bronchiolitis illness was important. He presented rather late as the parents were in a remote part of the country. He was admitted to intensive care, had a number of fits and was thought to be a bit floppy subsequently. His general development has been slow but he does not have signs to definitely indicate a cerebral palsy, his body righting reflexes are present but a bit weak. With the progress of time he developed a clearer picture of cerebral palsy with increased tone although he acquired independent walking. This boy has a chronic mild static brain disorder, which has presented as delay in walking as the main outward manifestation.

Management

He needs close developmental follow up but no specific investigations. He needs input from the physiotherapist and speech and language therapist.

Follow up

Following children up regularly enough to see progression towards walking is supportive. but the balance of control may lie with the therapists. A paediatric review would be important by 18 months to ensure all the medical causes are assessed for and investigated as appropriate.

Discussion

Although late walking is often less serious than language delay, it is usually the parameter that causes more concern.

Further reading

Horridge KA. Assessment and investigation of the child with disordered development. Arch Dis Child Educ Pract Ed 2011; 96:9–20.
Williams J. Global developmental delay – globally helpful? Dev Med Child Neurol 2010; 52(3):227.

Patient information

American Academy of Paediatrics
www.aap.org

Developmental delay

Dear Paediatrician,

I would be grateful if you could see this 19-month-old boy who I saw today with a cold. His mother noted that he wasn't yet walking and that his older sister walked at 14 months. He was born normally at term and there is no other past medical history. In clinic, he had a mild upper respiratory tract infection but otherwise seemed quite happy on his mother's lap. There is no other back ground history other than mild maternal postnatal depression.

I would be grateful for your assessment.

Dr Theo Davis

Case analysis

It is not unusual to pick up on parental concerns in an otherwise routine appointment. Trying to ascertain whether development is disordered or not can seem daunting considering the wide range of 'normal' for achieving milestones. The key is to recognising a few key milestones and remembering that skills are acquired sequentially and consistently (**Table 21.1**).

Differential diagnosis

The list of potential diagnoses when considering developmental delay is huge, and most children's delay remains unexplained. In all children with developmental delay, holistic management to improve outcome is essential whatever the underlying cause.

Trying to establish a diagnosis is important for two reasons:

1. The delay may be due to a treatable cause – such as hypothyroidism or a mucopolysaccharidosis, where early diagnosis and treatment will improve the outcome.
2. There may be an inheritable component to the problem, which may have implications if the parents are to have further children, or when the child or their siblings want to become parents.

The advances in genetic testing, means that an increasing number of children – albeit still only 10–20% – may have a genetic cause found to explain delay. Older children, who have had normal karyotyping, may have abnormalities detected in microarray.

Consultation essentials

History/examination

Getting a good developmental history is essential. Development starts from conception, so review of pregnancy is essential. This should include any medications taken, or drugs,

Table 21.1 Key milestones			
Age	**Gross motor**	**Fine motor and vision**	**Speech and language**	**Social/behavioural**
6 weeks	Head level with body In ventral suspension	Fixes and follows	Stills in response to sound	Smiles
3 months	Holds head at 90 In ventral suspension	Holds object placed In hand	Turns to sound	Hand regard, laugh, squeals
6 months	No head lag on pull to sit Sits with support Lifts up on forearms when prone	Palmar grasp of objects Transfers between hands	vocalisations	Start responding to facial expressions, copying noises. Like to be comforted
9 months	Sits unsupported Pivots around	Pincer grip Bangs objects together	Two syllable babble, mama, dada	Waves bye-bye, stranger awareness emerging, indicates want
12 months	Pulls to stand, cruises, may stand alone briefly	Puts blocks in cups, casts	One or two words Imitates adult sounds	Imitates activities, looks for lost items, points to indicate want
18 months	Walks well Runs	Builds tower 2–4 bricks, hand preference emerges	6–12 words	Uses spoon, symbolic/role play
2 years	Kicks ball, climbs stairs, 2 feet per step	Builds tower 6–7 cubes Circular scribble	Joins 2–3 words Knows some body parts, identifies object in pictures	Can remove some clothes
3 years	Climbs stairs 1 foot per step	Builds tower 9 cubes Copies a circle	Talks in short sentences	Eats with fork and spoon, puts on clothing. Toilet trained

especially alcohol. Trauma in pregnancy can cause fetal brain damage, and unfortunately domestic abuse often starts in pregnancy. It is rare for mothers to disclose this, and probably inappropriate to be over-inquisitive. Perhaps 'did you have any falls or major knocks when you were pregnant?' is as much as is reasonable to ask. Delivery, gestation, birth weight and neonatal issues may all impact on development. There is increasing interest in possible mild delay in the late preterm baby.

The letter focuses on one milestone, walking. There are a few helpful pointers – his age is right on the cusp of normal parameters. Alarm bells should ring if a boy isn't walking by 18 months (20 months for girls), the concern being a possible muscular dystrophy. Other useful information includes the age that he began to sit. Sitting is a more consistent milestone than crawling, which some children never do. It is useful to know whether he crawls or is a bottom shuffler. Bottom shufflers often have a family history of this.

Establish if the child vocalises and if so whether there are sounds or meaningful words. Parental assessment of children's hearing is often poor, but should be sought.

This mother has a past history of postnatal depression. Parents with depression may not stimulate or interact effectively with their child. This could impact on language development, play skills and social interaction. Children who are neglected can also present with developmental delay, so safeguarding issues should always be considered.

If the child has had significant medical illness this might also be expected to delay development – although there should be catch up as the child recovers.

Examination

Height and weight

Plot height and weight on centile charts: Significant short stature and failure to thrive are often to be associated with general problems. Alternatively, rapid weight gain is seen in Prader–Willi syndrome.

Head circumference

Plot head circumference on centile charts. Microcephaly would obviously raise concerns, as would an increasing head circumference that was crossing centiles. In this situation, an intracranial bleed or hydrocephalus is the most important differentials, and an urgent scan should be arranged.

Dysmorphic features

Dysmorphism can be difficult sometimes. Ask if the child looks like other family members. Remember to examine the eyes, ears, palate, hands and fingers.

Skin markings

Look for Café au Lait spots or axillary freckling suggesting neurofibromatosis or tuberous sclerosis.

Cardiovascular examination

Cardiac murmurs are common in many conditions, especially Down's syndrome, Williams' syndrome and 22q11 deletion syndrome.

Abdominal examination

Hepatomegaly may be found in metabolic disorders.

Neurological examination

An increased tone and spasticity are features of cerebral palsy whilst low tone and muscle weakness are more common in muscular dystrophies. Assessing swallowing and feeding may be essential for management.

Hearing and vision

Assessment of hearing and vision may need to be done by ophthalmologist/orthoptist and audiologist.

In most children the examination is essentially normal. Obviously any positive findings should trigger appropriate investigations. A specific developmental assessment should be performed by a person trained in the specific technique.

There are number of red flag presentations that should warrant a referral to a community paediatrician or paediatric neurologist (Table 21.2).

Table 21.2 Red flags for child development; referral to a community paediatrician or paediatric neurologist

Any age:
- Complex disabilities
- Developmental skill loss
- Floppiness or persistently low tone
- Head circumference above 99.6th centile or below 0.4th centile or has crossed two centiles (up or down) or is disproportionate to parental head circumference
- Hearing loss (simultaneously refer to audiology and/or ENT assessment)
  - Movement
  - Asymmetry or other features of cerebral palsy (e.g. increased muscle tone)
- Persistent toe-walking
- Uncertainty about any aspect of assessment but the assessing clinician thinks development maybe disordered
- Visual: problems fixing/following an object or confirmed visual impairment (simultaneously refer to paediatric ophthalmologist)

By 5 months (corrected for gestation):
- Unable to hold object placed in hand

By 6 months (corrected for gestation):
- Unable to reach for objects

By 12 months:
- Child unable to sit unsupported

By 18 months:
- Speech absent, especially in absence of communication by gesture or other means (simultaneously refer for urgent hearing test)
- Boy unable to walk – check creatinine kinase urgently

By 2 years:
- Girl unable to walk – check creatinine kinase urgently
- Unable to point at objects to share interest with others

By 2½ years:
- Unable to run

Data from Aicardi, 2009

Investigations

These will obviously be influenced by the history, examination and local policy. The list of potential investigations is endless, so should be discussed. Diagnosing muscular dystrophy early is important as many parents would contemplate having further children at around this stage. If this child has muscular dystrophy, this is likely to affect the parents pregnancy choices and hence the urgency to establish or exclude the diagnosis. Hypothyroidism may be insidious and checking thyroid function seems reasonable. If the child was not born in the UK they should have phenylketonuria testing performed as well.

Many children with developmental delay will have some form of neuroimaging, but this is rarely urgent.

Diagnosis

This boy could have isolated gross motor delay. It is important to examine him and identify significant conditions such as cerebral palsy or Duchenne muscular dystrophy. Consider whether there is specific or global delay. In this case, he was noted to be quiet, so could have language delay or social communication difficulties. Always listen to parents. They may be more or less concerned than the professionals involved. Understanding their reasoning is essential as is, occasionally, the need to challenge it.

Management

As this child is just within normal parameters it is reasonable to ask the health visitor to monitor the child's progress. The health visitor will be able to meet with the family, observe the child for a longer period and get a better idea of the family situation and their concerns. In the presence of language delay, a referral for a hearing test and speech and language therapy is reasonable.

Follow up

Some follow up is required. This can be in the general clinic, but if there are concerns, a referral to the community paediatrician should be made.

Discussion

The main points are to enquire about other aspects of development, examine and exclude any red flags. If these are present they need an urgent onward referral.

Further reading

Aicardi J. Diseases of the nervous system in childhood. Mac Keith Press 2009:243–380, 287–9, 891–893.
Bellman, et al. Developmental assessment of children. BMJ 2013; 346:e8687.
Horridge K. Assessment and investigation of the child with disordered development. Arch Dis Child Educ Prac Ed 2011; 96:9–20.

Patient information

Contact a Family
    www.cafamily.org.uk
Mencap
    www.mencap.org.uk
NHS Birth to Five Development Timeline
    www.nhs.uk

Diarrhoea: teenager

Dear Paediatrician,

Thank you for seeing Lianne who is 13 years old. She has a history of abdominal pain and diarrhoea which has been somewhat intermittent, but getting worse over the last 9 months. She sometimes needs to open her bowels 8 times a day. She is increasingly worried that she might have accidents, and this is causing her to miss a lot of school. Lianne says that sometimes her stool contains blood. She has few other symptoms, and does not appear to be losing weight.

Dr Michael Dobbin

Case analysis

Because these symptoms have been present for a long time, there is likely to be an underlying condition. The most serious possibility is inflammatory bowel disease (IBD). However, often the story given to the general practitioner is incomplete, so that this history could also be given with constipation/stool withholding and overflow.

Differential diagnosis

Inflammatory bowel disease

Although the exact diagnosis will need to be confirmed with a tissue diagnosis, if there is a strong suspicion of inflammatory bowel disease (IBD) referral for investigation should be expedited. Classically there is a history of diarrhoea – in colitis there would normally be blood in the stool, but in children with Crohn's disease, e.g. with terminal ileal disease, this may not be easily identified. It is imperative that a proper stool history is taken as this should suggest the diagnosis. Abdominal pain is again variable, and children diagnosed with IBD will usually have a history of persistent, recurrent abdominal pain which may have been present, and presumably misdiagnosed, for many years.

If the index of suspicion for diagnosing IBD is too low then many children will be subject to unnecessary investigations, whilst if it is too high there can be a significantly delayed diagnosis. Any or all of the symptoms of diarrhoea, abdominal pain and passing blood can suggest IBD, although there will be other causes as well. If the symptoms suggest an alternative diagnosis it is appropriate to treat the presumed diagnosis. If symptoms persist and the response to treatment is incomplete then at some time, as with all conditions there has to be a decision that the original diagnosis needs revisiting, and IBD needs more active consideration. Stool calprotectin is establishing a role as a screening tool to identify which children may need further investigation.

Other colitides

There are a number of other colitides, including eosinophilic colitis, these can present with similar symptoms, and the diagnosis is made on biopsy, as the symptoms should trigger a gastroenterology referral.

Coeliac disease

Coeliac disease can present at any age. Blood in the stool is unusual, and there is usually significant bloating. Many families will have identified a link to gluten containing foods.

Stool withholding and overflow

Significant stool withholding can occur at any stage, but transfer to secondary school with a stricter routine and less welcoming toilet is a common trigger. In this situation, the 'diarrhoea' will be small quantities of soft overflow stool. The diagnosis should be made on the history, and treatment is usually with an appropriate laxative regime.

Anxiety

Some children seem to develop an anxiety about not being able to get to the toilet, which causes urgency and diarrhoea when they leave their homes. However, at home they have no bowel symptoms at all. This can be very disabling, with children becoming effectively housebound. Again, a careful history should establish this diagnosis and management, and involve psychological support. Short-term use of antimotility agents such as loperamide may help – possibly as a placebo.

Irritable bowel syndrome

There is some debate about the existence of this as a separate entity in paediatrics, and the diagnosis should only, if ever, be made after serious consideration as it is often one that patients carry with them for a long time. The intermittent diarrhoea and constipation is often strongly linked to anxiety. Much of IBS is under-recognised constipation.

Pancreatic insufficiency

In many conditions, such as cystic fibrosis, pancreatic function will deteriorate over time so that symptoms become more marked. Usually there will be no blood in the stool, but there will be steatorrhoea and the stool will not flush easily. Pain may be less marked. Fecal elastase will suggest this as a problem but, if suspected, a referral to paediatric gastroenterology is required.

Drugs – laxative abuse

Many drugs cause diarrhoea as a side effect. If taking the medication for other purposes most families would report this to the prescribing doctor and alter the medication. In some instances the child may be taking the medication without the parents' knowledge, e.g. abusing laxatives or enemas in an attempt to lose weight. Often this does not become apparent till other investigations have been conducted and return as normal. Sometimes a period of close observation in hospital may help to suggest or confirm this diagnosis.

Infectious causes

Although these are worth thinking about, it is highly unlikely that an infection would cause such protracted symptoms.

Consultation essentials

History/examination

The most important fact to establish is what diarrhoea actually means – it usually means different things to different people, and many children seem happy to describe the nature of their stools without ever having seen them. It is therefore essential to ensure that the stool history is confirmed with proper descriptions. Diarrhoea is the frequent passage of large quantities of soft stool. A useful if crude question is to ask 'if you were to collect the day's stool in a bucket, how full would it be every day?' In a child with stool withholding and overflow, although the stool might be soft the usual daily quantity would be normal or small, with the occasional massive one. In genuine diarrhoea, the bucket would be overflowing every day.

Establish whether the blood is outside the stool, or only present on wiping suggesting a fissure, or mixed in with the stool as in colitis.

Tests/investigations

Although these are none specific, blood tests might include full blood count, erythrocyte sedimentation rate (ESR), clotting profile, liver function tests including albumin, amylase and a coeliac screen.

If there is a suggestion of steatorrhoea then fecal elastase may be useful and calprotectin – screening for inflammation – is increasingly available. These require soft stool – it is remarkable how many children with intractable diarrhoea seem to present a formed stool for analysis.

Further investigations should be discussed with a gastroenterologist or radiologist.

Diagnosis

Lianne had clinical features of colitis and was referred to the gastroenterologist for further assessment. She had a colonoscopy, the results of which confirmed Crohn's disease.

Management

She was started on a specific feed and her symptoms resolved well.

Follow up

Follow up would certainly involve the paediatric gastroenterologist, but in many places there would be shared care with a general paediatrician.

Discussion

Clinically it is important to distinguish between different types of colitis, as they will have different treatment strategies. Most children with IBD will have either Crohn's disease or ulcerative colitis – a further category of indeterminate colitis includes those children where it is hard to make either diagnosis. Overall, the incidence of IBD appears to be rising, about 25% of cases present in the paediatric age group. Although it is more common in older children, it is certainly not unheard of in the under 5 years.

IBD presents in myriad forms. There is still an unacceptable delay between onset of symptoms and diagnosis in IBD, with the mean time being around 2 years. Although the markers of colitis are pain and bloody diarrhoea, Crohn's disease may occasionally present with constipation or symptoms that are more vague. This always leads to a debate about how, and when, to investigate children. To make matters more complicated, although blood tests may suggest a diagnosis, e.g. anaemia, raised ESR, hypoalbuminaemia, they are neither highly sensitive nor specific. There is growing interest in the use of fecal calprotectin as a screening tool, but this has yet to find wide-scale acceptance in paediatrics.

Although endoscopic tissue biopsy remains imperative for confirming the diagnosis, there is also promising evidence that radiology – ultrasound, CT and MRI – may be useful as either screening tools or to quantify bowel involvement and thus limit the number of invasive procedures performed on children. Similarly, capsule endoscopy, where a 'camera' contained in a small pill-szied capsule is swallowed and transmits images from its journey through the bowel allows effective assessment, without the option of taking a biopsy.

Specific feeds that are used, particularly in Crohn's disease, have improved its management, so that relapses requiring hospital admission are less frequent.

Further reading

O'Gorman JR, Hussey S, et al. British Society of Paediatric Gastroenterology, Hepatology and Nutrition/British Paediatric Neurology Association: G192. The use of faecal calprotectin in paediatric inflammatory bowel. Disease Arch Dis Child 2013;98.Suppl 1 A87 doi:10.1136/archdischild-2013-304107.204

Fell J ME. Update of the management of inflammatory bowel disease. Arch Dis Child 2012; 97:78–83. doi:10.1136/adc.2010.195222

Patient information

Crohn's and Colitis UK
www.crohnsandcolitis.org.uk

Diarrhoea: toddler

Dear Paediatrician,

Thank you for seeing Albert who is two and a half years old. He seems to have permanent diarrhoea which is making toilet training almost impossible. He is otherwise well and thriving.

Dr Jo Fallowfield

Case analysis

Diarrhoea means different things to different people. Whenever there is a history of diarrhoea it is essential to understand exactly what this means. In a child this young, the parents will have seen the stool and should be able to report on it accurately. This would include the frequency, quantity, consistency and any abnormality, especially blood and mucus. Older children may report having diarrhoea, without ever looking at their stools. In true diarrhoea, there is an increase quantity of soft stool passed. Overflow incontinence is frequently mistaken for diarrhoea, because of its consistency, but in this case the child would be producing only very small quantities.

The presence of additional symptoms, especially a child who is not thriving, should arouse suspicions of a serious underlying cause. It is easy to shift focus from a child onto their stool, and there are many parents who worry about the nature of their child's stool, rather than accepting that their child is completely well.

Differential diagnosis

Pancreatic insufficiency/cystic fibrosis

Although in the UK the majority of children with cystic fibrosis should be diagnosed at birth, some will slip through the net. There are also other rare causes of pancreatic insufficiency. Children will usually present with failure to thrive, passing bulky, oily, foul smelling stool. The classic description of the stool not flushing will obviously not be given in a child who is still in nappies. The initial test would be a fecal elastase, but more specific pancreatic function tests may need be carried out by a paediatric gastroenterologist. Treatment depends on what the cause of the problem is.

Coeliac disease

This is another homogenous disease, with some patients presenting with florid signs soon after the introduction of gluten, whilst others wait many decades for diagnosis. Classically, there will be bloating and failure to thrive. Children with coeliac disease are frequently miserable, but their misery can be attributed to their diarrhoea. Because of its very presentation, it would be reasonable to suggest that any child with unexplained abdominal symptoms should have a coeliac screen performed.

Toddler diarrhoea (rapid gut transit)

Many children seem to have rapid gut transit, and this may be exacerbated by an overly active gastrocolic reflex. They open their bowels, frequently during the day, passing large quantities of soft stool which may contain the expected undigested foods of carrots and peas and raisins. Often there is a history of high fruit sugar intake, either in the form of fruits themselves or in fruit juice drinks.

Children with toddler diarrhoea are otherwise well, and rarely complain of other symptoms. The condition is usually diagnosed on history alone, and no tests are necessary. Reducing fruit-sugar intake may be helpful. The condition will improve over time, although some children will continue to have symptoms in primary school and beyond. In these situations, or when toilet training is difficult, loperamide can be of benefit.

Infectious/postinfectious diarrhoea

The commonest cause of diarrhoea in children would be infectious diarrhoea. Whilst the lining of the bowel is recovering from this, there may be increased stool production. Following severe bouts of infectious diarrhoea, it may take 3 months or so for the stool to return to normal. During this time, the stool sample would be normal – infection has cleared, but the healing process needs to complete. There may be accompanying secondary lactose intolerance.

Giardiasis is uncommon, but can cause persistent diarrhoea. An appropriate stool sample should be sent, and the child treated with metronidazole. This is sometimes prescribed empirically for prolonged unexplained diarrhoea. There are obviously advantages and disadvantages to this.

Immunocompromised

Children who are immunocompromised, either with a primary immunodeficiency or with HIV, are more likely to have infectious diarrhoea, and the infections can be serious. These children are usually unwell, and the underlying diagnosis should be obvious in light of their known immunodeficiency.

Wheat/milk intolerance

In some children with diarrhoea there is a clear link to the introduction of particular foods. Wheat and milk are the main culprits. If there is a suggestion that this may be the case, an exclusion diet is merited. This should not continue for more than 4-6 weeks. Any change should be challenged to ensure that the food is genuinely to blame, and clinical improvement was not just coincidental. Many parents are keen to pursue other exclusion diets, but there is little evidence that these make a significant difference, and it is important that the child is not deprived of vital nutrients or the enjoyment of a varied diet.

Inflammatory bowel disease

This is rare in children of this age. There would normally be a history of abdominal pain, blood and mucus in the stool and weight loss. However, as in older children, this is somewhat variable.

Disaccharide intolerance (sucrase isomaltase deficiency)

Disaccharide intolerances are also rare, and tend to improve with age. They present with a very acid stool, with a particularly offensive smell. The stool may be quite caustic, and cause significant nappy rash. Reducing substances would be present in the stool. Treatment is with an exclusion diet. It is possible that this is now simply diagnosed as rapid gut transit.

Lymphangectasia

An extremely rare cause of diarrhoea, usually there is malabsorption and protein loss with signs of peripheral oedema.

Medication

Many drugs are associated with gastrointestinal upset, and if the child is on any medication this should be considered – including herbal medicines. Occasionally, the child may be given medication inappropriately which may be as a result of a misunderstanding, e.g. uncertainty about dosage, or may have more sinister causes, such as intentional poisoning.

Fabrication/embellishment

Although this is a rare cause, most cases of fabricated or induced illness (FII) have a gastroenterological component. Parents have been known to download copies of bloody stool claiming it was their child's. If there is any suspicion, the child can be admitted to hospital for close observation, where the nursing staff can record stool output. FII clearly needs input from the safeguarding team.

Consultation essentials

History/examination

It is essential to establish the nature of the stool being passed, what it looks and smells like and any other particular features. This can help distinguish the normal from the abnormal. The duration of diarrhoea is also important. Diarrhoea of recent onset in a child of this age is more likely to be infectious or postinfectious rather than anything else. A longer history would suggest either toddler diarrhoea, or a problem with absorption.

Examination should include a good general examination, remembering to look in the mouth and around the anus. The child's growth parameters need to be plotted to check if they are thriving.

Tests/investigations

If the history is clear, often no investigations are required. The presence of fat, mucus, blood or undigested food other than peas, carrots, raisins, etc. should be taken as a signal that further investigations are necessary.

Most parents will expect their child to take a stool test. Most stool tests, surprisingly, require a liquid stool for analysis. The stool is then analysed to detect either a viral or bacterial infection. If Giardia is expected then a fresh sample will need to be supplied, asking specifically for giardia. More than one sample may be required.

Tests for malabsorption are expensive, and should only be undertaken on clinical grounds. Stool elastase will test pancreatic function, and reducing substances will identify any sugar malabsorption. There is growing interest in using fecal calprotectin as a screening tool for inflammatory bowel disease. Early studies are promising, but this is not yet accepted as a mainstream test. It should only be undertaken if there is a strong suspicion of inflammatory bowel disease

Blood tests are again of debatable value. If there is any uncertainty, coeliac screen seems reasonable. Undertaking basic blood tests to reassure is often suggested, but may provide false reassurance.

Other investigations, including imaging or endoscopy should be discussed with relevant specialists.

Diagnosis

From the history, Albert has had diarrhoea for some time. His stool was soft and brown, and he was opening his bowels 7 or 8 times a day. There was no undigested food in his stool. He was thriving, and ate well. He drank about two small cartons of fresh orange juice daily. It seems as if Albert has rapid transit/toddler diarrhoea.

Management

Albert's family were advised to reduce the orange juice, and this made a significant difference. He was still opening his bowels 3 or 4 times a day, and was struggling to be toilet trained. It was decided to try loperamide for a few months, and this was of benefit.

Follow up

Albert was followed up every 4 months. Before every clinic visit his family were advised to try him without the loperamide. He needed to continue this for 1 year or so, before his symptoms settled and he was discharged from clinic.

Discussion

Diarrhoea in global terms is a massive problem, accounting for millions of child deaths every year – largely preventable. The introduction of an effective rotavirus vaccine is encouraging, but more important would be the provision of clean water and sanitation. Another preventable cause in infant deaths related to diarrhoea is the marketing of powdered breast milk substitutes to poor countries. Whilst diarrhoea is rarely a cause of death in the UK, there is still considerable work to be done to make this the case globally.

Further reading

Powell CVE, Jenkins HR. Toddler diarrhoea: is it a useful diagnostic label? Arch Dis Child 2012; 97:84–86. doi:10.1136/adc.2010.191825

R Hastings ,Kolic I, et al. British Society of Paediatric Gastroenterology, Hepatology and Nutrition/Neonatal Nutrition Network: Can you diagnose coeliac disease without the need for a duodenal biopsy? Arch Dis Child 2012; 97:Suppl 1 A56-A57 doi:10.1136/archdischild-2012-301885.138

Patient information

Baby Milk Action
    www.babymilkaction.org
Coeliac UK
    www.coeliac.org.uk

Dizziness

Dear Paediatrician,

Thank you for seeing this 14-year-old girl who seems to be having recurrent episodes of dizziness. It often occurs in the morning and she needs to sit down to feel better. She has not had any blackouts. I wonder if she has postural hypotension?

Dr Neeru Kapur

Case analysis

The description favours a diagnosis of postural hypotension but there are other differentials. Families seek medical attention because of frequent episodes affecting schooling and daily routines. It is essential to exclude common causes of dizziness in order to offer appropriate reassurance and to advise on appropriate management. Serious causes for dizziness are uncommon in children, but they have to be considered.

Differential diagnosis

Postural hypotension

This is commonly seen in adolescents especially during a pubertal growth spurt. The main symptoms reported by the child or young person include light-headedness, vision going black for a few seconds, a feeling of subjective spinning (vertigo) and syncope. There may be visible pallor, sweating or abnormal gait or body movements reported by witnesses that may be confused as a seizure. The diagnosis is made from clinical history and by establishing a significant difference in systolic blood pressure (usually >20 mmHg) with changes in posture, when measured initially lying down and then having stood up.

Postural orthostatic tachycardia syndrome

A variant of postural hypotension is called postural orthostatic tachycardia syndrome, (POTS). It is referred to by some physicians and researchers as postural tachycardia syndrome, or just postural tachycardia. This condition is described when the normal physiological responses to going from supine to erect fail, and there are autonomic symptoms including tachycardia, sweating and dizziness. It is a type of dysautonomia. Diagnosis requires specific symptoms and confirmation of the response to a tilt test.

Vertigo/labyrinthitis

In true vertigo there will be an equilibrium disturbance associated with the dysfunction of either the central or peripheral vestibular system. There may be a preceding history of ear or central nervous system infection. Management could include anti-sickness medication and rest but it might be better to allow natural 'recalibration' of the vestibular apparatus in the cochlear to re-set balance. In time this should lead to a reduction of the dizziness symptom.

Underlying brain abnormality

Structural brain abnormalities are a rare underling cause of such a presentation in children. These include conditions such as cerebellopontine lesions, presenting with dysarthria, ipsilateral hearing loss and other cranial nerve deficits and posterior fossa lesions, presenting with cerebellar signs, and pyramidal signs affecting gait and coordination.

Migraine

This is common in children with up to 30% of adolescent girls experiencing migraine head aches. The estimated prevalence is reported to be around 5–10% in children. Dizziness or vertigo is associated with migraine, especially the basilar migraine, a rare type of migraine involving dysarthria, vertigo, tinnitus, diplopia, ataxia and syncope.

Epilepsy/seizure

See Cases on absence seizures and generalised seizures.

Cardiac causes

The possibility of arrhythmia or other cardiac abnormality should be considered. The absence of chest pain or palpitation would reassure against this as a cause.

Psychogenic

A psychological stress may be identified as a cause of dizziness in children. Ask about family dynamics and how things are at school. A mental health assessment may be indicated. In adolescents psychiatric co-morbidities like anxiety and depression is also common.

Chronic fatigue syndrome/ME

Dizziness may be a presenting feature of a chronic fatigue picture.

Medications and drugs

Both prescribed and recreational drugs could be a cause of such symptoms.

Systemic illnesses

Occasionally dizziness can be the presenting symptoms of a systemic illness, such as diabetes or Addison's disease. There would usually be other clues in the history and these two conditions are likely to be picked up on routine blood chemistry analysis.

Consultation essentials

History and examination

Clinical history should entail full personal and family details, and any possible triggers. Asking about diet and eating habits could uncover a body-image perception and possible eating disorder. Fluid intake should be assessed. Take a drug history to include any medications. A recreational drug habit could be relevant.

Perform a full cardiac and neurological examination. Measure blood pressure in supine and standing posture. Significant postural hypotension is diagnosed when a fall in systolic blood pressure of at least 20 mmHg and/or diastolic blood pressure of at least 10 mmHg is recorded within 3 minutes of standing. Check that hearing is not impaired; a hearing test may be indicated.

Investigations

If there is evidence of postural hypotension, and the story fits, no further investigation is necessary.

If the story does not fit, or there are some features pointing to a neurological or cardiac cause, consider an ECG which may be useful in excluding a cardiac conduction abnormality such as prolonged QT syndrome. This should this be done if there is any history of collapse. An EEG is not usually indicated; it needs specialist interpretation and could lead to a misdiagnosis of epilepsy.

Blood tests are not routinely indicated. If anaemia is suspected clinically or there is a history of a poor diet, a full blood count and ferritin levels help diagnosis. Blood sugar could be checked if there is clinical suspicion of diabetes. Dizziness and collapse due to low sugar will be difficult to pick up on without considering a controlled fast.

Brain imaging by MRI would only be considered if there are red flag signs, including: head trauma with new-onset vertigo with or without headache, associated complaints of double vision, difficulty swallowing, slurred speech, changes in vision, facial numbness (all concerning for cranial nerve deficits), difficulty with coordination, new-onset severe headache, progressive symptoms of vertigo, episodes of loss of consciousness, altered mental status, previous history of intracranial abnormality and abnormal examination findings (papilloedema, cranial nerve deficits, weakness or ataxia or sensory deficits).

Diagnosis

The diagnosis in this girl is postural hypotension. This diagnosis is made from the clear history and measurement of blood pressure, demonstrating significant postural changes in systolic blood pressure (lying 90/80 mmHg and standing 75/65 mmHg). No confirmatory tests were felt necessary.

Management

The management will be reassurance in the main. Usual advice is to counsel against sudden postural changes, i.e. care when getting up from lying or sitting down. Those with low or borderline blood pressure may benefit from adding salt to their diet. Making sure fluid intake is adequate will help. The symptoms of dizziness in postural hypertension in children of this age usually improve by the time they finish puberty. Anaemia can be corrected with dietary advice and iron supplements. Consider an ENT referral in severe cases or in those with hearing impairment or signs of labyrinthitis. If there are focal neurological signs or changes on the MRI of the brain, an urgent referral to a neurologist should be made.

Follow up

It is not necessary to offer routine follow up for postural hypertension.

Discussion

The family's differential

Some families may be concerned that this is a form of epilepsy. Epilepsy is often unprovoked rather than having a clear trigger and there should be additional clinical features in history. In clinical practice, dizziness or 'feeling dizzy' is a common complaint by children. This may present on its own or as part of other symptoms. For some children this may be a non-specific symptom with no underlying organic cause. When associated with other symptoms or with physical signs, this should be taken seriously. Detailed history and full clinical examination is mandatory and it will often provide the answer. Investigations should be targeted for an aetiology inferred from the history. Reassurance is usually all that is required after elimination of possible treatable causes. For most children they will grow out of the dizziness symptom with conservative management only.

Further reading

Taylor J, Goodkin HP. Dizziness and vertigo in the adolescent. Otolaryngol Clin N Am 2011; 44:309–321.
Eviatar L. Management of dizziness in children. In: Bernard LM, Ed. Current Management in Child Neurology, 3rd ed. Hamilton: BC Decker; 2005:370–376.

Patient information

www.healthychildren.org

Case 25

Down's syndrome follow up

Dear Paediatrician,

Thank you for seeing this 8-month-old child with Down's syndrome who has recently registered with us. His family have recently arrived from Poland and he does not appear to have had any regular medical assessments carried out to date.

His mother reports he was born at term and did not have any major neonatal problems. She is unaware of any blood tests that had been conducted on him.

On examining him, he shows some dysmorphic features suggestive of Down's syndrome. He is thriving well with the weight on the 25th centile but is developmentally delayed.

Both parents are in their thirties and healthy. The family is planning to stay in this country.

Please see him for further assessments and follow up.

Dr Jill Fenton

Case analysis

The parents and general practitioner (GP) are unaware of any previous investigation or screening carried out in Poland.

The child is developmentally delayed but the letter does not give more information of the level of delay.

One needs to assume that this child did not have the routine screening for Down's syndrome.

The GP is clinically confident that this child has Down's syndrome.

Consideration must be given regarding confirming the diagnosis, early screening test and planning future follow up.

Differential diagnosis

Down's syndrome (also known as trisomy 21) has distinct features including: brachycephaly, small palpebral fissure, antislant eyes, epicanthic folds, brushfield spots, low set ears, small chin, small oral cavity, protruding large tongue, single palmar creases, short fingers, wide gap between the big and second toes, joint laxity and hypotonia.

Mosaic trisomy 21 may have subtle dysmorphic features and is not common. This should be considered in children with mild developmental delay.

Other rare dysmorphic syndromes can present with some of the above features. Some can be diagnosed by chromosomal analysis and others by the geneticist.

Consultation essentials

History

Look for any complications of the syndrome:

Respiratory	Disturbed sleep, snoring, upper airway resistance syndrome/sleep apnoea
Haematology	Abnormal bleeding (indicator of underlying blood disorders)
Gastroenterology	History of altered bowel habit. Constipation is common due to sluggish peristalsis but Hirschsprung's disease must be considered in severe cases. Diarrhoea and abdominal distension may be due to coeliac disease
Cardiovascular	Symptoms such as breathlessness on feeding, cyanosis
Development	Child's ability to look and follow, hearing, motor development such as head control, rolling over, pull to sit, sit alone, bearing weight on both feet

Examination

General	Features of Down's syndrome; check length and weight and plot on the Down's syndrome chart
Respiratory/ENT	Upper airways for evidence of obstruction such as stridor, mouth breathing, and nasal flaring; ears for evidence of glue ear and discharge
Cardiovascular	Cyanosis, heart sounds and murmurs
Abdominal	Enlargement of liver, spleen and abdominal distension or lumps
Musculoskeletal	Hip and spine examination for dislocation
Neurological	Exclude spinal cord compression due to atlantoaxial instability (pay particular attention to reflex and ankle clonus)
Developmental	Assessment to include visual behaviour, presence of cataract, squint or nystagmus

Tests/investigations

Full blood count and blood film look for any abnormal blood cells to exclude any leukaemia, platelet reduction, and transient leukaemia (myelopoitic abnormality) which is usually present in the newborn period and resolves over a few months.

Thyroid function test – in UK this is routinely done at birth using Guthrie blood spot.

Chromosomal analysis to confirm the diagnosis of Down's syndrome.

Other investigations as directed by examination findings.

Referrals to other specialists

- **Cardiology:** Referral for echocardiogram. Even if clinical findings are normal (i.e. no murmur), every child with Down's syndrome must have an echocardiogram within 6 weeks of birth. Further cardiology follow up will depend on the findings.
- **Audiology:** UK born children are routinely screened as neonates for hearing loss. Children with Down's syndrome are 50% more likely to have hearing impairment than the normal population. This can be conductive, sensorineural or mixed hearing loss.

- **Ophthalmology:** Cataracts are common in children with Down's syndrome. Despite the general population screening programmes of neonatal and 6–8 week checks, cataracts may still be missed. It is essential that the eyes are examined by appropriately trained staff. Nystagmus and refractive errors are also common.
  Developmental delay is common in children with Down's syndrome. Their cognitive ability on average is 50 compared to normal of 100.
- **Physiotherapy:** Most children with Down's syndrome have motor delay. Early referral prevents parental anxiety as appropriate advice can be given on how to assist mobility.
- **Preschool advisory teacher:** Early referral to this service is recommended given the severity of cognitive delay. This will open up opportunities to attend local educationally run play groups where additional support is available to these children and their parents.

Diagnosis

The diagnosis can be made clinically but it is important to let parents know that confirmation will be made by the analysis of blood chromosomes.

Management

Ideally both parents should be present during this consultation and urgent appointments must be given with adequate time. Discuss your clinical findings and the probable diagnosis of Down's syndrome but emphasise that confirmation will be made by blood test. Discuss the need for regular follow up. Be empathetic and answer any questions. Offer to see them again soon to answer any further questions they may have. Inform the health visitor, if not present at the clinic to support the family.

Follow up

Further regular follow up is usually every 6 months by the community paediatrician in the first 2 years but may be more frequent if there are specific health issues. Paediatric follow up will be yearly after 2 years until adult-hood. Blood tests should be done for thyroid function and coeliac screen during each visit for the first 5 years and then 2 yearly (coeliac disease is prevalent in 4–17% of children with Down's syndrome). Type I diabetes can occur in children with Down's syndrome, and is common if the child also has thyroid disease. Blood glucose should be checked if symptomatic.

Follow-up appointments will focus on growth and look for evidence of complications:

- Look for specific neurological symptoms such as deterioration in gait, falling over, pain behind the ear or neck, abnormal posture of the head, torticolis, and loss of bladder or bowel control indicating cord compression. Clinical signs of spinal cord compression will need prompt referral to a neurologist or orthopaedic surgeon
- Specific attention must be made in children without cardiac abnormality as children may develop mitral valve prolapse or aortic valve incompetence during their adolescent years. Therefore, it is essential that these children are examined regularly by a paediatrician. Later in life they should have opportunistic examination by their GP
- Growth is monitored regularly by the use of Down's syndrome growth charts

Specific follow up includes:

Audiolog

Eighteenth months review, repeat yearly until 5 years and then 2 yearly.

Vision

Initially paediatricians will follow this up until the child is 18 months (look for visual behaviour such as fixing and following, squint, nystagmus). At around 18–24 months review is by a trained orthoptist /ophthalmologist as refractory errors are very common. This should occur again at 4 years and then they should be reviewed every 2 years by an orthoptist.

Speech and language therapist

There is usually a delay in saying their first word, which usually occurs around 30 months. It is important parents are aware of this but encourage communication. Referral to speech and language therapist may be considered at 2 years if there are significant concerns.

Occupational therapy

Only if there is a significant centred around the delay in hand function.

Discussion

Down's syndrome is a significant chromosomal abnormality, with important clinical manifestations. Screening for these complications is important as outlined above. Attention should be made to the social and educational issues. Families will likely need some emotional support. Regional support groups are accessed through the Down's Syndrome association.

Further reading

Bennett KC, Haggard MP. Behaviour and cognitive outcome from middle ear disease. Arch Dis Child 1999; 80:28–35.
Irving CA, Chaudhri MP. Cardiovascular abnormalities in Down's syndrome: spectrum, management and survival over 22 years. Arch Dis Child 2012; 97:326–330.

Patient information

Down's syndrome association
    www.downs-syndrome.org.uk

Case 26

Dribbling and drooling

Dear Paediatrician,

Please can you see this 3-year-old boy who is dribbling excessively. He has to wear a bib all the time which needs changing several times a day. His mother is concerned that children will not want to play with him. He seems to have a mild tongue tie. He was born at term and has developed normally.

Dr Karen Goodyear-Smith

Case analysis

Dribbling and drooling are both used to describe the uncontrolled release of saliva from the mouth – salivary incontinence or sialorrhoea. Any difference between the two terms is immaterial, and this chapter will refer to the condition as drooling. Drooling is normal in young toddlers but usually clears up well before pre-school and nursery, becoming unusual and abnormal after the age of 4 years.

The innate reflex governing salivary continence is linked to the acquisition of speech and is highly complex, requiring an intact neuromuscular system. Drooling can be a significant issue in children with profound neuromuscular problems. The overall prevalence of persistent drooling is about 0.6%. However in children with quadriplegic cerebral palsy it may be over 50%. Salivary incontinence causes social stigma, both with other parents and other children, including embarrassment isolation, smell and physical issues such as skin irritation and perioral rash.

Differential diagnosis

Physiological

Drooling is a part of normal development. Continence of saliva is usually acquired between 15 and 18 months, but may be delayed till about 4 years of age. Saliva production increases and swallowing back of saliva may decrease during teething. Children who dribble probably do not produce excess saliva but have poor oromotor and tongue control and a poor swallowing reflex.

Some children will continue to dribble beyond the age when it should have improved because they do not keep their lips closed, there is a problem with swallowing, or they do not swallow often enough, or they are not aware or more likely, not bothered by the dribble.

Swallowing involves a complex interaction of muscles and is a subconscious act under parasympathetic control. Adults will swallow once every minute. Although autonomic, it is dependent on the ability to be able to feel the build-up of saliva, and normal control and movement of the tongue to move it to the posterior pharynx for swallowing.

Neurological abnormality

Children with profound neurological abnormalities are at high risk of drooling and in this population it is a massive issue. Bulbar or pseudobulbar palsy may be part of a generalised neurological abnormality in quadriplegic cerebral palsy in combination with learning difficulties, or in isolation. This will compound the issue. These children will likely need medication. Secretions can go to the back of the throat and be aspirated, leading to respiratory problems.

Speech and language mal-development/ oromotor co-ordination issue

While most children are able to develop their oromotor skills in line with other areas of development, this is one area which can lag behind. Drooling can occur in combination with poor swallowing, feeding issues or difficulties coping with oral food boluses or textures. These children may have poor diction, delayed speech development, and recurrent ear or throat infections.

Other contributing issues

Poor dental hygiene, lack of concern by the child about being wet and macroglossia are other issues to consider.

Consultation essentials

History

The age of the child will depend on what further assessments to make. A child over 4 years old should be considered carefully. A drooling rating scale has been described by Thomas-Stonell and Greenberg, known as their classification for drooling (**Table 26.1**). The two grades are added to create the total score.

Various tools exist for assessing the extent of drooling:

- Salivary flow rate (mL/min) is the increase in weight of dental rolls kept directly at the orifices of large salivary glands divided by time of collection. Clearly this requires a degree of cooperation and is usually impractical
- Drooling quotient is a record of 40 observations every 15 minutes. The quotient is calculated by $100 \times$ number of drooling episodes/40

Table 26.1 Thomas-Stonell and Greenberg's 1988 classification for drooling				
Drooling severity			Drooling frequency	
Score	Description		Score	Description
1	Dry		1	Never
2	Mild – wet lips		2	Occasionally
3	Moderate – wet lips and chin		3	Frequently
4	Severe – clothing damp		4	Constantly
5	Profuse – clothing, hands and objects wet			

- The teacher drooling scale is a Likert scale from 1 to 5 where 1 = no drooling, 3 = occasional drooling and 5 = constantly wet saliva leaking on clothes and furniture
- Volume measurements for absolute quantity of saliva spill or intraoral pooling, obtained using an external collection device such as an intraoral suction hook

A less scientific approach is counting the number of wet bibs/bandanas a day. On a practical level the child's parents and carers will know if the drooling is problematic and how it responds to medication. Find out why the family are concerned about the drooling and what solution they are hoping for. Sometimes all they want to know is that it will improve over time.

Ask about any ENT symptoms including recurrent upper respiratory tract infections and tonsillitis. Identify any oral sensitisation, e.g. bottle aversion, food aversion, infants not placing objects in their mouths, and any neurological symptoms suggesting an issue with the swallowing reflex.

Consider oromotor control – which is important in dealing with different textures of food, avoiding choking especially when drinking. If the symptoms improve at night this is suggestive of lack of lip closure and reduced swallowing of saliva during the day. Check oral hygiene including teeth – a dental review may be needed. Dribbling will obviously be naturally worse if the child is always bent over a toy box, or computer keypad.

Some conditions, notably gastro-oesophageal reflux can make drooling worse as can some medications.

It can be helpful to observe feeding, drinking and swallowing, and watch the child at rest and when concentrating on a task or in play.

Examination

Examine the mouth including the teeth, how the lips close, tongue movement and swallowing. Assess the child's postural control, breathing and general neurology.

Tests/investigations

Any specific tests are best organised by, or in conjunction with, a speech and language therapist and/or ENT surgeon.

Diagnosis

This child had no predisposing neurological factors. He had poor lip seal and poor diction. His oromotor capabilities were delayed for his age and he was treated by the speech and language therapist with a specific programme to train his oromotor function. This, along with a behavioural approach reminding him to keep his lips together, brought a significant improvement over a few months.

Management

There are a number of approaches to management.

Nonpharmacological/conservative

Absorbent neck bandanas are marketed and can help soak up the saliva spill. For older toddlers using wrist bands rather than bandanas can be more appealing. Encouraging a dab rather than a wipe will prevent oral soreness.

Oromotor training including devices

Exercises can be taught to improve oral muscle tone, promote lip closure and good head and body position. Oral motor training is time consuming. The child needs to be able to understand the commands and the carers need to be motivated. There is little data on effectiveness. Intraoral devices exist to compliment oral-motor therapy promoting mandibular stability, lip closure, better tongue position and swallowing. They are best used during sleep, but have many practical limitations including compliance issues with younger children.

Behavioural

There are very few behavioural studies on drooling, but behavioural techniques include:
- Instruction, prompting, and positive reinforcement (verbal and auditory cues are used to attempt to increase the frequency and efficiency of swallowing)
- Negative social reinforcement (probably best avoided)
- Self-management procedures (such as chewing gum to stimulate swallowing in older children where there is no risk of aspiration, timed beeps to give a reminder to swallow, dab or wipe)

Pharmacology

Although excess saliva production is rarely the primary cause, reducing production will reduce drooling. Anticholinergic drugs inhibit activation at muscarinic receptors and may decrease the volume of drooling. Hyoscine is probably most commonly prescribed via the transdermal route. Glycopyrrolate is probably the next popular. Botulinum injection therapy is another option. These are usually reserved for children with underlying neurological abnormalities.

Surgery

Surgery to remove obstructing tonsils or adenoidal tissue to correct chronic open-mouth posture may be corrective. Other procedures include re-routing of ligation of salivary ducts and excision of salivary glands.

Follow up

Management may involve the wider team, and for children with significant disability, the community paediatric service would usually be the best place for follow up.

Discussion

The vast majority of children presenting to the general paediatric clinic with drooling are developmentally normal and reassurance and behavioural techniques are all that is required. Recognition of the problem, explanation of the natural history and a sympathetic ear are the mainstays of management in this situation.

Further reading

Fairhurst CBR, Cockerill H. Management of drooling in children. Arch Dis Child Educ Pract Ed 2011; 96:25–30.
Parr JR, Buswell CA, Banerjee K, et. al. British Academy of Childhood Disability Drooling Study Development Group. Management of drooling in children: a survey of UK paediatricians' clinical practice. Child Care Health Dev 2012; 38(2):287–291.

Patient information

The Royal Children's Hospital Melbourne
www.rch.org.au

Case 27

Dysmorphism

Dear Paediatrician,

Thank you for seeing this newborn girl. Mum had a normal pregnancy and delivery. However, at the newborn check, her daughter was noted to have a few unusual physical features, including unusually shaped ears, a small head size, fifth fingers are incurving and her eyes appear small.

Dr David Day

Case analysis

The unusual facial feature raises the possibility of a diagnosis of a genetic syndrome. Genetic testing is rapidly advancing, however basic principles still apply, namely a thorough clinical assessment in conjunction with the right test at the right time. The most likely diagnosis here is a chromosome abnormality, so chromosome tests (see below) should be sent. The possibility of a structural eye abnormality (microphthalmia) should prompt referral for an ophthalmology review.

Differential diagnosis

This child is likely to have a genetic syndrome. Sometimes a child has a recognisable facial appearance enabling a targeted diagnostic approach. For the majority, a systematic diagnostic approach is required. The number of described syndromic entities is enormous, and careful assessment of various organ systems as well as the facial appearance may be important.

Consultation essentials

History/examination

Ask about antenatal problems, including the 20-week anomaly scan. Were any invasive tests performed?

Is there a family history of children with congenital problems, a previous pregnancy with complications, or a history of multiple miscarriages? Has the child or another family member been seen by a genetics specialist previously (check for other family names)? Ask about parental consanguinity and ethnicity:

- Measure growth parameters including head circumference
- Are there multiple anomalies or a facial appearance suggestive of a specific diagnosis?

Perform a developmental assessment. Is there global or specific developmental profile (e.g. 'cocktail party' personality often seen in Williams' syndrome. This is a chatty, outgrowing persona typified in this condition).

- Are there any behavioural problems? Are they unusual? (e.g. sleep disturbance and self-harming behaviours in Smith–Magenis syndrome)
- Are there any congenital structural abnormalities which may be associated with a particular syndrome (e.g. pulmonary stenosis and Noonan syndrome)?
- Are there CNS features suggestive of a neurometabolic diagnosis (e.g. developmental regression, epilepsy). If so, discuss with your regional neurology or metabolic unit.

Tests/investigations

This child needs genetic analysis. As with all tests there is a balance between speed, information gathered and cost. Not all conditions will need chromosomal analysis and consider whether there may be a simpler investigation that will make the diagnosis (e.g. X-rays for suspected skeletal dysplasia).

Array comparative genomic hybridisation

The first line chromosome testing at most UK centres now is array comparative genomic hybridisation. This is a detailed chromosome test, using EDTA blood test, able to detect most aneuploidy, small, medium or large chromosome deletions or duplications as well as mosaicism for some chromosome abnormalities. It is also able to detect some small deletions within a single gene, but not single nucleotide mutations.

Chromosome variants detected may be of unknown clinical significance, and in that case parental samples may then be requested. A child with a seeming genetic abnormality may share the same chromosomal changes with relatives who are 'normal' in which case the chromosome changes may be coincidental. Some chromosome variants have extremely variable effects in different family members (variable penetrance).

Rapid aneuploidy

A rapid aneuploidy test is a florescent in-situ hybridisation (FISH) test available for chromosomes 13,18, 21, X and Y, this can give results rapidly (within hours) and is useful in a neonatal situation, e.g. making a diagnosis of Down's syndrome, Edward's syndrome, Patau syndrome, or sex chromosome aneuploidy as quickly as possible. The test is only able to identify aneuploidy for these chromosomes.

Karyotype

This remains useful in confirming the structural basis of chromosome abnormality, e.g. the mechanism of aneuploidy (i.e. Down's syndrome caused by a Robertsonian translocation or simple trisomy), and identifying balanced chromosome translocations and abnormalities of the X-chromosome (e.g. Turner syndrome).

Single gene tests

Other syndromic entities may be caused by mutations in single genes and/or imprinting disorders. If a particular syndrome is suspected, consider sending EDTA blood for testing, or discuss with your regional genetics service. Information about which specific gene tests available in the UK can be found online at (www.ukgtn.nhs.uk/gtn/Home). Current UK reporting time for a single gene test is 8 weeks. Many syndromes have more than one known genetic cause, so a negative test does not necessarily rule out the diagnosis.

Genetic test results are carefully worded and often have useful suggestions for on-going referral and cascade screening.

Diagnosis

This girl has significantly unusual facial features to warrant further investigation. Her karyotype showed an unbalanced chromosome translocation with a duplication/trisomy of a segment of chromosome 9p and a deletion of a segment of chromosome 1q. The imbalance was large and cytogenetically visible, i.e. could be seen under the microscope after staining.

Management

A specific genetic diagnosis may facilitate management, prognosis, counselling for a future pregnancy and anticipation of complications. Accuracy and compassionate communication are vital, a syndrome diagnosis is rarely good news, but many families benefit from receiving a named diagnosis.

Does the child need a review in the clinical genetics clinic? Children with a significant chromosome imbalance may need further investigations for structural abnormalities (consider echocardiogram, ophthalmological review and renal ultrasound scan). A chromosome imbalance may contain a gene associated with a specific abnormality or syndrome: seek appropriate advice.

Genetic test results may have implications for the child, parents and siblings. They may reveal paternity, predict future health problems, may have financial implications and affect career choice. For the family receiving a genetic diagnosis it is a life-long process, not a one-off event. A cautious and thorough approach is necessary. For detailed management advice: Dyscerne (www.dyscerne.org/dysc/Guidelines), Genereviews (www.ncbi.nlm.nih.gov/sites/GeneTests/review).

Follow up

There may be a national specialist clinic for children with a rare diagnosis – contact the regional genetics service for advice. Refer the family for a genetics assessment and counselling; discuss why this is recommended with the family. Families need support and in the event of no apparent diagnosis a support group exists called SWAN (syndrome without a name), at www.undiagnosed.org.uk.

Discussion

Responses to a genetic diagnosis may vary considerably; ethnicity, education and cultural background are important considerations. A large proportion (60% or more) of children with a syndromic diagnosis currently remain undiagnosed because of the complexity of human development. Teratogens (e.g. fetal alcohol exposure) or antenatal infection also need to be considered.

Advances in DNA technology have revealed multiple novel genes for various syndromes, but have also shown the complexity and variability of all our genomes. Whole exome testing (all coding genes in genome) is likely to be introduced to clinical practice over the next few years. This may help to increase the rate of diagnosis.

Further reading

Reardon W. The Bedside Dysmorphologist. Oxford: Oxford University Press, 2007.
Cassidy S, Allanson J. Management of Genetic Syndromes, 3rd edn. Wiley; 2010.

Patient information

www.rarechromo.org.
www.cafamily.org.uk.

Eczema

Dear Paediatrician,

I would be grateful if you would see this 5-month-old boy who has had severe eczema since 3 months of age. It is not settling with 1% hydrocortisone and emollients. He is itchy with sleep disturbance and his parents are very worried about allergies.

Yours sincerely,

Dr Nigel FitzGerald

Case analysis

This is likely to be atopic eczema. The child is itchy and has had visible dermatitis from the age of 3 months. Many parents are convinced that allergy is the cause of their child's eczema but it is important to find out if there is any history of food reactions. Parents are often worried about using topical corticosteroids and may be using none, or inadequate amounts, of prescribed treatment.

Differential diagnosis

Atopic eczema

This usually starts at 3 months with dry skin and poorly defined itchy erythema on face, scalp, which spreads to extensor surfaces and trunk. It usually follows an episodic pattern with flares and remissions. At 2–3 years of age the pattern changes to affect flexural areas of the front of the elbows, the back of knees, around neck and in front of ankles (**Figure 28.1**). Lichenification, thickening of the skin due to chronic scratching, typically occurs in the antecubital and popliteal fossae. In severe cases it may be generalised with lymphadenopathy.

Seborrheic eczema of infancy

An erythematous, shiny well demarcated eruption in the nappy area and flexures along with scaling in the scalp (cradle cap), presents in first 3 months of life. Child is usually non-itchy and happy. This has a good prognosis and usually clears by 12 months of age. It may be treated with emollients only. Mild topical steroids either alone or combined with antifungals (e.g. Daktacort) may be helpful.

Scabies

Children may present with an eczematous rash on the entire body. Burrows and pustules on the palms, soles, genitalia and between the fingers in the web space will help establish

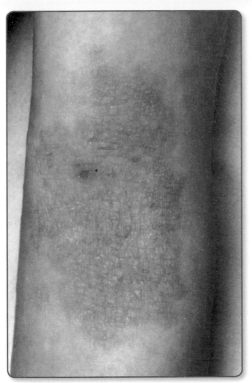

Figure 28.1 Licenification of flexural eczema at the elbow.

diagnosis. Other family members may be affected by an itch rash of the forearms, lower legs or ankles, and may have the classic burrows of the web spaces.

Immunodeficiency disorders

Infants may present with severe eczematous rash with failure to thrive, recurrent infections and petichae, e.g. hyper IgE syndrome, Wiskott–Aldrich syndrome.

Consultation essentials

History/examination

Enquire about family history of atopy, triggering and relieving factors, diet and infant feeding including any food reactions and avoidance diets already tried, the impact on the child's and the family's quality of life including everyday activities and sleep, current and past treatments, quantities used and their effects including any alternative therapies. Consider food allergy if a child has an immediate reaction to food (lip swelling, facial redness, itching, vomiting, anaphylaxis), late reaction (worsening of eczema within 24–48 hours of food ingestion) and in infants and young children with moderate or severe uncontrolled eczema, particularly with reflux, colic, diarrhoea or failure to thrive.

Examine extent and distribution of involved skin. Look for evidence of secondary bacterial infection usually by *Staphylococcus aureus* with yellowish crusting, weeping,

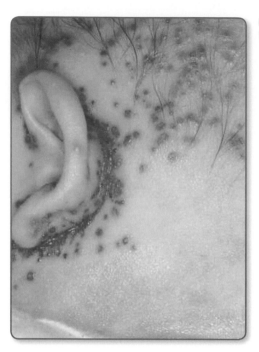

Figure 28.2 Multiple 'punched out' erosions of eczema herpeticum.

pustules and folliculitis. Eczema herpeticum due to herpes simplex virus usually presents with widespread umbilicated vesicles which often become eroded and pustular (**Figure 28.2**). Record growth parameters to check for failure to thrive.

Tests/investigations

Usually no investigations are required. Take skin swab for bacteriology/virology if infection clinically suspected. The majority of children with mild atopic eczema do not require allergy testing. Specific IgE antibodies, skin prick tests and open food challenges may be helpful in suspected food allergy but require expert advice to interpret test results.

Diagnosis

The diagnosis in this case is atopic eczema.

Management

Education and practical demonstration of topical treatment by a health care professional such as specialist paediatric dermatology nurse will have the greatest impact. It is important to explain that the eczema will wax and wane. They should follow the stepped care pathway where treatment is tailored to severity. Information should be provided in verbal and written forms covering how much treatment to use, the frequency of application, when and how to step it up or down and, how to treat infected atopic eczema.

Emollients

These should be used liberally and frequently – at least twice daily – and be continued even when the eczema is clear. Sufficient quantities should be prescribed, aiming to use 250–500 g weekly. The choice depends on the severity of the eczema and patient's and parent's preference. Greasy emollients such as emulsifying ointment and 50:50 mix of liquid and white soft paraffin are best for very dry skin and for application at night time before sleep. Less greasy, water based creams include Cetraban and Doublebase creams. Encourage parents to bathe children daily with an emollient soap substitute such as emulsifying ointment or Dermol 500 lotion which allows debris and skin scales to be removed.

Topical corticosteroids

Steroids should be used once or twice a day to red inflamed eczema and for 2 days after the skin has cleared to reduce flares. Ointments are more effective preparations than creams as they are greasier. Creams often contain preservatives which can irritate or cause contact allergy. A reluctance of parents to administer steroids results in under-treatment in many children. Explain to parents that thinning of the skin is rare with sensible use, and that the benefits outweigh the risks if used correctly. Explore what the parents' concerns are. Topical corticosteroids (TCSs) are divided into four groups:

Mild
>   Hydrortisone 1%, synalar 1:10

Moderate
>   Eumovate, Betnovate-RD, synalar 1:4
>   With antimicrobials: Trimovate (oxytetracycline, nystatin)

Potent
>   Betamethasone 0.1%, Betnovate, elocon, synalar
>   With antimicrobials: Betnovate-C (clioquinol)

Very potent
>   Dermovate

The potency of TCS is tailored to the severity of the eczema and may vary according the body site. Certain body sites such as the face, neck, axillae and groins are more prone to skin thinning, particularly with potent TCS.

General advice is:
- Use mild TCS for mild areas and face and neck
- Use moderate TCS for moderate atopic eczema short term (3–5 days) on the face and neck
- Use potent TCS for severe eczema (excluding face) for up to 2 weeks only
- Do not use very topical TCS in children
- Reduce frequency and/or potency as the inflammation settles

The finger-tip unit (FTU) can be used as a guide for appropriate steroid quantities. 1 FTU = the quantity of steroid squeezed from a standard tube in a line from the distal crease to the tip of the index finger. One FTU should be used to treat an area of skin equivalent to twice the flat area of the same adult hand with the fingers together.

Antihistamines

Sedating antihistamine such as hydroxyzine can be used in acute flares where there is significant sleep disturbance.

Treatment of infections

Bacterial

Bacterial infection is common, usually *Staphylococcus aureus*, or occasionally *Streptococcus pyogenes*. The treatment for localised areas is to use a topical steroid-antimicrobial combination for 7–14 days (e.g. Benovate-C ointment). If the infection is severe or generalised, use an oral antibiotic such as flucloxacillin or erythromycin.

Herpes

Eczema herpeticum is herpes in infection of eczema (**Figure 28.2**). The treatment is systemic acyclovir. Ask for ophthalmological advice if the infection is around the eyes because involvement of the surface of the eye may result in corneal scarring.

Diet

The National Institute for Health and Care Excellence guidelines recommend that in children under the age of 6 months with uncontrolled moderate or severe atopic eczema, a trial of an extensively hydrolysed protein formula or amino acid formula (e.g. Nutramigen Aptamil Pepti, Nutramigen AA or Neocate) should be offered in place of cow's milk formula for bottle-fed infants.

Second line treatments

If the above does not control the eczema, topical calcineurin inhibitors are indicated. There are two preparations currently available: Pimecrolimus (Elidel) 1% cream and Tacrolimus (Protopic) 0.03% and 0.1% ointment. Both are recommended for moderate or severe eczema where there is a serious risk of adverse effects from TCS, and can be used on the face in those requiring long-term TCS treatment. They are licensed from 2 years of age and above (0.1% tacrolimus is licensed from 12 years). They should be used like TCS, being applied once or twice daily. The application can be reduced with improvement.

Bandages or stockinette garments (wraps)

Using wraps can protect the skin from scratching and will aid healing. It can also help the penetration of topical treatments. There are a wide variety of products available, e.g. Tubifast and Comifast, as well as medicated bandages such as Ichthopaste. They can be worn on top of emollients and topical corticosteroids for short-term treatment of flares and for chronic lichenified eczema.

Follow up

This depends on severity and support required by the family. Many children with mild/moderate eczema can be discharged following education, demonstration of topical treatments and written management plan of stepping up and down of topical treatments depending on severity. Children with more severe eczema and associated food allergies will require longer term follow up.

Discussion

Atopic eczema can cause much distress to the whole family, particularly with the associated sleep disturbance. It is important to allow adequate time for explanation and discussion, preferably with a trained nurse. The aim is to clear the eczema quickly and then adopt an effective maintenance regime, depending on severity, to treat the eczema. Parents can be reassured that most cases of eczema will clear, 50% by age of 5 years and 60% by age of 10 years.

Further reading

National Institute for Health and Care Excellence Clinical Guideline No. 57. Management of childhood atopic eczema. www.nice.org.uk/CG057
Harper J, Giehl K, Bingham A. Guidelines to Management of Atopic Dermatitis. In : Irvine A, Hoeger P, Yan A, Eds. Harper's Textbook of Paediatric Dermatology 3rd edn. Oxford: Blackwell Publishing Ltd, 2011: 30.1–30.14.

Patient information

The National Eczema Society
    www.eczema.org
The Nottingham Support Group
    www.nottinghameczema.org.uk
The British Association of Dermatologists
    www.bad.org.uk

Epistaxis

Dear Paediatrician,

Thank you for seeing this 6-year-old boy who is suffering from nosebleeds.

He has been having them recurrently over the winter usually when he has a cold, but recently the frequency has increased to several times a week.

His mother tells me that he doesn't pick his nose and that his sister used to suffer with the same thing.

Dr Christopher Fouin

Case analysis

This is a typical case of a young child suffering from nosebleeds. At this age, they may be habitually nose-picking, often associated with nasal vestibulitis, or be getting frequent upper respiratory tract infections (URTIs), which are both common causes. However, less commonly there are other causes, e.g. foreign body, neoplasms, coagulation disorders and hereditary conditions.

Children tend to bleed from the anterior nasal cavity. Usually, the bleeding comes from the caudal part of the anterior nasal septum. This region is known as Little's area and is the confluence of several feeding arteries. As this region is relatively exposed both to environmental effects and to direct trauma, it has an increased susceptibility to mucosal damage and bleeding. There is also often a leash of vessels that is easily visible under a thin mucosal layer in this region which contributes to the likelihood of bleeding from the area.

Nasal mucosa has a mucociliary clearance mechanism that causes mucous to be wafted backwards to be swallowed. Inflammation and trauma may cause this system to stop working and increased amounts of secretions may dry and crust in the nose. This sets off a vicious cycle of nose-picking trauma and recurrent crusting, punctuated by traumatic bleeding. Recurrent bleeds over periods of days usually represent a single bleed that does not get the chance to heal before being set off again.

Differential diagnosis

Idiopathic

There is often no clear cause identified for nosebleeds in children. However, the likelihood is that it is in some way related to trauma or inflammation.

Trauma

Nose-picking trauma to the nose is very common. Parents are sometimes unaware of the habit and can often be understandably reticent to admit that their child has it, so a delicate approach is recommended. Other kinds of trauma, for instance falling onto the nose or inadvertent knocks are also common causes of usually self-limiting nosebleeds. Environmental trauma can also be a predisposing factor, from drying due to air-conditioning or central heating, or from high altitude.

Inflammation

Upper respiratory tract infections, allergies and non-allergic aetiologies cause rhinitis with associated increased nasal congestion, rhinorrhoea, crusting and mucosal fragility. Blowing the nose and attempts to relieve nasal irritation then lead to bleeding and nasal vestibulitis which may be associated with infection, e.g. by *Staphylococcus aureus*. Chronic rhinitis and sinusitis are also predisposing conditions.

Foreign body

In the younger child infection or trauma in relation to a foreign body is another, not uncommon, cause of unilateral nosebleeds. Bleeding is usually light and associated with an offensive ipsilateral rhinorrhoea.

Systemic causes

Coagulation or bleeding problems (e.g. haemophilia, leukaemia, platelet disorders, liver failure), hypertension, persistent cough.

Neoplasm

Tumours as a cause of nosebleeds in children are very rare. Of particular note, juvenile nasopharyngeal angiofibroma should be considered in male adolescents with nasal obstruction.

Congenital causes

Hereditary haemorrhagic telangiectasia or Osler–Weber–Rendu syndrome is an autosomal dominant defect in the contractile elements in the walls of precapillary arterioles that results primarily in mucosal and cutaneous telangiectasias in the respiratory and gastrointestinal systems. Patients may be recognised by telangiectasias on the lips, tongue and face. The condition may be complicated by haemoptysis, haematemesis and intracranial bleeding. The condition is managed by fibrin glue application, laser coagulation, oestrogen treatment and grafting of the affected area in the anterior nose.

Consultation essentials

History/examination

Anterior bleeding is often unilateral and with simple measures stops quickly. Posterior bleeding is more likely to be bilateral. Pain and obstruction may indicate uncommon pathologies. Length of history and frequency of bleeds may rarely indicate that a significant quantity of blood may have been lost since the nosebleeds began. A history of easy bruising or prolonged bleeding, or a family history of either should be asked about. Examination may reveal a recent bleeding point, obvious vessels in Little's area, evidence of trauma and vestibulitis or rarely, a nasal mass. Examination of the nose soon after a bleed is unlikely to reveal any useful information.

Tests/investigations

Blood tests

In an uncomplicated case these are rarely necessary. Where clinically indicated, full blood count and clotting studies may be helpful.

Diagnosis

The diagnosis is anterior nasal vestibulitis that has become established following on from an episode of URTI.

Management

The family were reassured that the nosebleeds were not due to anything worrying and that they would settle with the twice daily application of an antiseptic nasal ointment for a week and if the nose were otherwise allowed to settle without interference.

Sometimes reassurance and advice will suffice but if there are any worrying or unusual features in the history or examination, or if the nosebleeds do not settle, a referral to ENT is appropriate. The child may then need endoscopic examination, cautery or packing of the nose or go on to have further blood tests or imaging.

Follow up

This is not strictly required. If there is significant anxiety, an appointment a little while after the end of any therapy may be reasonable, e.g. in 4 weeks' time.

Discussion

Nosebleeds can be dramatic and frightening but in children are rarely causes for serious concern. Simple measures such as sitting calmly, local pressure on both alae for a few minutes and application of a cold compress almost always resolve bleeding. Afterwards, the patient ought to be discouraged from physical interference with the nose both in the immediate aftermath and the longer term.

Further reading

Brown NJ, Berkowitz RG. Epistaxis in healthy children requiring hospital admission. Int J Pediatr Otorhinolaryngol 2004; 68:1181.

Bernius M, Perlin D. Pediatric ear, nose, and throat emergencies. Pediatr Clin North Am 2006; 53:195.

McGarry G. Nosebleeds in children. Clin Evid 2005; 14:399–402.

Pope LER, Hobbs CGL. Epistaxis: an update on current management. Postgrad Med J 2005; 81:309–314.

Patient information

NHS Choices
   www.nhs.uk

Case 30

Excessive blinking

Dear Paediatrician,

Thank you for seeing this 7-year-old boy who has excessive blinking episodes at school and at home.

He has been assessed by an optician who suggested that his long eyelashes were collecting dust and causing irritation and contributing to the blinking.

Dr Sandeep Kumar

Case analysis

Causes of increased frequency of blinking can be categorised into several groups, including eye blinking tics; blepharospasm (uncontrollable muscle spasm/contraction causing the eye to close) and excessive blinking due to habit, ocular surface disorders such as blepharitis (inflammatory condition of the rims of the eyelids) or dry eyes. In the main the condition is benign; however there are reports of more serious diagnoses. In young children up to 4 weeks, of age, the normal blink rate in is 1–4 per minute, increasing to 10–12 per minute in older children and adolescents. Blinking will increase during conversation and will reduce when reading.

Differential diagnosis

It is debatable whether the first three are the same or different diagnoses.

Habit/tic

This is the most common and is benign. There is rapid, exaggerated contraction of the orbicularis oculi muscles. Generally tics are difficult to control although some control may be possible. They can become more marked in certain situations such as anxiety, or focussing on them. There is not usually any visual impairment. Habit tic can affect children from 2–13 years and can last from 1–52 weeks (median 9 weeks in one study). However, the exclusion of some of the other important eye-related conditions is necessary.

Psychogenic

The possibility of psychogenic blepharospasm can be considered if there are no other diagnoses apparent after neurological assessment and ophthalmology review. There is usually an anxiety trigger which may become apparent during the discussion in clinic. One study suggested the mean age in the 10 patients with psychogenic blepharospasm was 7.3 years (2.5–11 years). In each case, there was a stress or specific situation which was identified as contributing (e.g. potty training, or attending a new school).

Blepharospasm

This is a condition characterised by repeated and forceful involuntary sustained closure of the eyelid with contractions of orbicularis oculi. The 'benign essential' form is of unknown aetiology and is more common in adults. Dry eyes can also cause blepharospasm, usually in the context of an arid environment (central heating/ceiling fan).

Uncorrected refractive error

The need to refract the incoming light to compensate for a refractive error, either long or short sighted, might contribute to a habitual symptom which becomes more frequent in an attempt to see better. Other eye conditions such as strabismus might be apparent.

Ocular surface abnormalities

Blepharitis is rare in children. It causes burning, soreness or stinging in the eyes, which leads to blinking. There may be crusty eyelashes and itchy eyelids. It can be caused by a bacterial infection, or complication of a skin condition such as seborrhoeic dermatitis. Another ocular surface problem is dry eye when the layer of tears is not sufficient to coat the surface which is not common in young people.

Allergies

An allergic conjunctivitis can occur with seasonal or perennial rhinitis which may cause blinking.

Epilepsy

Blinking can occur in seizure disorders, both partial and generalised and absence seizures. In particular can present with blinking, but this is likely to be sporadic rather than continuous.

Consultation essentials

History/examination

Identify if the blinking is continuous or sporadic and whether it is situational, depending on where the child is and what they are doing. Most children can discuss tics in the form of compulsions, whereby they feel tense prior to the tic, which itself brings some calm.

Many patients will already have had eye tests. Ensure that visual acuity is normal, and there are no obvious visual field defects. A full visual/eye assessment is important, including looking at the globe, lids and fundi.

Tests/investigations

No specific tests are indicated. Fluorescein examination of the cornea is necessary if the history is relatively recent, to exclude a corneal abrasion or foreign body on the surface of the cornea.

Diagnosis

Diagnosis in this case is a benign tic.

Management

Tics need no specific treatment and if all ophthalmological assessments are normal reassurance would be all that is required.

Follow up

No specific need for routine follow up.

Discussion

A summary of two prospective studies on referred patients can be found in **Table 30.1**. These confirm that the majority are due to habitual tics or anterior segment/eyelid abnormalities.

Table 30.1 Summary of excessive blinking in childhood studies			
Study	**N**	**Ages**	**Causes**
Aghadoost and Talebian, 2004	60	2–16 years 39 (65%) were male and 21 (35%) female	Habitual tic in 25 (41.7%) Uncorrected refractive error in 20 (33.3%) Ocular surface abnormalities such as blepharitis in 6(10%) Psychogenic in 6(10%) Central nervous system diseases in 3(5%)
Coats, Paysse, Kim, 2001	99	Twice as many boys as girls presenting. The most common causes were anterior segment and/or lid	Anterior segment and/or lid abnormalities (37%) Habit tics (23%) Uncorrected refractive errors (14%) Intermittent exotropia (11%) Psychogenic blepharospasm (10%) Other details: • Bilateral in 89% of children presenting • A history of neurologic disease was present in 22% of the patients but was not causally related to the excessive blinking in most cases • Vision-threatening disease was noted in 6% and was easily detected on standard clinical examination (one with trichiasis, three with foreign bodies on the ocular surface, one with chronic keratitis due to ocular rosacea and one with acute microbial keratitis) • Life-threatening disease was the cause in 4% of the children, but the presence of life-threatening disease was already known in all such patients (two children with brain tumours, one with acute disseminated encephalomyelitis, and one with an uncontrolled seizure disorder).

One study of 50 children <16 years assessed the presence of a psychiatric issue in children seen and treated by the ophthalmologist for excessive blinking, and reported that most of the children with frequent eye blinking had a transient tic disorder.

Further Reading

Aghadoost D, Talebian A. Evaluation of excessive blinking in childhood. Acta Medica Iranic 2004; 42(6):455–457.
Coats DK, Paysse EA, Kim DS. Excessive blinking in childhood: a prospective evaluation of 99 children. Ophthalmology 2001; 108(9):1556–1561.
Jung HY, Chung SJ, Hwang JM. Tic disorders in children with frequent eye blinking. J AAPOS 2004; 8(2):171–174.

Case 31

Failure to thrive

Dear Paediatrician,

Please would you see this 4-week-old baby who was born at term by normal delivery? His birth weight was 2.85 kg and today the health visitor asked me to see him as his weight was only 3.01 kg. He is fully bottle fed and seems otherwise well on examination.

Thank you for your help.

Yours sincerely,

Dr Stuart Finnikin

Case analysis

It is difficult to make any assumptions about the possible diagnosis from this referral letter; however it is clear that the baby is failing to gain weight and due to his young age should be seen as a matter of urgency.

Differential diagnosis

The possible causes of poor weight gain include malfunction in any of the organ systems of the body as well as nutritional, environmental and social factors.

'Failure to thrive' or 'weight faltering' is a description of the growth rather than a diagnosis; there is usually an underlying cause. As a marker for further assessment, a drop in weight of more than two major centile spaces downwards on the UK-WHO growth chart is often used (a centile space is the distance between two major centile lines). The trend in growth is the key and it is important to differentiate true weight faltering from those infants who are genetically small.

The causes of failure to thrive can be divided into three categories: inadequate calorie intake, inadequate calorie absorption and excessive caloric consumption. These are summarised in **Table 31.1**.

Table 31.1 Differential diagnosis of failure to thrive		
Inadequate calorie intake	**Inadequate calorie absorption**	**Excessive calorie consumption**
Breastfeeding problem	Food allergy/milk intolerance	Congenital heart disease
Improper formula preparation	Pyloric stenosis	Thyroid disease
Gastroesophageal reflux	Metabolic	Respiratory disease
Neglect		
Cleft lip or palate		

Inadequate calorie intake

Over 80% of cases of failure to thrive are due to inadequate calorie intake. Calculation of the feed volume in formula fed infants and details, and difficulties with breastfeeding may suggest this as the cause. Determining feed volume in breast fed infants is a challenge. Advising the mother to express and feed with expressed breast milk for 2–3 days will give some idea of the volume of milk available. Weighing the infant just before and straight after a feed can also be used to estimate feed volume. Breastfeeding technique should also be assessed. Likewise for formula fed infants, the type of formula and preparation should be checked as well as how it is being made up.

Usually gastroesophageal reflux is more of an inconvenience than a medical problem. However, for some infants the amount of feed vomited or regurgitated is significant enough to affect weight gain.

It is always important to consider psychosocial aspects of failure to thrive. Postnatal depression and neglect are uncommon but important causes. Maternal wellbeing, mother-baby interaction and the general condition of the infant should be determined during the history and examination. In such cases admission of the infant to hospital where adequate feed volumes are administered is often the only way to make this diagnosis.

Inadequate calorie absorption

Cow's milk protein allergy is the commonest cause of malabsorption. Often there will be a history of bloody stools, diarrhoea or constipation, eczema or an unsettled baby.

Metabolic causes are rare. The infant may be unwell at presentation with a low blood sugar or acidosis. There may be a family history of unexpected infant death.

Excessive calorie consumption

An underlying physical problem will put increased metabolic demands on the infant leading to an increased calorie requirement. The situation may be further complicated by the infant struggling to feed because of the underlying problem. Physical examination is the key and will give the clue to the diagnosis.

Consultation essentials

History

The most important part of the consultation is to obtain an accurate account of the infant's feeding. If milk feeding, ask about the type of milk used, feed frequency, volume taken with each feed, vomiting and effort to feed. If the child is weaned, ask about age of weaning, range and types of food eaten now, mealtime routine and behaviour around eating. A 3-day food diary can be helpful if this can be requested before the child is seen. Observing feeding or mealtimes either at home, nursery or in hospital would be helpful in further assessing the issue.

Antenatal, birth and neonatal history is important to help rule out any organic pathology. Maternal wellbeing is important as a difficult postnatal course or postnatal depression may affect milk production. Attention should also be paid to the social history to look for any risk factors for neglect.

Examination

A top to toe examination should be performed noting the presence of red flag signs which would suggest an underlying medical condition. These are shown in **Table 31.2.**

Plotting weight, length and head circumference on a growth chart and comparison with previous weights is essential.

Tests/investigations

There is no clear consensus on investigations. They should be reserved for secondary care. If there is concern about a medical cause with symptoms and signs of a disease, then test as appropriate. **Table 31.3** is a suggested screen in the presence of persisting or significant faltering growth.

Diagnosis

This infant was initially breast fed. Formula was introduced 1 week ago and for the last 3 days had been fully formula fed. He is described as a hungry baby and often wants more than the 90 mL per feed offered but he often vomits after a feed if he takes that amount. His intake was 180–220 mL/kg/24 hours. Between feeds he was sleepy. His parents have two

Table 31.2 Red flag signs and symptoms suggesting medical causes of failure to thrive
Cardiac findings suggesting congenital cardiac disease or heart failure
Developmental delay
Dysmorphic features
Failure to gain weight despite adequate calorie intake
Organomegaly or lymphadenopathy
Recurrent or severe respiratory, mucocutaneous or urinary infection
Recurrent vomiting, diarrhoea or dehydration

Table 31.3 Suggested investigation for faltering growth in secondary care
Blood tests
Full blood count
Ferritin
Renal function tests
Thyroid function tests
Coeliac tests
Vitamin D levels
Chromosomes in girls
Sweat test – especially if respiratory infections
Urine (mid stream)
Chest X-ray – especially if respiratory infections

other children. His mother was well and she has a supportive partner. This baby looked thin with muscle wasting. His weight had crossed two centile spaces and was clearly failing to thrive. He was not dysmorphic and the rest of the examination was otherwise normal.

The most likely cause in this case is inadequate calorie intake from breastfeeding. The baby is now hungry and feeding well but is demanding so much feed for catch-up growth he is vomiting with the excess volume.

He was seen by the dietician and put onto a high energy formula to allow adequate calories within a manageable milk volume. Once he has caught up with his weight he can return to normal formula.

Management

This depends on the cause and the first issue to address will be feeding if this is identified as the problem. Specific input in the community would be the ideal set up to support feeding. There is evidence that such interventions are effective. A rise up through the centiles (the beginning of catch-up growth would be expected within 4–8 weeks of the instigation of a feeding regimen). The dietician is best placed to advise on high energy formula milks which contain more calories per mL, and allow better growth with less volume.

Follow up

Babies with faltering growth need close monitoring. As a guide, monthly before 6 months and every 2 months between 6–12 months and every 3 months after that. The aim is get them to within 1–2 centile spaces of their previous measurement. Some children do not get back to where they were but remain growing along a lower centile. If this is appropriate for their genetic predisposition, then this could be a normal variant. A team approach is best with a combination of dietician, health visitor and medical follow up depending on the availability of services.

Discussion

Poor weight gain in infants is a cause of anxiety and stress to parents. The majority of cases are simply due to inadequate intake and once this is addressed the infant will start to gain weight. In breast fed-infants increasing calorie intake can be problematic. Mothers should be reassured that formula top up feeds may be required in the short term but this does not mean that breastfeeding will not be successful in the long term. Domperidone can be offered to the mother to help increase the milk supply.

There are many ways to feed a baby. Feeding should be a pleasurable experience for mother and baby. Ensuring the baby receives adequate nutrition to thrive is key.

Further reading

Cole SZ, Lanham JS. Failure to thrive: an update. Am Fam Physician 2011; 83(7):829–834.

Wright CM. Identification and management of failure to thrive: a community perspective. Arch Dis Child 2000; 82:5–9.

Shields B, Wacogne I, Wright CM. Weight faltering and failure to thrive in infancy and early childhood. BMJ 2012; 345:5931e.

Case 32

Foreskin problems

Dear Paediatrician,

Please see this 3-year-boy who has had two episodes of balanitis. He has a whitish discharge which has failed to respond to Canesten cream. His foreskin balloons when he passes urine. On examination, the foreskin is very tight with a pinhole meatus and I think he needs a circumcision.

Yours sincerely,

Dr Santhanam Tak

Case analysis

The crux of this consultation is to know the natural anatomical development of the foreskin. The essential anatomical point is that the inner layer of the foreskin and the outer layer of the glans are usually physically fused at birth. The two layers can be physically forced apart which is what happens during neonatal circumcisions. The two layers naturally separate in the majority of cases by round about 5 years of age; however, a small percentage will separate later with the true post-puberty congenital phimosis rate being approximately 1%. Many of the signs and symptoms relate to the degree of separation of the foreskin from the glans.

Differential diagnosis

A number of differentials should be considered:

True bacterial balanitis

This results in a grossly swollen penis when florid – the shaft can look grossly swollen and bruised. There may be systemic symptoms.

Separation of adhesions

Commonly, young children experience irritation and soreness which probably relates to separation of adhesions between the foreskin and the glans. The prepuce naturally looks a little red and is consequently diagnosed as balanitis.

Smegma

Usually there may be a whitish discharge which is mistaken for candida when actually it is just a dribble of urine trapped under the foreskin mixed with penile secretions, known as smegma. Thrush medication will be ineffective. Smegma secretions can build up under the foreskin and when large enough can give the impression of a sometimes quite large cyst. This is a physiological process aiding separation of the glans and inner prepuce. Reassurance is all that is needed.

Habit

When out of nappies, young boys 'discover' their penis and will often hold it. The holding is construed as being due to pain.

Ballooning

When the foreskin fills with urine whilst voiding, it 'balloons'. It is actually helping to separate the adhesions internally and is a normal physiological process that does not affect flow. It is not usually painful but looks disconcerting.

Congenital phimosis

It is possible to have a genuine congenital phimosis.

Lichen sclerosus

This is rare before 5 years of age and usually presents later in childhood when the foreskin is completely scarred with a pinhole meatus, consistent with the manifestation of lichen sclerosus, balanitis xerotica obliterans (BXO).

Consultation essentials

History

It is important to quantify the problem with the parents: how many general practitioner (GP) visits have there been with this problem, how many courses of antibiotics have been prescribed, how many days off school, and how long has it been an issue? Check the family history. Often the child's father or siblings have had circumcisions. Religious beliefs and attitudes may also affect the referral from the GP and the family's expectations.

Examination

Examine the child in the supine position. Firstly, look carefully at prepucial opening. It is normally a little pink as it is a soft mucosal skin. Look for scarring or the white thickened skin of lichen sclerosus. Check for smegma build up around the corona. Check that both testes are present.

Gently retract the foreskin and it should 'flower' or 'pout' if the prepucial opening is still tight; if it is loose it may open to reveal some persistent adhesions around the glans. Do not force the glans through as this will cause pain. Pull the foreskin forward off the glans and this will often demonstrate a reasonable opening – not the pinhole basis of the referral.

Diagnosis

This child has a physiological phimosis. The ballooning is not affecting the stream, and there was a reasonable meatus when assessed. Reassurance was all that was necessary with specific advice not to try and retract the foreskin as it will occur naturally as the boy gets older.

Management

There is no advantage in having a retractile foreskin aged 3 years as opposed to 7 years. Circumcision is painful whatever age it is carried out. Circumcision is not a benign operation; it involves a general anaesthetic, has a 1: 200 re-operation rate for bleeding, and has a 2–3% meatal stenosis rate which can lead to long-term voiding issues.

Genuine recurrent balanitis with proven multiple infections is best treated with circumcision.

The more common irritated phimosis can usually be treated with topical steroid cream. Trimovate applied topically at bedtime is effective as it also contains antibacterial and antifungal agents which help prevent infection. The steroid reduces inflammation, helps separate adhesions and softens the skin to allow retraction.

Lichen sclerosus, if caught early, can be treated with topical steroid cream, but more advanced cases will need circumcision and possibly ongoing steroid treatment if there is meatal involvement. If the glans is involved then it is essential to have follow up to ensure complete resolution of lichen sclerosus to prevent long-term meatal stenosis.

Follow up

Physiological phimosis and smegma pearls do not need follow up, unless there is significant parental anxiety. Lichen sclerosus should have follow up if steroid cream is being used. In cases of BXO it is advisable to follow up and treat any residual lichen sclerosus on the glans.

Discussion

Parents and young boys need to understand the natural history of the foreskin. A significant proportion of children in early childhood do not have retractile foreskin (**Figure 32.1**).

Nontherapeutic circumcision

Male circumcision performed for any reason other than physical clinical need is termed non-therapeutic (or sometimes 'ritual'). Parents will have their own views on what they want for their son; people see it as a desirable health benefit. It is essential in some cultures and religions. The British Medical Association has produced guidance on the law and ethics of male circumcision. The best interests of the child should always be central and they should be able to express their wishes if they are old enough. Nontherapeutic circumcision should not be carried out if one parent disagrees.

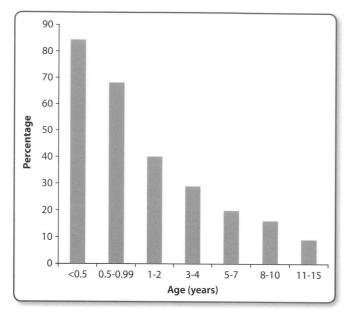

Figure 32.1 Percentage of nonretractile foreskin according to age.

Further reading

British Medical Association (BMA). The law and ethics of male circumcision, Guidance for doctors. London: BMA, 2006.

Patient information

www.caringforkids.cps.ca/handouts/circumcision
www.healthychildren.org

Gait abnormalities and limping

Dear Paediatrician,

Thank you for seeing Liam, who is 22 months old. His parents have noticed that he walks with an in-turned right foot. His running is better but he often trips and falls. He started walking at 17 months.

Dr Philip Fraser

Case analysis

The anxiety of a skeletal, developmental or neuromuscular disorder is usually unfounded in toddlers with unusual walking styles since there are common normal variants which describe the position of legs and/or feet in children. Knowing these variants and the time at which to expect improvement can help parents understand the natural process of acquiring a normal childhood gait.

Differential diagnosis

Toddler gait patterns

On acquiring the skill to walk upright without support, not unsurprisingly, the toddler uses a wide-based gait, with high steps and a flexible, flat foot. The tibias look bowed and the femurs are rotated. The vision of a toddler walking with arms outstretched in this fashion, for added stability, is classical for a toddler who has recently learned to walk. The heel strike does not appear until 15–18 months. Runing is a 2-year-old skill. As the child gets older, the step frequency reduces and the length of step increases up to adult gait by 8 years.

Normal variants

Bow legs

Bowed legs (known as genu varus) describes outward curving of the legs and is common in almost all children <18 months of age. It is part of normal development. It is due to the folded position in the uterus, so most babies and children are bow legged at birth and this persists until about age 2 or 3 years.

Knock knees

At the age of 3 or 4 years, children develop knock knees, which describes the legs turned inwards. This improves by the time the child is 6 years.

In-toeing (pigeon-toed)

A combination of the above can cause an 'in-toeing' appearance where the feet point towards each other. There is often a history of trips and falls, which is common in toddlers as their immature gait matures and becomes more confident. The position of the foot when flat on the ground will point inwards. It can be due to metatarsus adductus or metatarsus varus which is due to intrauterine position. Flexible forefoot abduction on the lateral aspect of the foot is common in newborns, but improves in the majority of children as they get older. It can persist and cause a transverse crease on the plantar aspect of the foot which may need treatment. Internal tibial torsion is characterised by the child walking with their patella facing forwards and toes pointing inwards. This is common from when the child starts to walk until 3 years of age. In contrast, in persistent femoral anteversion, in-toeing will persist and is manifest by the child walking with patellae and feet pointing inwards. This commonly occurs between 3 and 8 years of age. The cause of in-toeing can be detected easily by examining the child in the prone position with knees flexed. In either case the child can move freely with no functional abnormalities, has no pain and the appearances are symmetrical. The gait may look worse after prolonged activity or at the end of the day when the child is tired. Gait will improve as the child develops further and the appearance will improve as the skeleton matures. The tibia will 'untwist' by the age of 3–4 years and the femur by 7–8 years. Orthopaedic referral is indicated if the appearances are asymmetrical or there is progression of the appearances. Surgery will be deferred until later in childhood if indicated.

Out-toeing

This is less common than in-toeing but is more common in younger children, and can be one of the reasons a child's walking is delayed. The gait is often unstable but it will improve in time.

Flat feet (pes planus)

Flat feet describe a foot with the medial arch on the ground or close to the ground. This will put the heel in an outward (valgus) position. The infant has a flexible, mobile foot, and the toddler's foot is also fairly flexible but in adults it is less common. Flat feet are usually asymptomatic. While intervention with orthotic supports has not been shown to resolve the position, in order to improve comfort, a support is indicated. It may be familial. Flat feet usually resolve by the age of 6 years. Jack's test (or the big toe extension test) is a test to show whether the foot is flexible. When the big toe is extended, or the child stands on their tiptoes, the medial longitudinal arch appears.

Toe-walking

This is commonly seen as the mature gait pattern develops. If it is unilateral, it is usually abnormal. If the Achilles' tendon is tight, a surgical release may be required.

Abnormal gait patterns

Spastic gait

This gait is stiff with dragging of the inverted foot and is seen in conditions with upper motor neuron abnormalities such as diplegic or quadriplegic cerebral palsy, and cerebrovascular disease.

Antalgic gait

This is a unilateral gait with less time spent in weight-bearing on the affected side. There is reluctance to weight bear. There are many causes including juvenile idiopathic arthritis (JIA), trauma to the sole of the foot or osteomyelitis of the spine. Trauma may be unwitnessed.

Circumduction gait ('peg leg')
Typically seen in restricted, stiff movements in arthritis, unilateral spacitisity in cerebral palsy, especially hemiplegia. The hip is abducted outwards in an excessive way as the leg swings forward to gait.

Ataxic gait
This is an unsteady gait with wide base as the legs are widely spaced. This is seen in cerebellar abnormalities.

Trendelenberg gait
Normally, the contralateral hip rises while weight bearing on the ipsilateral side. In Trendelenburg gait, the contralateral hip falls. If bilateral, the gait is seen as 'rolling' with externally rotated hips, knees, and feet. It is caused by many conditions including developmental dysplasia of the hip, Perthes disease, slipped capital femoral epiphysis, JIA of the hip joint, muscle disease and neurological conditions.

Toe-walking (equinus)
While habitual toe-walking is a common and normal variant. It can usually be overcome by asking the child to walk with their heel flat on the ground. However, if persistent, it is abnormal and may be associated with spastic upper motor neuron neurologic disease such as cerebral palsy.

Stepping gait
An exaggerated stepping motion occurs as the foot is lifted off the ground to cause a stepping gait. It is a sign of weak ankle dorsiflecors and the excessive knee flexion compensates for this. It occurs in lower motor neuron conditions such as spina bifida and peripheral neuropathies such Charcot-Marie-Tooth disease.

'Clumsy' gait
Poor fine and gross motor skills resulting in 'clumsiness' manifest as problems with motor co-ordination. There are reports of trips and falls and difficulties with tasks such as feeding and dressing. School may report untidy handwriting. Neurological assessment should be able to determine an underlying muscle abnormality, arthritis, orthopaedic problem or neurological abnormality.

Developmental dysplasia of the hip

This is a condition which used to be known as congenital dysplasia of the hip. It affects 1–3% of newborn infants. The condition can manifest as mild acetabular dysplasia or a dislocated hip with an abnormal femoral head and acetabulum. If diagnosed early, outcome is better than if diagnosed late. Neonates are screened during their postnatal examination, but some cases are not apparent at that age. Ultrasound can confirm diagnosis in children <6 months. Late diagnosis has a worse prognosis. Dislocation if untreated causes soft tissue contractures and joint relocation will not be achievable without surgery. There are changes to the femur and acetabulum if the hip is left dislocated and surgical correction is required. To assess for developmental dysplasia of the hip (DDH), the Galeazzi test is done. With the child supine, the relative heights of the knees are observed with the hips and knees flexed at 90°. A lower knee suggests shortening of the thigh because of the dislocated hip on that side. Other signs suggestive of DDH include discrepancy in leg length, a widened perineum on the affected side, flattened buttock and asymmetrical thigh skin folds. Neither of these are a good discriminator and abnormal skin creases are seen in 25% of normal babies. In an older child limited hip abduction when the hips are fully flexed will be seen in older children with DDH. The child is likely to have developed to independent walking but will likely have a toe-walk on the affected side or a painless limp due to unequal leg lengths.

Osgood–Schlatter disease

This is an inflammatory condition of the insertion of the patellar tendon on the tibia tuberosity. It affects boys and girls during their growth spurts (8–13 for girls and 10–15 for boys). It is associated with exercise. The key to treatment is rest, despite this condition affecting more active children (boys more than girls). It usually improves by the age of 18 years.

Perthes disease (Legg–Calvé–Perthes)

This is a condition of children usually boys aged 4–8 years, affecting the blood supply to the femoral head. The exact cause is not known. Management includes analgesia, maintaining movement and preventing additional hip deformity. While surgery may be required, most children improve without needing it.

Cerebral palsy

Upper motor neuron lesions, manifesting with a movement disorder can present with limp as the child becomes independently mobile. Multiple aetiologies are possible including premature birth, meningoencephalitis in infancy, anatomical abnormalities and metabolic conditions.

Muscular dystrophy

Weakness due to a muscular dystrophy may manifest as a gait abnormality. Gower's sign (where the child 'climbs' up their legs in order to get up from sitting on the floor) in an ambulant child will be positive in proximal muscle weakness prompting further assessment. Calf hypertrophy is often seen in toddlers. There are many different types and further assessment by a neurologist is indicated if there is concern about this diagnosis.

Differential leg length

While DDH is a cause of leg length discrepancy, there are other causes such as previous fracture, osteomyelitis of the growth plate and neuromuscular problems.

Blout's disease

This is a dyschondrosis of the medial epiphysis of the proximal tibia. Leg bowing is seen from about 2 years old. The exact cause is unknown. To correct the problem, children may need bracing or surgery when they are between 3 and 4 years old.

Rickets

Rickets, caused by lack of vitamin D or calcium in the diet causes severe bowing of the legs. Classical radiographical appearances show splaying of the epiphyses. Treatment is vitamin D replacement and usually will result in resolution of the bowing over time.

Slipped upper femoral epiphysis

This is a condition where the epiphysis of the femoral head separates and slips away from the rest of the bone. It presents with limp, groin, knee or hip pain. It occurs most commonly in boys who are on a higher weight centile, at the time of puberty. Diagnosis can be made on X-ray. A surgical correction with nailing the epiphysis back into place is usually required.

Trauma

Toddlers fracture is a spiral fracture of the lower tibia in children under 5 years of age. It is commonly causes by a twisting injury and may have seemed innocuous at the time.

Consultation essentials

History/examination

Watching the child walk, usually with and without shoes can be helpful. Give them a long area, e.g. down the corridor. If they can be encouraged to run that can further help assess their gait and look for a latent hemiplegia. Assess for hypermobility. Examine the hips to look for range of movement, skin creases and symmetry of groins, buttocks and perineum. Measure leg length from bony landmarks on each side. Look at the back for scoliosis.

Gross motor development should be assessed. Walking begins with 'cruising' around furniture while holding on, or with hands being held, usually by 1 year of age. If a child is not walking by 18 months of age, referral to a paediatrician is indicated, unless the child is bottom shuffling, in which case referral could be a bit later.

Tests/investigations

If there is any suggestion of a bony abnormality, X-rays of the limbs should be performed. Any suggestion of DDH requires a hip X-ray in an older child. Ultrasound is reserved for younger children < 6 months.

Diagnosis

Liam had a slight in-turning of the right foot. It was less obvious when he ran. His leg length was equal and his hip movements were normal and symmetrical, particularly abduction. His tibias were slightly bowed.

Management

In younger children under 5 years with bow legs or knock knees, as long as the deformity is symmetrical and there is nothing in the history to suggest underlying disease (i.e. no history of illness or injury), then reassurance is all that is needed. This was the case for Liam.

Follow up

Routine review to endure resolution is not strictly necessary but may give the parents some reassurance. Usually, the parents will notice improvement in the appearance over time in line with the continuing development towards a more stable and confident gait.

Discussion

If the normal variants described above persist beyond the ages expected, or if there are changes which are progressive or asymmetric, pain or neurological disease then further assessment is warranted.

Further reading

Bannon M, Carter Y. Practical paediatric problems in primary care. Oxford: Oxford university press, 2007.
Sewell MD, Rosendahl K, Eastwood DM. Developmental dysplasia of the hip. BMJ 2009; 3 39:4454b.
Evaluation of gait disorders in children
www.bestpractice.bmj.com

Patient information

www.patient.co.uk

Generalised seizures

Dear Paediatrician,

Thomas is a 4-year-old boy who was seen in your children's emergency department last week. He had an afebrile generalised seizure that lasted for 3 minutes from which he has recovered fully. This is his second afebrile seizure in 2 months. His mother who is a nurse in ITU in the same hospital informs me that he had five febrile convulsions up until he was 3 years old. There is no family history of febrile convulsions, epilepsy or learning difficulties. Clinical examination is completely normal with no neurological findings. There is no concern about his development and he is in full time nursery.

Many thanks for seeing him,

Dr Michael Goodare

Case analysis

This young boy has been referred following two afebrile seizures with a history of febrile convulsions. This is a common scenario and his parents are almost certainly worried that he may have epilepsy.

At first it is essential to establish that the seizures are true seizures. There are many non-epileptic seizures that mimic epileptic seizures. Distinguishing between the two may be difficult and require experience. Misdiagnosis of epilepsy is common and up to 30% of patients are treated unnecessarily with antiepileptic drugs that can be associated with morbidity. Detailed history of the events from an eye witness or video footage is invaluable in the diagnosis of epilepsy.

Differential diagnosis

In simple terms, 'epilepsy' means recurrent seizures. Epileptic seizures are caused by abnormal and excessive synchronised neuronal discharges resulting in different clinical manifestations that could range from motor, sensory, autonomic or psychic symptoms with or without loss of awareness.

It is important to know some of the common epileptic conditions in children. Epilepsy is broadly classified as generalised, focal (partial) and focal (partial) with secondary generalisation. In generalised epilepsy, epileptic discharges originate from both cerebral hemispheres and are associated with loss of consciousness. Seizures may be clonic, tonic, tonic-clonic, atsatic (drops), myoclonic or absences. Focal seizures may be simple or complex, where consciousness is generally maintained at the onset but lost by secondary generalised seizures. There may be predisposing symptoms of sensory aura such as smell, taste, visual and auditory symptoms.

In this case, it is important to establish that this is definitely an afebrile seizure. Risk of developing epilepsy following simple febrile convulsion is low (1–2%), unless associated with complex seizures and neurodevelopmental abnormality when the risk rises significantly along with increasing age.

Consultation essentials

History

As with any medical consultation, a detailed history forms an important part in the management of anyone presenting with seizures. Obtain a detailed description of the events from an eye witness. Getting the necessary details may pose difficulty as they might not have seen it or may not remember the details in what was likely a stressful situation. It is important to gather information step-by-step from the beginning of the event to set the chronology of the seizure:

- Events prior to seizure: ask what the child was doing prior to the seizure. Was he unwell? Did he have fever or other illness?
- Events during seizure: what exactly happened during the seizure? Get all the details in a chronological order
- Events after seizure stopped: what did he/she do after the seizure? Did the child became confused or sleep? How did he recover? How long did it take for him to recover?
- What was the duration of seizure from beginning to end? Witnesses may sometimes exaggerate the duration and therefore this has to be clarified in seconds or minutes
- Events during seizure: details of salivation, tongue biting, incontinence, nausea, vomiting or other symptoms should be recorded

Take a clear account of the child's general development, behaviour and social interactions.

These days, capturing the events on a video camera is possible and this would be a useful tool in the diagnosis. However, there are practical difficulties and this may not be possible in all cases.

Examination

A thorough clinical examination is important in all children presenting with a seizure, although the examination is likely to be normal in the majority. Physical signs include skin lesions such as depigmented macules, café au lait patches, conjunctival telangiectasia may point to possible diagnosis such as neurocutaneous syndromes. Look for facial dysmorphic features. Examine the pupils and fundi. Do not forget to measure head circumference, weight and height and check blood pressure.

Tests/investigations

Blood tests

Children attending the emergency department with seizures have blood tests routinely, to check full blood count, kidney function, calcium and magnesium levels, liver function, C-reactive protein, blood sugar and acid base status. If the child is pyrexial a blood culture is carried out. The value of routine blood tests other than doing a blood sugar level is questionable, particularly in those presenting with simple, short seizures. Blood investigations should be selective and individualised to clinical need, rather than routinely sent.

Electrocardiogram

A standard 12-lead electrocardiogram (ECG) and rhythm strip is essential in any child with afebrile seizures. Cardiac conditions such as prolonged QT syndrome may be a cause for the seizures.

Electroencephalogram

An electroencephalogram (EEG) is not indicated following a simple febrile convulsion. However, this may be useful in children with complex febrile convulsions. General recommendation is to wait for at least 2 weeks after the seizure. There is controversy among experts on performing EEG after the first unprovoked (afebrile) seizure as by definition this is not epilepsy. It is recommended in those with suspected focal onset or prolonged seizures.

Following a second or third afebrile seizure a routine standard EEG is recommended in all children. You may consider referring these children to the paediatrician with specialist interest in epilepsy or to a paediatric neurologist. Sometimes, the EEG is requested when 'sleep-deprived'. It can uncover EEG abnormalities not seen when awake.

Brain imaging

Epilepsy is a functional disturbance of the brain. Therefore, functional imaging modalities like PET and SPECT scans are more sensitive than CT or MRI. MRI is the preferred imaging for structural abnormalities in the brain. The practical difficulty in performing an MRI is that children need to be sedated or anaesthetised to keep them still for the required time. Facilities for this may not be available locally and these children may need to be referred to the regional neurology centre.

Cerebrospinal fluid studies

Metabolic and genetic tests are not routinely done in all cases unless specifically indicated.

Diagnosis

Thomas' clinical presentation was suggestive of a generalised tonic-clonic seizure. Thomas was examined and no abnormality found. His general behaviour, development and cognitive function were appropriate for his age. Parents reported no concerns from the nursery. His standard EEG was normal as was a MRI of the brain. A sleep EEG was also unremarkable. The family were reassured about the normal investigations. They were informed of the diagnosis of epilepsy and the treatment options outlined. Antiepileptic treatment with either sodium valproate or carbamazepine was discussed. It was agreed to wait and observe him for a few months and not to start antiepileptic medication immediately.

Management

The family and the child should be fully informed and should be involved in decision making and management plans, once the child is old enough. Important issues about living a normal life, and specific restrictions as well as the use of rescue mediations in the event of a prolonged seizure.

The following is a list of issues to discuss relating to management:

- Management during a seizure – advice the family about positioning their child in the recovery position during and after a seizure and ensure they are free from any nearby danger.
- Monitor breathing and colour closely
- If the seizure continues beyond 3 minutes:
  - call for emergency help (999 or 911)
  - administer buccal midazolam
- Antiepileptic treatment needs to be discussed. The side effects and duration of treatment need to be explained.
- Information about reasonable precautions during high risk activities such as tree-climbing, swimming and cycling
- Information about sudden unexpected death in epilepsy should be given

Follow up

All children with a diagnosis of afebrile seizures should be reviewed regularly in outpatient settings to monitor their seizures, general health, development and cognitive function.

Discussion

Epilepsy is not easy to diagnose despite the availability of diagnostic investigations. Clinical symptoms and seizure events may change or evolve. If uncertain, it is advisable to wait or refer for expert advice. Misdiagnosis has devastating consequences including the stigma, effect on school, education, family and social life and the unnecessary medical interventions.

Further reading

Sadlier LG, Scheffer IE. Febrile seizures. British Medical Journal 2007; 334:307–311.

The epilepsies: the diagnosis and management of the epilepsies in adults and children in primary and secondary care. National Institute for Health and Care Excellence (NICE) Clinical guideline 137, 2012.
    www.nice.org.uk /CG 137

Wallace SJ, Farrell K. Epilepsy in children, 2nd ed. London: Arnold publishers; 2004.

Patient information

Epilepsy action
    www.epilepsy.org.uk
Epilepsy society
    www.epilepsysociety.org.uk
Young epilepsy
    www.ncype.org.uk

Case 35

Growing pains

Dear Paediatrician,

Thank you for seeing this 5-year-old girl who has been waking almost every night for the last year with severe leg pains. Her parents massage them and often give her some paracetamol. The pains seem to settle and she eventually goes back to sleep, and is fine the next morning. Generally, she is very fit and healthy and there is no significant past history. Her maternal grandmother has arthritis.

Yours,

Dr Sarah Hawkes

Case analysis

Causes of musculoskeletal pain can be divided into mechanical or inflammatory. The former respond to physical treatments, such as physiotherapy and appropriate supports, the latter require medication. Both types may cause pain and swelling which should respond to anti-inflammatory medication. The story in this referral letter is classic for 'growing pains'. The duration of the symptoms, which of themselves are short lived, makes a serious underlying cause unlikely. This should not serve to belittle the distress and upheaval which they cause to the child and family.

Differential diagnosis

Juvenile idiopathic arthritis

This is suggested by a history of inflammation, pain and swelling in one or more joint usually for some weeks. In children there is usually systemic-onset presenting with symptoms such as fever, lethargy, rashes and lymphadenopathy. The usual age of onset is under 5 years. There is often a delay in diagnosis, with children receiving plaster instead of physiotherapy. In this situation, the pain is too short lived to be juvenile idiopathic arthritis (JIA).

Osgood–Schlatter syndrome

This affects young teenage boys who play a lot of sport. The action of kicking, running, or jumping cause repeated and vigorous use of the quadriceps muscles. However, it can also occur in children who are not all that sporty. The main symptom is pain just below the patella. The severity of the pain fluctuates but is usually worse during and just after activity. The pain tends to improve with rest. The pain typically lasts a few months, but can last up to 2 years. A tender, bony bump may develop a few centimetres below the patella over the tibial tuberosity where the patella ligament attaches to the tibia. The small bump is permanent, and in time it becomes painless. Knee movements are normal. X-rays are not normally required; the diagnosis is often clear from the clinical presentation. Physiotherapy may be useful.

Hypermobility

Benign joint hypermobility syndrome is said to affect about 10% of the population. The classic description is of children who are 'double-jointed' or who have lax ligaments. The terminology in this field is rapidly changing, and children are now being given a diagnosis of Ehlers–Danlos syndrome type 3. In the majority of cases, hypermobility causes no pain or problem.

Hypermobility can cause many symptoms, which are linked to joint laxity and associated mechanical stress. Leg pains are common, and hypermobility is often associated with fallen arches. Correcting this with supportive footwear is helpful, and should be the first area that is checked. Occasionally, a podiatry referral may be required. Children with hypermobile upper limbs may have difficulty at school, due to pain on writing. Symptoms are usually worse after exercise – although they may be delayed by a few hours. Hypermobility can also cause swelling and tenderness of the joints. Sometimes distinguishing it from JIA can be difficult, especially as both may be present in the same child. Physiotherapy is the treatment of choice. Girls are usually more affected than boys. Joint hypermobility is commonly diagnosed using the Beighton's modification of the Carter and Wilkinson scoring system. This gives indication of widespread hypermobility. A high Beighton's score by itself does not mean that an individual has hypermobility syndrome, it simply means that the individual has widespread hypermobility. **Table 35.1** shows how to calculate Beighton's score. If 4 or more joints are hypermobile and there is a history of pain in the joints for 3 months or more, then benign joint hypermobility syndrome is likely.

Growing pains

This is a diagnosis of exclusion. Studies estimate prevalence as wide as 2–50%, but probably about 37% is most accurate. They occur most commonly in 4–6 years old. The pain usually appears late in the day or at night, often waking the child. It can last from minutes to hours. It can be mild or very severe. By morning the child is almost always pain free. **Table 35.2** details some criteria on which to base a clinical diagnosis. Theories abound as to the aetiology including anatomical variants, muscle fatigue, psychological effects, lower

Table 35.1 Beighton's modified criteria for hypermobility: each positive result scores one point (maximum score nine points)
• One point for each thumb that can be flexed backwards by the examiner to touch the forearm
• One point for each hand in which the little finger can be extended back beyond 90° by the examiner
• One point for each knee that can be extended backwards by the examiner
• One point for each elbow that the patient can extended backwards
• Patient can bend forwards and place the hands flat on the floor without bending at the knees (one point)

	Inclusion criteria	Exclusion criteria
Onset	Afternoon (late)/evening	Persists to next morning
Duration and nature	Intermittent, with some pain-free days/nights	Persistent, with increasing intensity
Location	Bilateral Muscles – anterior thigh, calf, posterior knee	Unilateral Joints
Physical activity	No change	Reduced
Physical examination	Normal	Swelling, erythema, tenderness; local trauma/infection; reduced range of motion (joints); limp
Investigations	Normal	Positive findings on radiography, bone scanning, erythrocyte sedimentation rate, etc.

Table 35.2 Criteria on which to base a clinical diagnosis of 'growing pains' – inclusion and exclusion criteria.

Modified from Evans 2008.

pain thresholds, altered bone strength, local overuse 'syndrome', noninflammatory pain 'syndrome' and hypermobility. In fact the contribution of hypermobility to what could be considered 'growing pains' is significant and it is certainly true that some children with growing pains are also significantly hypermobile. However, the lack of a validated tool for assessment of hypermobility in children makes specific diagnosis a challenge. In terms of treatment, despite the literature parading many different options (muscle stretching programmes, leg rubs, in-shoe wedges and foot orthoses) physiotherapy is likely to be the best and most successful treatment option.

Acute leukaemia

An acute leukaemia can present with bone (marrow) pain. This is in the context of a child who by the time of presentation has been generally unwell for a number of weeks – lethargy, tiredness, bruising and may be some cough and/or cold type of infection. Localised bone tumours can also cause pain and can be insidious in onset. If there are persisting features of the pain then an X-ray will be required to rule out a solid bone tumour. The lower limb is an unusual site for an osteosarcoma; usually seen at lower femur in older, teenage children.

Musculoskeletal pains

Young children will run around and engage in rough and tumble play. They often have no sense or limit on their activity, and do not seem to fatigue. This is evidenced by the many hours in a 'soft play' activity centre, jumping on the trampoline or from the sofa onto the floor. While no immediate injury is often apparent, such activity inevitably takes its toll. Sometimes, a seemingly innocuous fall can be the cause of a limp or pain. There is not always a good history of sustained activity or an injury although it can come out in retrospect. If a sprain is likely it will get better with rest and analgesia.

Rickets

Vitamin D deficiency can cause bone pain. Usually due to a dietary deficiency or lack of exposure to sunlight, the clinical signs would give some indication: swollen wrists, bowed tibias and rachitic rosary on the chest.

Consultation essentials

History

Ascertain if there is any history of trauma or sustained physical activity. If the symptoms are at night time only, this is more reassuring than if they are present in the daytime as well.

Examination

Look for swelling, flexion deformity, and limited movement due to pain. Look for rashes, signs of rickets. Check Beighton's criteria.

Tests/investigations

If there is doubt, a check of inflammatory markers [erythrocyte sedimentation rate (ESR)], and ANA will suggest an underlying inflammatory or rheumatoid cause. Beware the nonspecific nature of ESR and false positive ANA. Probably no tests are indicated in the majority of cases.

Diagnosis in this case

This child is a keen trampoline jumper and spends lots of time jumping on the trampoline in the garden. The days she does more jumping seem to correlate with her complaints of pain. She has a 'full house' of Beighton's criterion (nine out of nine) which suggests she is hypermobile. Input from the physiotherapist and limiting the trampolining should help.

Management

The physiotherapists will manage hypermobility by teaching core muscle group strengthening exercises and avoiding activities which will stress the joints in preference for ones which will not, such as swimming.

Follow up

No specific medical follow up is required.

Discussion

Symptoms for hypermobility can vary greatly. Younger children are more naturally hypermobile and this may be given as the reason for the pains. The theories for growing pains abound yet there is no single test and diagnosis is a clinical one.

Further reading

Evans AM. Growing pains: contemporary knowledge and recommended practice. Foot Ankle Res 2008; 1:4.

Murray KJ. Hypermobility disorders in children and adolescents. Best Pract Res Clin Rheumatol 2006; 20(2):329–3251.

Uziel Y, Hashkes PJ. Growing pains in children. Review Pediatric Rheumatology 2007; 5:5.

Viswanathan V, Khubchandani RP. Joint hypermobility and growing pains in school children. Clin Exp Rheumatol 2008; 26(5):962–966.

Patient information

The Hypermobility Syndrome Association
   www.hypermobility.org/
Arthritis Research UK
   www.arthritisresearchuk.org

Haematuria

Dear Paediatrician,

I would be grateful if you could review Jack, a 6-year-old boy, who was detected to have 3+ blood on urine dipstick testing, when he presented with a fever with unknown focus 2 months ago and was treated with antibiotics on suspicion of urinary tract infections? However, the urine culture was negative and subsequent urine dipsticks have shown 2+ and 3+ blood on two occasions, when he was well.

Please could you see him with a view to investigating the cause of his haematuria?

Many thanks,

Dr Fiona Hayes

Case analysis

Microscopic heamaturia is known to occur with fever, illness, after vigorous exercise, or urethritis in children who don't drink adequate fluids. It is important to distinguish between intermittent and persistent haematuria. The latter needs investigation, especially in the presence of proteinuria, hypertension and/or impaired renal function. Urine dipsticks are extremely sensitive, and can be positive in the absence of significant haematuria – this can only be confirmed by microscopy. Conversely red blood cells (RBCs) will lyse when there is a delay in specimens being processed and may give a false negative result.

Infection, the commonest cause of haematuria, has been excluded in this case by the negative cultures.

Differential diagnosis

Microscopic haematuria associated with fever/intercurrent illness

It is common to have some RBCs in the urine associated with fever or with an intercurrent illness, but this should clear. The current findings are somewhat unclear. In order to ascertain what is going on, it is best to collect some specimens for urgent microscopy over the next few months, especially over a period of a few weeks or months of wellness. With this information, it should be possible to confirm or exclude this diagnosis. If this diagnosis is confirmed, no further action is required and the child will not need repeat urine tests for other illnesses, unless there is a suggestion of a urinary tract infection (UTI).

Urethritis/cystitis – lower urinary tract infections

These present with dysuria and microscopic/macroscopic haematuria. If urine culture is negative and there is no significant proteinuria or hypertension, urethritis is the most likely diagnosis. This is especially common in children with poor fluid intake or an excess of acidic drinks, and this is often linked to constipation/stool withholding. However, this should resolve with appropriate measures, but often recurs.

Henoch–Schönlein purpura nephritis

This presents with a characteristic palpable purpuric rash on the extensor surfaces of the lower limbs and buttocks and may be associated with abdominal pain, joint swellings and blood/protein in the urine. The rash may be mild or florid and may precede the haematuria by up to 6 months, so it is essential to ask specifically about previous rashes. Exacerbations of the rash with any intercurrent illness up to 6 months after the initial episode are also well known and may be associated with haematuria and proteinuria suggestive of nephritis. Blood pressure, urine microscopy, urine microalbumin:creatinine ratio and serum albumin, urea, creatinine and electrolytes must be checked.

If there is significant proteinuria then blood pressure and urine microalbumin:creatine ratio should be measured weekly in the initial stage. If these are improving, monitoring can be reduced but, if worsening, urgent referral for consideration of a renal biopsy should be made.

Immunoglobulin A nephropathy

Gross haematuria associated with an intercurrent illness, which resolves quickly once the child gets better suggests immunoglobulin A (IgA) nephropathy. Usually, these patients would be seen as an emergency and would have had blood pressure, renal function and urine dipstick checked. There may be a history of previous episodes and a positive family history.

IgA is only raised in 15% of cases at the time of gross haematuria, but if present is highly suggestive. Complement C3 level is normal, as opposed to lower levels in post-streptococcal nephritis.

If the blood pressure, renal function and urine protein level is normal in clinic, these patients would not need further investigations but 6 monthly follow up in a renal paediatric clinic would be ideal to see if further episodes occur. Parents should be instructed to seek medical attention if gross haematuria does not settle after resolution of intercurrent illness.

Familial causes

Ask for a history of haematuria/renal problems in either parent and check their urine for blood. If positive, may indicate familial or thin basement membrane disease or Alport syndrome (if the mother's urine is positive for blood). This child would then require a renal biopsy, if the patient shows persistent haematuria.

Alport syndrome is usually seen in boys and may present with macroscopic or microscopic haematuria with proteinuria. Female carriers may only show microscopic haematuria. Hearing loss and ocular problems usually develop in adolescence.

Ask for family history of polycystic kidneys as this is a known cause of haematuria and can be easily ruled out by an ultrasound of the renal tract.

Systemic lupus erthymatosus is less likely in this age group.

Hypercalciuria

This is also known to cause haematuria and would need to be considered. A fresh urine specimen must be sent to biochemistry for urine calcium:creatinine ratio but you will need to inform the lab that the specimen is being sent as urine needs to be acidified.

Renal calculi

Generally, this is a less common condition in children but may be seen in Middle Eastern or Asian families, or in certain metabolic conditions. It may be considered if abdominal or loin pain was associated with haematuria. An ultrasound to check for renal or bladder calculi would be a useful investigation. A radio-opaque ureteric calculus can be seen on a plain kidneys, ureters and bladder X-ray provided the bowel is clear.

Wilm's tumour

Although less likely in this age group, a Wilm's tumour can present with haematuria. More commonly it presents as a rapidly expanding mass.

Drugs

Some drugs may cause haematuria – a good history should identify this.

Schistosomiasis

Schistosoma haematobium causes a terminal haematuria. If the specimens have been mid-stream specimens with haematuria at the end of the stream then the schistosomes may not be detected.

Consultation essentials

History

The history should focus on the duration and severity of the haematuria. Ask if there has been gross haematuria which suggests either nephritis if the urine is brown in colour or calculi, crystalluria cystourethritis if red. The presence of pain suggests inflammation or calculi. Poor fluid intake or excess of acidic drink suggests urinary irritation as a likely cause. The presence of rashes or sore throat in the preceding weeks makes post-streptococcal nephritis or Henoch–Schönlein purpura nephritis more likely. Ask if there is a difference in the colour of the urinary stream or symptoms. In renal pathology the stream and any pain should be uniform, in bladder pathology symptoms and haematuria are more evident at the end of micturition.

A family history of renal disease or hypertension makes a familial condition more likely. Ask about foreign travel and whether the child is taking any drugs, e.g. high dose non-steroidal anti-inflammatory drugs or cytotoxics, although other drugs can also be implicated.

Examination

This should include ballottement of the kidneys. If there is any concern then an urgent ultrasound scan should be arranged. A blood pressure performed manually with an appropriate sized cuff is the most useful, and perhaps the only useful measure.

Investigations

A urine specimen must be tested in clinic and if positive for blood, should be sent for urgent microscopy. If there are > 50 red cells/mm³ then a further three specimens must be sent at different times over the next few months to see if it is persistent. In persistent haematuria the parents' urine needs to be checked for familial conditions. If there are < 50 red cells/mm³ no further tests are indicated, unless the urine looked red as in haemaglobinuria or myoglobinuria.

In the presence of haematuria, perform blood tests for, full blood count, urea and electrolytes, bone chemistry, bicarbonate, parathyroid hormone, C_3, C_4, antistreptolysin O titre (ASOT) and immunoglobulins. If sickle cell disease is possible perform haemoglobin electrophoresis as well. Urine should be tested for the albumin:creatinine and calcium:creatinine ratios.

Also a renal tract ultrasound looking especially for calculi or polycystic kidneys or a tumour should be considered.

If subsequent urine specimens are negative for RBCs, no further investigation follow up is indicated.

Diagnosis

This child had a history of a sore throat in the few weeks prior to the initial consultation with the general practitioner. The fact that ASOT remained high and the C_3 level was low confirmed a diagnosis of post-streptococcal nephritis. He had developed mild proteinuria and had a normal blood pressure.

Management

Continue monitoring the urine and blood pressure on a weekly basis till the proteinuria resolves. Blood pressure, renal function and complement levels should be checked after 8 weeks. If the blood pressure rises or proteinuria increases or persists, the complement levels remain low, or renal function is impaired, then a specialist opinion will be required.

Follow up

If all the tests are normal, persistent haematuria without proteinuria or hypertension and normal renal function would need follow up in a renal clinic 6 monthly with a consideration for renal biopsy if proteinuria or hypertension or impaired renal functions develop later. Persistent microscopic haematuria becomes a hindrance in later life, as it is detected at every medical and can lead to raised insurance premiums and exclusion from activities on medical grounds. Confirming a diagnosis allows young people to continue living normally. A biopsy is often necessary but would be delayed until school leaving age.

Discussion

Most haematuria is due to cystourethritis secondary to poor drinking habits, and/or secondary to fever or intercurrent illness and resolves when these improve. Dipsticks are highly sensitive and can over detect haematuria, especially if they are old. Any diagnosis of haematuria needs to be substantiated by microscopy.

In haemaglobinuria or myoglobinuria, the sticks will register blood but the microscopy will be negative. In these conditions there should be macroscopic urinary changes. There are foods and drugs which alter urine colour and can be mistaken as haematuria, such as beetroot and rifampicin.

Further reading

Webb N, Postlethwaite R. Clinical Paediatric Nephrology. Oxford: Oxford University Press, 2003.

Eison TM, Ault BH, Jones DP, Chesney RW, Wyatt RJ. Post-streptococcal acute glomerulonephritis in children: clinical features and pathogenesis. Pediatr Nephrol 2011; 26(2):165–180.

Hicks J, Mierau G, Wartchow E, Eldin K. Renal diseases associated with hematuria in children and adolescents: a brief tutorial. Ultrastruct Pathol 2012; 36(1):1–18.

Welch TR. An approach to the child with acute glomerulonephritis. Int J Paediatr 2012:426192.

Patient information

www.kidney.org.uk
www.gosh.nhs.uk

Case 37

Headaches

Dear Paediatrician,

Thank you for seeing Abigail. She is a 11-year-old previously well girl. In the last few months, she has been complaining of severe headaches and has had to miss quite a lot of school. She finds some relief with ibuprofen.

She is a very bright girl, hoping to join her older sister at the local grammar school. There are no health issues in the family, although mum said that she had migraine when she was a teenager.

Many thanks,

Dr Howard Collins

Case analysis

Headaches affect up to 10% of children of all ages. As well as worrying about the impact of the headache itself, families worry about the underlying causes, specifically brain tumours. In children as in adults, the overwhelming majority of headaches are caused by stress/tension, migraine or a combination of the two. In Abigail's case the letter is not specific enough to narrow down the diagnosis.

A common error is to consider stress/tension headaches to be caused by emotional or psychological stress and tension. Although these can be the cause, it is better to think of these headaches as being due to muscular stress or tension caused by numerous factors, of which psychological stress is only one. Abigail is at an age when she will be in the process of changing schools with the implied added pressure of trying to follow in the footsteps of her sister. This may be something that Abigail feels she can take comfortably in her stride.

A positive family history increases the likelihood of migraine, but it is always worth establishing how the diagnosis was made in other family members.

Differential diagnosis

Brain tumour (space occupying lesion)

These are extremely rare, whilst 1 child in 10 will have headaches, only 1 in 20 000 will have a brain tumour. There are a number of features which increase possibility of a tumour: Worrying symptoms include:

- Pain present on waking
- Headache worsening over time or changing in nature
- Personality change – can be difficult in children with previous behavioural disturbance
- Deteriorating school performance – can be subtle
- Change in headache with postural changes
- Seizures

- Diabetes insipidus
- Nausea/vomiting
- Auras that are always unilateral or last < 4 mins or > 1 hour

Worrying signs are:

- Hypertension
- Altered visual acuity, fields or fundoscopy
- Focal neurological signs
- Cranial bruit
- Change of head posture

Growth failure, a short history (less than 6 months), pre-school age group and a child not well in between headaches, increase the concern but are not as worrying as the bulleted features.

If any of these are present then urgent imaging is required. Whilst MRI is the optimal scan, in some hospitals it will be easier to arrange an urgent CT – the case should be discussed with a consultant and radiologist.

Stress/tension headaches

These are the commonest headaches in all age groups. Classically there is a long history, the headaches are often persistent ('all the time') and although they vary in severity rarely interfere with desired activities. They can co-exist with other headache types, especially migraine. In stress/tension headache, whilst the pain may limit some activities, notably school, it does not normally interfere with desired activities such as going to parties. Sometimes this is attributed to martyrdom 'he puts on a brave face and just goes'.

Stress/tension is more accurately applied to the nature of the muscles in the neck and skull. Common triggers or contributing factors include:

- Poor eating and drinking during the day – breakfast is considered a decidedly optional meal by most secondary school pupils, who may eat or drink nothing till the early afternoon
- Ingestion of alcohol, nicotine or caffeine
- Poor posture – made worse by hours on a laptop, or using a mobile phone
- Heavy schoolbags
- Uncorrected visual disturbances – teenagers may need reminding to wear their glasses, if their eyesight requires glasses
- Dental issues – braces or decay
- Tiredness
- Hair tension – excessive use of straighteners, etc
- Lighting – some lights seem to cause headaches – especially computer screens

Addressing these factors will often eliminate the headaches.

If the headaches are due to psychological or emotional stress, this needs further elucidating. Sometimes the fear that the headache may be caused by some terrible disease may be feeding into the anxiety. Merely reassuring that it is 'nothing serious' can alleviate much of the pain. Anxiety may be specific or non-specific. Specific anxieties need to be identified and addressed. More commonly the anxiety is general, self-help books, or a school counsellor may help; occasionally more formal psychology input is required.

Although stress/tension headaches often respond to simple analgesics, most likely a placebo effect, avoid analgesics where possible, partly because this 'medicalises' a simple problem, and partly to avoid overuse which can in itself cause headaches. Ideally, identify and rectify any causative factors first. Otherwise simple measures like going for a walk or head and neck massage may be beneficial.

Migraine

A significant number of children have migraine, which can probably present from babyhood. The classic triad of an aura heralding unilateral severe pain, visual symptoms and vomiting will occur in some children but it is rarely this straightforward. Younger children in particular may have milder symptoms of shorter duration – sometimes even less than an hour.

There are numerous migraine variants, but each person's migraines appear formulaic, with every attack similar to the one before. The symptoms are invariably disabling, so in contrast to stress/tension headaches significant events will need to be cancelled because of migraine. There is overlap between migraine and stress/tension headaches, and certainly psychological stress can make migraines worse.

Trying to identify the trigger for migraine is usually fruitless. Less than 10% of children have a dietary trigger, with the commonest culprits being, chocolate, cheese or citrus fruits. Because the severity of migraine waxes and wanes over time, if a child is forced to undergo dietary exclusion which appears successful, it should be challenged a few times.

Treatment of migraine consists of:
1. Identifying and removing obvious triggers.
2. Treatment of individual attacks-
   a. Non-steroidal analgesics work very well. They should be given as soon as an attack starts. Children may need letters for school to give them ready access to medication.
   b. Anti emetics may be needed if vomiting is a major feature.
   c. Triptans have shown little benefit over conventional treatment, but are often easy to administer, especially in children who vomit early in an attack. In the UK, they are only licensed for older children.
3. Prevention: If the headaches are frequent and/or very severe, a preventer may be indicated. Evidence of efficacy is hard as there is a significant placebo effect. Basic preventers are:
   a. Pizotifen – which can cause sleepiness and weight gain
   b. Propanolol – causes Beta-blockade
   c. Others – such as coenzyme Q10 for which there are some encouraging trials, but it is not available on prescription

Hemiplegic migraine can be mistaken for stroke, especially the first episode. In girls who have migraine with aura/hemiplegic migraine, there is some concern that the oral contraceptive pill may increase the risk of stroke and they should receive appropriate advice.

Sinusitis

The diagnosis of sinusitis is quite contentious. ENT surgeons feel that paediatricians diagnose this too readily. If a child has tenderness over the sinuses, and especially if there is a history of nasal discharge, then a trial of antibiotics may be useful, macrolides being the antibiotics of choice.

Analgaesic headache

This has many features of stress/tension headaches. A history of analgesic overuse should provide the vital clue to diagnosis,

Idiopathic intracranial hypertension

Idiopathic intracranial hypertension is more likely to present as an emergency than in clinic. Extremely severe headache with symptoms of raised intracranial pressure and papilloedema are apparent. The diagnosis is currently made by measuring cerebrospinal fluid pressure at lumbar puncture.

Consultation essentials

History

A pain history suggests the diagnosis in the vast majority of cases **(Figure 37.1)**. Pain severity can be assessed by simple questions regarding the effect of pain on the child, taking into account the child's stoicism. Standardised pain scales or children's drawings of their pain can be useful.

The amount of school missed is an unreliable measure of pain as there are many reasons why children will not go to school, particularly if school is the cause of the headache (always establish how long into the day the headache lasts). A more useful question being 'Is there anything that you really wanted to do that you could not because of the pain?' If the summer holidays are pain free, the pain could well be related to school, although children who are worried about things at school don't stop worrying just because they are not presently there.

Explore possible trigger factors, physical or psychological. Ask about any changes, however subtle, that have occurred. A good question is 'If you went to a family party and

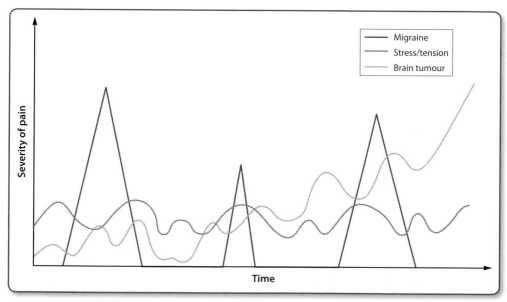

Figure 37.1 A scheme to show the severity of different causes of headache pain.

somebody who knew your son well but had not seen him for 6 months saw him again; would they think that there was anything wrong with him?'

As combination headaches are common, ask if all the headaches are the same.

Examination

Examination must include blood pressure, pulse, height and weight. Textbooks ask for a full neurological examination, but in reality this needs to be focussed. Fundoscopy and visual field testing can be hard to perform with an uncooperative child, but should always be attempted. If possible, a brain scan as an alternative to a physical examination, could be beneficial.

Tests/investigations

Scans (CT/MRI)

In a few cases a scan will be requested to confirm pathology- such as a brain tumour. In most cases it will be to reassure that no such pathology exists. Most families can be reassured without the need for a scan – make sure that the families anxieties are articulated and addressed. It is very easy to sell investigations as tools for reassurance, but this overlooks important costs including:

- The impact of the investigation:
  - It would be impractical, and costly, to give every child with a headache a CT scan. Also, in young children CT scans have some neurotoxicity
  - MRI scans often require sedation or even anaesthetic
- The inconvenience of scanning – time off school and parents' time off work
- Scans can pick up incidental findings, generating further anxiety
- Scans may not be the right test, and using them as tools of reassurance is not advisable
- Scans should be viewed as a scarce resource

The two commonest scans are CT and MRI; availability will vary in different hospitals, and it is worth discussing each case with a radiologist.

Other investigations are rarely required initially.

Diagnosis

A good history suggested that Abi was having a combination of stress/tension and migraine headaches.

Management

Features that contributed to her headaches were identified and Abi and her family will address these. The migraine component was infrequent enough to continue with symptomatic treatment only.

Follow up

This depends on the clinic and family. Sometimes a follow up appointment after 3-6 months is helpful to reassess the situation. Unless there is a specific reason, prolonged follow up should not be necessary.

Discussion

Although there are numerous differential diagnoses, the overwhelming majority of headaches seen in clinic are stress/tension headaches or migraine. As many headaches improve with placebo, it is important not to prescribe analgesics unnecessarily.

Further reading

RCPCH, The Diagnosis of Brain Tumours in Children: An evidence-based guideline to assist healthcare professionals in the assessment of children presenting with symptoms and signs that may be due to a brain tumour, Version 3, 2011.

Patient information

The Migraine Trust
www.migrainetrust.org

Case 38

Hearing impairment

Dear Paediatrician,

I would be very grateful if you could see this two and a half-year-old boy whose parents and nursery are worried about his language development and hearing.

He has only a few words and many of these are difficult to understand. His parents have been concerned that he is not able to hear properly and his nursery also noticed a possible problem. He is otherwise developmentally normal.

Dr Samuel Hamilton

Case analysis

While speech acquisition follows the normal temporal acquisition of other developmental skills, there are some specific issues which need consideration for a child referred with this issue. Firstly where should he be seen? The general acute hospital paediatric service rarely has a developmental paediatrician. More usually this work is done by the child development centre, which houses all the specialists and therapists required to manage this case. Clinicians need to be sensitive to the fact that autistic spectrum disorder can present with speech delay, and skilled assessment must ensure all the possibilities are picked up.

All newborn infants are screened for hearing deficit in the UK within 4 weeks of birth. One to two babies in every 1000 are born with a hearing loss in one or both ears. The newborn hearing screening programme in the UK aims to identify moderate, severe and profound hearing impairment in newborn babies. The screening aims to pick up children with hearing problems as young as possible, since early identification and treatment is important for the ongoing development of the child.

Differential diagnosis

The differential can be classified as follows (**Table 38.1**):

Hearing impairment

The most important medical cause of this presentation would be hearing loss. Humans have an innate propensity to vocalise and develop spoken language. This is greatly dependent on hearing it spoken. For this to mature, the child must be able to hear sufficient vocal characteristics of those around them to perceive the changes of pitch, volume, stress and syllabic patterning in their voices. These features are highly salient, in perceptual terms to the young child and are readily incorporated into their own voice. But not if he or she is deaf. Significant sensori neural hearing loss will halt the whole of this complex neurodevelopmental process.

Table 38.1 Classification of hearing loss
Lack of language input
Environmental factors
Hearing loss
Central processing difficulties
Global delay
Autistic spectrum disorder
Specific speech and language disorder
Output problems
Disorders of control of speech muscles (Oromotor dyspraxia)
Structural abnormalities cleft palate, lip, etc.

Lack of input – under stimulation

Development of speech and language is greatly dependant on hearing it spoken. Factors that interfere with the child hearing spoken language, e.g. in an unstimulating environment, could reduce the development of speech. This is usually a psychosocial issue and information may, or may not, be obvious from the consultation. Good practice would be to obtain objective correlating information from the multidisciplinary team, including the child's health visitor and social services if they are known to the family.

Global developmental delay

Speech and language delay could be part of a general developmental delay. There will be other clues in the history and a quick developmental screen of major milestones will reveal how 'on track' a child is for their chronological age.

Autistic spectrum disorder

As assessment of whether the child is keen to communicate, should be made. Does he use his own signs and gestures to make himself understood, or is he not interested in communicating with people around him, in which case he may prefer to play mainly with inanimate objects and appear to be in his own world? Children with autism do not have good eye contact with people around them and do not relate to people well. Speech and language delay is one of the main presenting symptoms of this condition, but if there is no interest to communicate by other means, this would be a further sign of this as a possible diagnosis.

Specific developmental language disorder

This should be considered if none of the above applies. One theory of aetiology is an abnormality in auditory premotor cortex of the brain. In this group of children the ability to hear voice and to perceive the temporal changes of pitch and volume are intact but they are unable to transform the sounds they perceive into the motor activity which drives the mechanics of respiration and of the larynx into reproducing these sounds for themselves.

Articulatory dyspraxia

In this situation, the child understands speech very well without lip reading and communicates back but the articulomotor effect is too great .The muscles of articulation may be faulty or delayed in maturation and therefore these muscles that work together in an intricate manner to produce clear articulation of words do not function effectively in a coordinated manner. Therefore, the child really tries hard but the effort is so great that they give up and stick to just saying single words. The fault may be in the efferent motor innervations to these muscles or weakness of the muscles itself although a pure muscular problem is very rare. Words are used sparingly and clarity of speech is greatly reduced so that often only the child's parent is able to understand what the child is so determined to tell them. In severe cases, not even the parents can understand what the child is saying. If you ask the child to say a word in isolation, he may be able to with perfect clarity but clarity drops off sharply because effort cannot be sustained in connected speech. This clearly has important implications for communication and referral to a speech and language therapist would be recommended.

Consultation essentials

History/examination

History should include pre-pregnancy, pregnancy and perinatal history in case there are any relevant issues which are impacting development. Asking where the child was born is important, to know whether newborn screening was done. A full developmental history of skills in other areas of development should be made, as well as an assessment of understanding of language. What are the sounds in the environment he responds to? Does he respond to 'soft' sounds, e.g. cat mewing, front door being opened, etc? Ask about a history of repeated upper respiratory infection which may affect the ears. Check for a family history of speech and language delay or hearing loss.

Tests/investigations

Assessment in the outpatient clinic can be done both with and without specialist equipment. Some of the tests will depend on whether the child has developmental and cognitive capacity to perform the test. McCormick's Toy Discrimination Test is widely used. If done with and without lip reading, it will give information immediately on hearing status of speech frequencies. Clinical examination of the upper respiratory tract, including otoscopy of the ears for effusion, looking into the nares and visualising throat is essential. It might be possible to determine whether the child is a mouth breather, or if there are upper airway issues from the quality of speech (e.g. nasal in adenoidal hypertrophy).

Diagnosis

This child was born in Italy to English parents, so never received postnatal screening. Based on the referral details and clinical history, it is crucial to test his hearing across the speech frequencies and refer to a paediatric department for detailed assessment and immediate management since the child is already delayed in diagnosis, they have lost 2 and a half

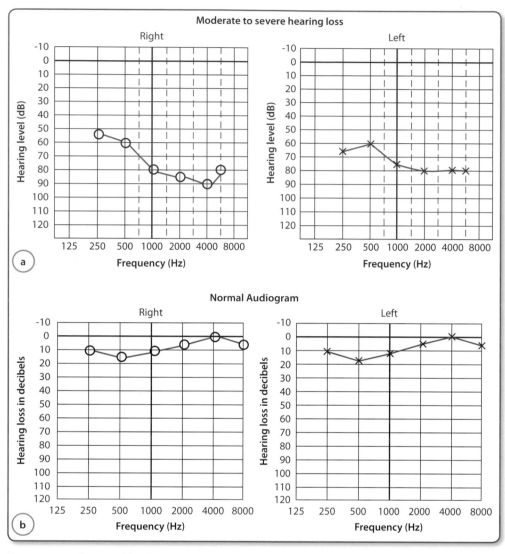

Figure 38.1 Audiogram of this child.

years of auditory deficit resulting in such a delay in speech and language. There is only a small window of opportunity as the central auditory pathways are maximally plastic for stimulus driven development up to 3 and a half years of age. Aiding or cochlear implanting after this age results in poor results and the child will have long term consequence of under developed central auditory pathway. Babies having cochlear implants < 1 year of age perform well above those who have had their implants after this age. The hearing test shows that he had a bilateral moderate to severe sensorineural hearing loss diagnosed on audiogram (**Figure 38.1**).

Management

A multidisciplinary management programme is used for the hearing impairment. This may include grief counselling to support the parents in coming to terms with this diagnosis. As well as help during this period to deal with the shock of the diagnosis, support will enable them to adopt a positive approach and to accept the hearing loss and hopefully reduce the disability caused by the impairment and prevent handicap.

This boy needs amplification by hearing aids, which are necessary to monitor his own voice and so he can access all the frequencies in the speech spectrum. This is a balance because the output needs limiting so that we do not cause over amplification damage of the residual hearing the child has. There are specific prescriptive rules to help the child to access optimal access to the entire speech spectrum without damaging his own residual hearing. Paediatric amplification considers the necessity for the child to monitor his/her own voice and thereby to develop speech production.

The involvement of a specialist teacher will play an important role in auditory training for speech and language development, hopefully contributing to general developmental progress. Pre-school and nursery will need to be involved.

If managed closely at an early age, within the age of cerebral plasticity, i.e. up to 3 and a half years, children can do well. The earlier the diagnosis, the better the outcome. If speech development of a child is considered, it takes 10 months to 1 year to say the 1st word (e.g. Mummy) with meaning. The earlier the diagnosis and management, the better the outcome.

A speech and language therapist may be needed in some cases if no progress is made. Social services support may be necessary to support the family through difficulties following the hearing impairment, especially if there are financial implications including regular attendance to the audiology department.

Follow up

Lifelong follow up is essential with repeated audiological assessments and retuning of hearing accordingly. The transitional period from paediatric to adult needs to be carefully managed.

Discussion

When there is a hearing loss as in this case, aetiological investigation should be considered. These are very specific based on clinical history, clinical examination, and laboratory investigations which will depend on the clinical history and clinical examination. Other investigations may include TORCH (toxoplasmosis, rubella, cytomegalovirus, herpes simplex, and HIV) screen, including blood spot for CMV, MRI of the temporal bone with specific attention to the anatomy of the cochlea, family audiograms, ophthalmological referral to make sure the vision is good so that lip reading is not hindered and to exclude usher's syndrome, ECG (to exclude Jervell and Lange-Nielsen syndrome a condition involving long QT syndrome, associated with severe, bilateral hearing loss in profound deafness), genetic referral as it has now been possible to identify certain genes that causes non-syndromic hearing loss and this will be useful for genetic counselling.

In this child aetiological investigations have drawn a blank so far and he is awaiting genetic investigations.

Further reading

NHS National Hearing Screening Programme
www.hearing.screening.nhs.uk

Patient information

National Deaf Children's Society
www.ndcs.org.uk
Action on Hearing Loss
www.actiononhearingloss.org.uk

Case 39

Heart murmur

Dear Paediatrician,

I would be grateful for your opinion on Alan, a 4-week-old boy who presented today with feeding difficulties and inadequate weight gain. He was born at term and was initially solely breastfed. Because of poor weight gain the health visitor advised top up formula feeds from 2 weeks of age but he still feeds poorly and his rate of weight gain has not improved. On examination today, I could detect a loud systolic murmur all over the chest and the baby also appears to be tachypnoeic. His discharge examination from the hospital was normal. Thank you for your expert review.

Yours sincerely,

Dr Matthew Innis

Case analysis

Because the letter doesn't give an indication of how well or unwell Alan is, he should be seen as soon as possible. With the above information the likely scenario is that Alan is in heart failure due to a structural heart defect associated with a significant left to right shunt. This is causing a secondary failure to thrive. If Alan was well at hospital discharge with no murmur apparent then it is likely that with the physiologic drop in pulmonary vascular pressures over the first few weeks of life the shunt has increased. A murmur is now evident with subsequent pulmonary congestion leading to breathlessness and poor feeding.

However an open mind needs to be kept during evaluation as there are other causes of breathlessness and failure to thrive in early infancy and the murmur may be physiological and a 'red herring'. Regardless of the final anatomical diagnosis, he will need medical treatment of the breathlessness and nutritional support.

With all murmurs, an echocardiogram will provide a definitive diagnosis. In most centres these should be fairly easy to access. Other tests such as ECG and chest X-ray are of limited benefit in diagnosing a cardiac defect, unless there are specific indications, e.g. if there is a suspicion of an arrhythmia (such as supraventricular tachycardia) then an ECG is essential. Similarly with respiratory symptoms a chest X-ray is helpful.

With lesions that cause cardiac failure, definitive treatment involves interventional cardiology or surgery. In life-threatening situations, this will have to be done urgently (sometimes a temporary procedure is used before the definitive one). However, as surgery becomes safer and easier as the child grows, surgeons will try to delay surgery until a baby has reached a specific weight. This entails ensuring optimal nutrition, usually requiring dietetic input. As cardiac failure is a high energy state, high energy feeds are often necessary and because feeding exacerbates breathlessness, tube feeding is often employed. At the same time, most children will be on diuretics to control the cardiac failure.

Differential diagnosis

Large septal defects (or combinations thereof)

A large perimembranous ventricular septal defect (VSD) or smaller muscular VSD, if multiple or in combination with an atrial septal defect (ASD), or as a complete endocardial cushion defect, are the most likely cause of Alan's problems. As it is a left to right shunt problem, the saturations should be normal, and there will be a loud early or pansystolic murmur – loudest at the left sternal edge. Secondary features of cardiac failure may be present.

Large patent arterial duct (patent ductus arteriosus)

The arterial duct usually closes in the first few days of life, but may remain patent. This will cause a high output cardiac failure. There should be the classic machinery murmur loudest at the second intercostal space and a wide pulse pressure. At this stage, medical attempts at closure are not likely to be successful. If the cardiac failure can be controlled, the baby may be able to tolerate the patent duct until he is large enough for transcutaneous closure, otherwise surgical ligation will be required.

Duct dependant lesions

A number of cardiac abnormalities will have their symptoms masked by a patent arterial duct, and as the duct closes, the symptoms will become more significant. These children usually deteriorate rapidly as the duct closes in the first 72 hours of life. Immediate management includes prostaglandin infusions to keep the duct open. Treatment is with interventional cardiology or emergency surgery.

Alan has symptoms that are more chronic so are unlikely to fall into this category.

Left ventricular outflow tract obstruction

Aortic stenosis or other more significant obstruction, including a coarctation of the aorta can be unmasked as the arterial duct closes. There is a harsh systolic murmur at the right second intercostal space. The resulting decreased blood supply to the peripheries causes a metabolic acidosis. In a coarctation there will be a significant drop in systolic blood pressure (usually >20 mmHg) before and after the coarctation. Coarctation of the aorta and significant aortic stenosis will need intervention. Milder forms of aortic stenosis may be managed conservatively initially.

Pulmonary outflow tract obstruction (pulmonary stenosis, tetralogy of fallot)

The murmurs associated with pulmonary outflow tract obstruction are early systolic, loudest at the left second intercostal space and should be evident at birth but may be missed as the initial intensity may be low. The severity of the obstruction can be measured by echocardiogram. Mild or moderate stenoses can be managed conservatively. In severe cases dilatation and stretching of the valve or, more rarely, valve replacement may be required.

Cardiomyopathy

Cardiomyopathies are rare in children. The most common type is a dilated cardiomyopathy, which usually has a viral cause. Presentation is with initial fever, tachycardia, tachypnoea, hypotension and poor perfusion. A murmur may be present. The diagnosis is made by echocardiogram, treatment is supportive, but many of these children will require transplantation.

Innocent/physiologic

These are present due to the dynamic circulation of infancy. If Alan's murmur is innocent, then an alternative cause for his symptoms must be found.

Noncardiac causes

Cardiac failure can be secondary to nonstructural causes of heart failure. such as anaemia thyroid disease. Also, bronchiolitis can present in a very similar way (or at the same time) and the two can be easily confused.

Consultation essentials

History

It is important to consider 'old' and 'new' information.

'Old' information includes a history of the pregnancy and the results of any antenatal scans. Also, whether there is a family history of heart disease or a maternal history of illness that could have a cardiac impact on the baby, such as systemic lupus erythematosus or thyroid disease. Alan's condition at birth and results of the newborn investigation are also helpful. The most useful information will be from the parents. Unfortunately, it is not uncommon for the baby to have a seemingly normal neonatal course, yet the parents say 'I was always worried about his breathing/feeding/colour and I told the midwives/doctors but they told me it was normal'.

'New' information includes a chronology of the breathing and feeding difficulties.

Examination

This should include looking for dysmorphic features. Chromosomal problems may be first detected after the presentation of a murmur, and it is not unheard of for trisomy 21 to present late in this way. An assessment of cardiac failure should include heart rate, respiratory rate, blood pressure and checking for radiofemoral delay. Examination of the heart includes precordial activity and defining and grading the murmur. Innocent/flow/ functional murmurs are usually soft, heard only at the left sternal edge with no significant radiation and an intensity that changes with a change in position or activity. They are usually not present or much less evident when the infant is quietly asleep. Pathologic murmurs are fixed in intensity with no change when posture is altered, are easily heard and may radiate widely. Early assessment with echocardiography is suggested. The liver should be palpated to check for hepatomegaly.

Tests/investigations

In clinic the oxygen saturations should be measured – both pre- and post-ductally – and blood pressure recorded in all four limbs. Most children will need a chest X-ray to exclude a respiratory cause of the symptoms, and possibly an ECG.

The most useful test is an echocardiogram which should be arranged as soon as possible. Further tests may be indicated, e.g. Fluorescent in-situ hybridisation (FISH) for 22q deletion (DiGeorge, Velocardiofacial syndrome).

Diagnosis

Alan was clearly in cardiac failure.

Management

He was admitted and started on diuretics. An echocardiogram confirmed the presence of a large VSD. He was treated conservatively. The VSD persisted and he had a surgical closure at 9 months of age.

Follow up

Initial cardiac follow up may be at the tertiary centre, before returning to a local outreach clinic. Local close paediatric follow up will be required to monitor the cardiac failure.

Discussion

Heart murmurs are common findings in infancy and childhood. Congenital heart disease (CHD) occurs in 8/1000 live births and innocent/functional/flow murmurs are at least 5–10 times more common. The direct cause of innocent murmurs is unknown but may represent infant/childhood flow characteristics and the proximity of the heart to the chest wall surface.

Antenatal screening in the UK means it is unusual now to encounter lethal and severe forms of congenital heart disease not previously diagnosed or suspected. Babies born with CHD are therefore more likely to be amenable to surgery. It is important that those missed antenatally are diagnosed early in the postnatal period to allow optimal outcomes from surgery.

Screening at birth currently consists of a physical examination. Babies with murmurs will have their oxygen saturations (SaO_2) measured and an ECG. Large cohort studies support the introduction of universal SaO_2 screening of infants at birth but, to be useful it has to be done after duct closure. In the current climate of early discharge and a push towards nonobstetric unit births, there are real practical difficulties to be overcome to make this achievable. Repeat examination of infants with soft murmurs, normal SaO_2 and ECG at birth is suggested at 2 weeks to weed out those with benign murmurs of early infancy.

Delayed presentations of murmurs – after 2 weeks – occur with lesions that give rise to significant left to right shunting once there has been a physiologic fall in pulmonary vascular pressures. Ductal closure may also unmask new murmurs from the closing duct itself or as the infant exhibits the physiologic effects from a duct-dependent structural heart lesion.

Murmurs that are newly identified outside the period of infancy tend to be benign and not representative of significant structural heart disease and the routine timing of their assessment is reflective of this. Murmur as a cause of acquired heart disease is uncommon in children, except in the case of extensive tooth decay or previously known cardiac pathology, and tend to occur in the older age group. Multiethnicity and migration however mean that rarer causes of acquired heart disease should not be overlooked and sought in the history of at risk groups.

Antibiotic prophylaxis

The National Institute for Health and Care Excellence guidelines no longer recommend the routine use of prophylactic antibiotics for any procedures. Patients with the following lesions are at increased risk of developing infective endocarditis and should be advised about risks, symptoms and signs and advised to seek prompt treatment if required.

- A prosthetic valve
- A past history of infective endocarditis
- Unrepaired cyanotic congenital heart disease
- Repaired congenital heart disease with prosthetic material or device – for 6 months post surgery
- Repaired congenital heart disease with residual defects at the site or adjacent to the site of a prosthetic patch or prosthetic device (which inhibits endothelialisation)
- Cardiac transplantation recipients

Remember to reinforce the necessity of good dental hygiene.

Further reading

National Institute for Health and Care Excellence. Prophylaxis against infective endocarditis, 2008. www.nice.org.uk/CG064

Patient information

British Heart Foundation
http://www.bhf.org.uk

Case 40

Hoarse voice

Dear Paediatrician,

Thank you for seeing 9-year-old Adam who has presented with a hoarse voice for 6 months. He tends to shout a lot.

He has no breathing difficulties or developmental abnormalities and is in good general health with no relevant family history.

Dr Thomas Hunt

Case analysis

Paediatric hoarseness is common in prepubertal children and more common in boys. The age of the child suggests a hyperfunctional disorder. The commonest cause is vocal nodules secondary to vocal abuse.

Differential diagnoses

Vocal nodules and functional voice disorders

Vocal nodules are the result of phonatory trauma and pathologically consist of subepithelial fibrovascular depositions in the superficial layer of the lamina propria of the membranous vocal fold. Generally, they are symmetrical at the junction of the anterior and middle third of the vocal fold. The aetiology can be multifactorial including genetic predisposition, behavioural factors, and laryngopharyngeal reflux. A laryngoscopy is essential to obtain a diagnosis.

Functional disorders

A wide range of functional disorders can occur in children without demonstrable nodules. These children may present with dysphonia or aphonia with a normal laryngoscopy, which suggests psychological factors at play. A normal cough or laugh adds support to this contention. Highly specialised voice and psychological therapy is recommended.

Laryngeal papillomatosis

This is caused by human papilloma virus infection. They are the commonest benign tumour of the paediatric larynx and the second commonest cause of chronic hoarseness. As disease progresses there may be symptoms of airway obstruction. Early symptoms such as chronic cough may initially be misdiagnosed as asthma, croup or bronchitis. Late symptoms include recurrent pneumonia, failure to thrive, dyspnoea and dysphagia. A comprehensive history of the time of onset of symptoms, prior airway trauma, previous endotracheal intubation and specific characteristics of voice and cry are important. Progressive inspiratory or biphasic stridor suggests an expanding lesion of the glottis or subglottis. A laryngoscopy is essential.

Laryngopharyngeal reflux

Gastro-oesophageal reflux of acidic stomach contents can reach the posterior pharynx and irritate the larynx causing hoarseness. Empirical treatment with antireflux medication is usually given to mitigate this.

Vocal cord paralysis

Generally, bilateral vocal cord paralysis results in a good voice and cry, but airway issues; unilateral paralysis presents with aspiration and a weak cry. It is the second commonest cause of infant stridor after laryngomalacia. A thorough history, including history of birth trauma or cardiac surgery, congenital neurological disorder, e.g. Arnold–Chiari malformations are important. Laryngoscopy with acoustic measures if feasible is useful. A CT of brainstem to mediastinum along the entire course of the vagus nerve is recommended.

Intubation injuries can cause voice disorders. Examples range from minor scarring of the vocal folds, intubation granuloma, and cricoarytenoid joint fixation subglottic stenosis. History and careful laryngostroboscopy and/or examination under anaesthesia are essential for diagnosis.

Consultant essentials

History and examination

Ask about onset and duration of hoarseness, characteristics of cry and laugh, breathing difficulties and stridor, history of intubation, surgery and trauma as an infant, behavioural characteristics, and psychological issues.

Investigations

Laryngoscopy is essential. In older and more co-operative children this can be achieved with a fibre-optic nasal endoscope in ENT outpatients. In younger children a direct laryngoscopy under anaesthesia is usually required. For complex voice disorders, video-stroboscopy and objective acoustic measures jointly with a paediatric voice therapist can be helpful.

Diagnosis

This patient is very likely to have vocal nodules with the short history and the age of the patient, though laryngoscopy is important to exclude other less common causes.

Management

Many voice disorders can be expected to improve at puberty. This is a time for great change in the larynx with tremendous growth of the membranous vocal fold in the male and, to a lesser extent, in the female. Studies have shown that only 10% of nodules do not improve at puberty and vocal hygiene advice alone does not improve nodules. Voice therapy (VT) showed some benefit with the degree of benefit related to the number of sessions with the therapist. The essentials of voice therapy include reduction of vocal strain; reduced shouting, whispering, coughing and throat clearing. Periods of quiet play after noisy activity (e.g. football) are recommended.

Surgery for nodules is rarely recommended in children due to the natural resolution at puberty and the risk of scarring. If long-term VT fails and the nodules harden or a co-existing polyp develops, microsurgical excision has a role. As a technical point, it is important for the surgeon to preserve the medial phonatory margin to promote a good fluid mucosal wave postoperatively as much as possible.

Follow up

This child would be followed up until puberty or resolution of symptoms. This occurs in the vast majority of children by the age of puberty. Any child with persistent dysphonia lasting over 2 months should be referred for laryngoscopic assessment.

Further reading

Mori K. Vocal nodules in children, preferable therapy. Internal Journal of Pediatric Otorhinolaryngology 1999; 49:303s–306.

Infections: recurrent

Dear Paediatrician,

Thank you for seeing James. He is 2 years old and his parents are concerned about the number of infections he seems to be getting. Going through his records, he has had five courses of antibiotics in the last 6 months for respiratory infections. He has had many more infections than his older sister had when she was his age.

Otherwise he seems to be thriving, but he does have a tendency towards constipation.

Dr Yannis Samaras

Case analysis

The letter is nonspecific. The amount of antibiotics received is rarely an indication of how often they are required – a comment that holds true in all paediatric practice. It is important to ascertain the reason for each course of antibiotics, clearly if they were prescribed for recurrent pneumonia this would be more alarming than if they were prescribed for upper respiratory infection with anxiety.

The hallmarks of significant immunodeficiency are: poor weight gain, diarrhoea and recurrent chest infections.

Differential diagnosis

Normal childhood infections

Children in the first few years of life may have 10–20 viral infections per year. As each infection can last for a week to 10 days, they can literally spend most of their life being unwell. Obviously, the number of infections will be linked to the number of viruses that the child encounters. Children, who are at nursery or at child-minders, will have more exposure to infections than those that are at home. Similarly, children with older siblings will have their brothers and sisters bringing back infections from their friends as well.

Normally, these infections are likely to be mild and self-limiting. There is some currency in the idea that some infections may be immunomodulatory, and reduce the effectiveness of the immune system. This leads to the child acquiring another infection before they have fully recovered from the first one, making them more vulnerable. Many children seem to go through a stage of 6 months or so when they seem permanently unwell.

If the child has only viral infections, and in the absence of systemic symptoms, reassurance is all that is required. This can be augmented with the idea that early antigen exposure may 'train' the immune system to deal with challenges later on – and therefore multiple minor infections are beneficial in the long-term.

Immunodeficiency

Significant immunodeficiency is likely to present with significant infections or a significant response to minor infections. A history of his previous infections is essential. If there is any doubt then further investigations may be helpful. The number of tests available and their complexity means that a discussion with the laboratory or an immunologist is likely to be useful, as tests of function – such as a vaccine response test – are of more value than absolute numbers.

IgA deficiency

This is common and in most children is transient, but in a few cases it may progress to a more generalised immunodeficiency. Children present with repeated respiratory or sinus infections, but are otherwise well. Diagnosis is confirmed by low serum IgA levels. Treatment options include using prophylactic antibiotics and prompt antibiotic treatment for future infections. Children with IgA deficiency are at a higher risk of having coeliac disease. This is made more complicated, because the coeliac blood test measures an IgA antibody so is of little value in IgA deficiency.

Rhinitis

This is often overlooked in children, especially of this age. Allergic symptoms are easily misinterpreted as being infectious ones. On direct questioning there is often a history of nasal or ophthalmic irritation, with nose and eye rubbing and frequent nasal discharge; at night this will cause coughing. Treatment is often difficult at this age. Identifying and eliminating allergens has more theoretical appeal than practical application. Antihistamines are relatively easy to administer but may have limited effectiveness, whilst steroids given intranasally and any form of eye drop may be effective, they are often difficult to administer.

Cystic fibrosis

With universal screening it is unusual to detect new cases clinically. However, the screening does not detect 100% of cases. It identifies the common cystic fibrosis (CF) mutations so, for example CF in a child with consanguineous parents from the subcontinent would be less likely to be detected. If there is any doubt a sweat test should be performed. Although pancreatic insufficiency is associated with diarrhoea, some children with CF will have significant constipation – distal intestinal obstruction syndrome.

Primary ciliary dyskinaesia

This is another condition with a spectrum of severity. In 50% of cases there is situs inversus. Symptoms can be subtle, but would normally include sinusitis (uncommon in children this young whose sinuses have not yet formed), repeated pneumonia (often starting in the neonatal period), otitis media, wheeze and persistent nasal discharge. If there is a history of persistent nasal discharge from birth, then primary ciliary dyskinaesia must be considered. Investigations and management should be guided by a respiratory paediatrician.

Respiratory

Other rare respiratory causes might include tuberculosis, bronchiectasis and bronchiolitis obliterans. If there is any doubt, a plain chest X-ray will help to decide if any of these are a possible diagnosis.

Recurrent fever

Recurrent infections tend to occur with a set frequency and each episode has a predictable presentation. Unfortunately, these are often diagnosed rather late. Inflammatory conditions are unlikely to have a respiratory presentation.

Metabolic

Children with mild metabolic abnormalities may not have more infections than others, but because they have faulty homeostatic mechanisms, each infection may cause metabolic decompensation, so the child will seem more ill and for longer than would be expected. If there is any question of this, it is worth asking for the child to present at the time of an illness so that blood glucose, blood gas and possibly ammonia can be checked.

Consultation essentials

History/examination

Clearly, the most important part of the history is establishing the nature of the infections. If they all seem low grade and most likely to be viral, then no further action is required. If all or some of them seem to be more significant then this needs more consideration.

Systemically, if he is thriving this makes significant underlying illness less likely, so plotting height and weight is essential.

Tests/investigations

Often, no tests are required. This would be the case if the child was thriving and seemed to have had a series of clearly viral illnesses. If there seems to be anything more sinister, then tailored investigations are indicated. Immune investigations, other than the most basic ones, should be discussed with an expert.

Diagnosis

James was thriving. The antibiotics were given with a low threshold, and were almost certainly not necessary. There was a history of atopy in the family and James exhibited features of rhinitis.

Management

James was given a trial of antihistamines. The family were reassured about the normal frequency of infections. They had read about IgA deficiency and wanted immunoglobulin levels measured. This showed a slightly low IgA level. As he seemed to be getting fewer infections, no action was required. He remained well and his levels were presumed to have risen to normal.

Follow up

Minimal follow up is required. The family may be offered an appointment in 4–6 months to review the situation, but this monitoring could take place in primary care. A safety-net procedure would include encouraging them to seek a sooner review if the symptoms change or if James were to develop features of any of the specific conditions highlighted above.

Discussion

The recurring challenge in paediatrics is determining the normal from the abnormal. In medical terms, the hallmark of early childhood is repeated minor infections. As passive immunity wanes, and exposure to infectious agents increases, children of this age group can be expected to have 10–20 viral illnesses a year. As each can last for up to 10 days, it is not uncommon that they spend most of their time unwell. There are some children who seem to be particularly vulnerable and suffer 6 months or so of almost constant infections – perhaps some of the infections have immunosuppressant qualities. A second child will invariably have more infections than a first one, because the older child will bring their infections home and is likely to pass them on.

Further reading

Stiehm RE. The four most common pediatric immunodeficiencies. Adv Exp Med Biol 2007; 601:15–26.

Patient information

Immune Deficiency Foundation
   www.primaryimmune.org

Infections: lower urinary tract infection

Dear Paediatrician,

Please could you see Sarah, a 4-year-old girl who has frequent lower urinary tract infections, presenting with pain, mild fever, dysuria, and frequent wetting. Her urine specimens have shown either coliforms or a mixed growth. I have given her about six courses of antibiotics over the last 6 months and the parents and myself want to make sure that we are not overlooking another underlying medical issue.

Many thanks,

Dr Brian Jaidev

Case analysis

The letter fairly clearly describes intermittent lower urinary tract symptoms. The diagnosis seems clear and the main issue will be management.

Differential diagnosis

Recurrent lower urinary tract infection (cystitis/urethritis/vulvovaginitis)

This is the most likely diagnosis. Sarah is at an age where her oestrogen levels will have reached a nadir, between birth and puberty. Oestrogens help protect the lower urinary tract from irritation and infection. Coupled with this she will be achieving independence without responsibility. So she will go to the toilet and wipe herself afterwards without being observed, and is likely not to be doing this well.

The exact anatomical location of the problem is often hard to pinpoint and not relevant to the treatment plan. However, it seems that urethritis or vulvovaginitis is more common than cystitis. In either scenario, it is likely that initially there is some irritation or inflammation which can cause dysuria and incrase the vulnerability to superadded infection. Frequency can be due to bladder sensitivity or more likely because only a small amount of urine is passed when necessary, with pain limiting emptying; this results in a much distended bladder with small amounts of urine being passed when it 'bursts'. Not surprisingly this can cause suprapubic pain as much as an inflamed bladder can. Wetting can be due to failed urine withholding, or the negative effect of inflammation on the urinary sphincter function.

There are a number of lifestyle factors which can make children prone to recurrent lower urinary tract infections (UTIs). The level of lifestyle changes necessary depend on the severity of the symptoms. It seems unnecessarily draconian to ban bubble bath for a girl who has had two minor episodes in the last year, although this may be appropriate if they are occurring every week.

- **Constipation/stool withholding:** This impacts on bladder function. The presence of stool in the rectum increases the chances of vulvovaginitis, especially with coliforms. It is difficult to treat any urinary problem in the presence of untreated constipation and/or stool withholding. It is important to enquire about this in detail.

- **Poor wiping:** The ideal way for a girl to wipe after passing urine is 'front-to-back'. This is actually counterintuitive and 'back to front' is a more natural movement. If further wiping is required, a clean tissue should be used. It is essential to establish how she wipes but, rather than asking her, it is better to ask her to demonstrate how she wipes. If she is bashful then show her both options (if you are bashful this will be a challenge to overcome). Some girls rather than wiping will just dab. If she is wiping the wrong way, this will need correcting, and as it is likely to have become a habit and the parents will need to reinforce this. Generally children understand up and down better than back and front. For those with good English skills the lesson is 'wipe doWn after a wee – uP after a poo'.

- **Washing:** It is important that good local hygiene is maintained, and this should include a good daily wash. Soap or bubble bath may add to the irritation because, as detergents, they remove the protective oils on the skin. A shower, which sprays water from above the head, will not adequately clean the necessary area. Therefore, enquiring as to what method is used, and how often washing happens is essential.

- **Poor drinking:** There does seem to be a link with poor fluid intake and lower urinary symptoms. In practice this can be hard to change as most children drink very little at school. The nature of the drink is a little more contentious, it is possible that sugary or fizzy drinks exacerbate the problem.

- **Inadequate ventilation:** Keeping the area dry and well ventilated is important, skirts and cotton knickers are better than tight lycra leggings.

- **Foreign body:** This is unlikely, and there would usually be a persistent vaginal discharge.

- **Sexual abuse:** In the absence of a disclosure, establishing sexual abuse is difficult. Explicit images, sexually transmitted infections, sperm and pregnancy are the only pathognomonic clinical signs of sexual abuse. Not only is it effectively unheard of for abuse to present exclusively this way, it would be next to impossible to prove it. Although most books raise the possibility, in practical terms it is often offensive rather than helpful to even mention it. A common presentation, however, is the child whose parents are divorced who returns from her father with some vulvovaginitis and the mother wants a medical opinion to establish if her daughter has been abused. Not only is this impossible to determine – and any accusation must be processed through the appropriate multiagency channel – but it highlights the father's dilemma. If he pays attention to his daughter by cleaning and changing her, on her return her mother asks if Daddy touched her, to which she replies 'yes' and triggers the accusation. Alternatively, if he leaves her alone, she returns home with some vulvovaginitis and the outcome is the same. These situations are always difficult.

Consultation essentials

History and examination

Distinguishing between upper and lower urinary tract symptoms should be straightforward (**Table 42.1**). Some children will have both upper and lower urinary tract problems, in which case they each need to be dealt with appropriately.

It is helpful to ascertain how the urine was collected. It is a rarity to obtain a clean catch from a child that has been washed with water. Often the specimen or child is not properly prepared. A potty will be full of organisms and cleaning it with bleach before collecting the sample will not only kill all resident bacteria but also kill any that might be present in the urine.

Many specimens in this scenario may have few white cells, or have epithelial cells, which will suggest a contaminated specimen. It is doubtful that repeated urine testing plays any major role in the practical management of lower urinary problems.

Lifestyle factors as mentioned above need to be explored and explained in some detail.

Investigations

These are rarely, if ever required. The National Institute for Health and Care Excellence guidelines recommend an ultrasound and DMSA scan for children with more than three episodes of lower UTI. This seems excessive, particularly if there are clear untreated risk factors such as poor wiping, constipation and poor drinking.

Diagnosis

Sarah has had recurrent lower UTIs. From her results, there is evidence of a clear infection on only one occasion; the other samples seemed to be contaminated specimens.

Management

She was given advice about lifestyle changes. A discussion followed about treating any future episodes. As the family found it difficult to get to their general practitioner they were given a prescription of antibiotics to use if she had symptoms which did not improve spontaneously after 48 hours.

Table 42.1 Differentiating between lower and upper urinary tract infection (UTI)		
	Upper UTI	**Lower UTI**
Pain	Loin pain (less localised in younger children	Suprapubic, may be mild
Fever	Often very high >39 degrees Centigrade (burning up)	Mild or absent
Rigors	Often present	Absent
Vomiting	Often present	Absent
Urinary symptoms	Mild or absent – may have slight dysuria	Frequency/wetting/dysuria – common
Urinary nature	May look cloudy	Usually clear, may have blood on tissue after wiping

Follow up

No follow up is strictly necessary, unless investigations have been planned. A single follow up to ensure that changes have been implemented and are successful may be valuable.

Discussion

Although these symptoms may be given the abbreviation UTI, there is some debate as to whether the 'I' stands most correctly for infection, inflammation or irritation. Some people suggest that UTI should be dropped and replaced with lower urinary tract symptoms.

There is an essential distinction to be made between upper and lower urinary tract conditions. In the former there is an association with long-term renal problems and usually further investigation and monitoring are required. The strength of this association and the need for intervention is a matter of some controversy. The National Institute for Health and Care Excellence guidelines provide a framework, but these guidelines are not without their critics.

There is general agreement that lower urinary tract symptoms are more of a nuisance than anything else, and are only rarely associated with underlying problems, and rarely require further investigation. In recurrent cases, where no obvious 'lifestyle factors' are identified then some imaging – such as an ultrasound scan may be helpful. When discussing lifestyle issues, be careful not to sound judgemental. It is better to use the term 'lifestyle' rather than 'hygiene' as the latter can appear derogatory. Also, the girls that are prone to these symptoms, probably do things no differently to their peers, they merely have vulnerability, which is likely to be constitutional. This means that they have to be more conscientious with their hygiene to prevent further episodes.

Further reading

National Institute for Health and Care Excellence. Urinary tract infection: diagnosis, treatment and long-term management of urinary tract infection in children. Clinical guidelines, CG54 - Issued: August 2007. www. nice.org.uk/CG54

Patient information

Education and Resources for Improving Childhood continence (ERIC) www.eric.org.uk

Case 43

Labial adhesions

Dear Paediatrician,

I wonder whether you could advise me on Sophie who is 4 years old. Mum reports that Sophie is wet every day. She described a sensation of 'bubbling' as she passes urine. Her urine dipstick is negative. I would value your opinion.

Thank you,

Dr John Shaw

Case analysis

The first issue is to manage the incontinence and day wetting. Consider poor voiding and bladder instability and anatomical problems, such as adhesion of the labia minora, commonly known as labial adhesions, fusion or synechia vulvae or labial agglutination.

Differential diagnoses

Labial adhesions

These are a benign condition reported in about 2% of girls in the first few years of life. Peak incidence is around 2 years of age. Labial adhesions are usually noted as an incidental finding or because of parental concerns regarding appearance of labia. However, they can also be found 'incidentally' when assessing for urinary symptoms in a presentation such as this. Occasionally, they can be severe and cause partial obstruction to urine flow and result in urinary tract infections, urinary retention and/or day wetting. With labial adhesions the wetting occurs after micturition, where urine is retained behind the adhesions and then leaks out afterwards. In the majority of cases, the adhesions will respond to topical oestrogen cream – although this is invariably effective, it is debatable whether it is always indicated as the labia will usually separate with age. Sometimes a single course is helpful in reassuring the family that the underlying anatomy is normal. They do have a tendency re-adhere after treatment and repeated courses are of more dubious benefit. Advice on genital hygiene is important.

Vulvovaginitis (see Case 79)

Lower urinary tract infection (see Case 42)

Congenital absence of hymen

The appearance known as 'congenital absence of the hymen' is unlikely to exist as a congenital abnormality on its own. Studies have failed to demonstrate the absence of a hymen at birth in a large series of newborn girls. While the size of hymenal opening will vary with position, examination technique and how relaxed the child is, it will only be absent as part of a congenital agenesis or other anatomical abnormality of the genitalia.

Vaginal agenesis

This is reported to affect 1 in 5,000 to 7,000 female infants. It can be part of a rare syndrome (Mayer-von Rokitansky-Küster-Hauser syndrome) with congenital abnormalities such as an absent vagina or an incomplete vaginal canal, absent uterus and cervix, kidney abnormalities, hearing loss, and scoliosis. Girls with this condition will go through normal puberty since their ovaries are present.

Scarring from sexual abuse

Despite the examination of young children in cases of alleged abuse being left to the community paediatric doctors, a general paediatrician needs to be aware of the signs to look out for. If there is any possibility of child sexual abuse causing the symptoms, further assessment and escalation is warranted. Without an allegation or disclosure, an urgent second opinion concerning physical signs might be a more sensitive way to approach the situation.

Consultation essentials

History

A history of when the symptoms started is important. Check if the parents describe normal looking genitalia. Assess for underlying lower urinary tract infection or constipation which may be contributing to the symptoms.

Examination

Genital examination is essential to this assessment. Performing this in a sensitive way with a chaperone will help the child feel at ease. Explain what you are about to do in simple terms: 'I just need to have a look 'down below' at where the wee comes out to see if there is a reason for the problems you are having'. Ask the child to remove their trousers/skirt and underwear, and lie on the examination couch; offer them a blanket or sheet to retain modesty. Roll the sheet up over their knees and ask them to put their knees up. When their heels are near their buttocks, ask them to gently part their knees down to each side exposing the introitus. It may be necessary to gently part the labia to see the vestibule. This can be the time to notice the 'keyhole' appearance of the posterior fusion of the labia, or the slit-like appearance of complete fusion. Sometimes there is a flat appearance or the impression of a film across the vulval opening (**Figure 43.1**). Assess the skin for excoriation and irritation. Bruising or other marks may necessitate further assessment, as would an unexpected hymenal opening for a prepubertal child. Any secondary sexual characteristics or precocious development will need further assessment.

Diagnosis

Sophie's description of dribbling and bubbling on micturition led to a suspicion of labial adhesions. This was confirmed on examination. The wetting was because of a 'dam' effect of trapped urine behind the adhesion which was incomplete but with a very small opening.

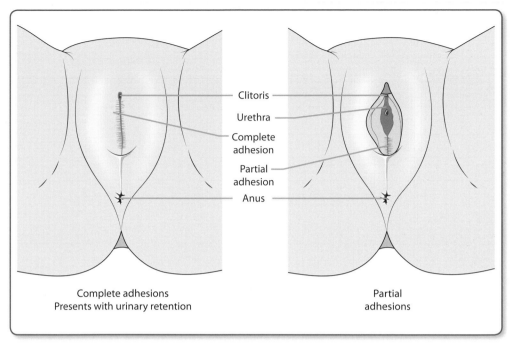

Figure 43.1 Labial adhesions.

Management

In some cases no treatment is necessary. Advice on genital hygiene, paying attention to all the measures for vulvovaginitis will reduce any irritation. However in symptomatic cases, a topical oestrogen cream [Gynest (estriol) 0.01 %] may be used. Topical treatment should be applied twice a day for 6 weeks. The oestrogen mimics the changes in the vulval skin at puberty and the adhesions release. They can reform when the cream stops. Surgical treatment should be reserved when urinary retention is associated. An urologist may be able to divide the adhesions in clinic under topical local anaesthetic. Sometimes formal surgical division is required under anaesthetic. Vaseline applied to the area can help prevent adhesions re-forming.

Follow up

Usually, the parents can monitor the response to oestrogen cream and advice be given to the general practitioner for urological/paediatric gynaecology referral if the adhesions persist.

Discussion

Other skin conditions such as lichen sclerosis can present with irritation and skin changes of the vulva. Any vaginal discharge needs further assessment but in young girls is likely to be due to vulvovaginitis.

Further reading

Davis VJ. What the paediatrician should know about pediatric and adolescent gynecology: perspective of a gynaecologist. Paediatr Child Health 2003; 8:491–495.

Eroglu E, Yip M, Oktar T, Kayiran SM, Mocan H. How should we treat prepubertal labial adhesion? Retrospective comparison of topical treatments: estrogen only, betamethasone only, and combination estrogen and betamethasone. J Pediatr Adolesc Gynecol 2011; 24:389–391.

Anogenital Findings – Sexual Abuse in Prepubertal Children and Adolescents

Lymphadenopathy

Dear Paediatrician,

Please could you see this 4-year-old boy who has had swollen glands in his neck for a couple of months? He is otherwise very well. The parents are concerned about the prolonged persistence of these lumps.

Dr Karen Neoh

Case analysis

In the majority of cases, persistent lymphadenopathy is due to a response to local or systemic infection. However, a misplaced anxiety about the possibility of malignancy means that these children are often asked to be assessed urgently, e.g. via the '2-week' cancer referral pathway. It is important to address this anxiety if it has been raised, but more important not to raise it in the first place unless there are other concerning features. It is very rare for children with a malignancy to present in this way.

Most commonly the child with persistent lymphadenopathy will be well, and although the nodes may increase and decrease in size as the child has subsequent infections, as long as they are not persistently growing then the family can be reassured that malignancy is not a consideration.

Differential diagnosis

Normal anatomy

It is normal for children to have several tiny pea-sized glands palpable in the anterior and posterior triangles of the neck and behind the mastoid process.

Reactive lymph nodes

Reactive lymphadenopathy is the most common cause of lymph node enlargement and is often secondary to common paediatric infections and inflammatory conditions such as recurrent tonsillitis, eczema, and cradle cap or head lice. These glands tend to increase in size in response to local infection and although they may reduce in size when the child is well they may not completely disappear.

Atypical mycobacterial infection

This causes slow growing, persistent lymphnode enlargement in the neck. Occasionally, these nodes may become chronically indurated and ulcerated with a draining sinus. Treatment is by excision biopsy of the entire gland.

Lymphadenitis/ abscess

This is an inflammatory process which often presents acutely with rapid lymph node enlargement over a few days and accompanying redness, pain and tenderness. The gland may be firm initially and later becomes fluctuant as it progresses to abscess formation. Management is with antibiotics – oral or intravenously – and surgical drainage if an abscess is formed. Initially no investigations will change management. If the swelling persists despite treatment then an ENT opinion should be sought.

Lymphoma

These may present with an isolated palpable lymph node which steadily increases in size. Non-Hodgkin's lymphoma usually arises in the abdomen or chest and there may not be palpable peripheral lymph nodes. These tumours grow relatively rapidly and would not present with a history of several months. Hodgkins lymphomas may be slower to grow and can present over a few months with progressive increase in the size of the nodes. However, this is predominantly a disease of adolescents and adults, and is highly unlikely in a 4-year old. In lymphoma the nodes are often rubbery or hard.

Leukaemia

Isolated lymph node enlargement is not a feature of leukaemia which usually presents with the triad of anaemia, thrombocytopaenia (bruising and bleeding) and infection. The child is usually unwell, lethargic, miserable and may have bone pain.

Consultation essentials

History/examination

Identify all of the lymph nodes of concern. It can be hard to find them, but the parents usually are very aware of their presence, so ask the parents to point them out. Establish the duration of lymph node enlargement and whether there is a change in size: either a steady increase or waxing and waning.

Ask about symptoms of a precipitating cause, such as sore throat, enlarged tonsils, scalp eczema, postauricular rash and head lice infestations.

Look for signs of the above problems and more generally for pallor, bruising or mucosal bleeds.

Examination of the nodes should include size, consistency and presence of redness or tenderness. This should be recorded, ideally on a body map, but certainly with a clear indication of location and nature.

Nodes that are >2 cm in diameter, painless and non-tender and have steadily increased in size are of concern. A hard or rubbery gland may indicate a malignancy. Examine the axilla, and inguinal region for lymphadenopathy, and check the liver and spleen.

Tests/investigations

Usually no investigations are required. A full blood count is of minimal value in a young child who has small cervical lymph nodes as it does not help to rule out malignancy and causes pain and anxiety rather than providing reassurance. Frequently, there may be minor abnormalities such as lymphocytosis or a mild neutropenia which are a reflection of an underlying infection and tend to exacerbate unnecessary anxiety and precipitate further unnecessary tests. Erythrocyte sedimentation rate, C-reactive protein, lactate dehydrogenase measurement can be raised, but are non-specific inflammatory markers and do not aid management.

Ultrasound is helpful if the gland is tender and inflamed and may aid in decisions concerning surgical intervention.

Large lymph nodes and those with concerning features of a malignancy should be referred to a tertiary paediatric oncology centre for a biopsy. Fine needle aspiration is not performed for the diagnosis of paediatric malignancies.

If there are features of a possible atypical mycobacterial infection, an excision biopsy needs to be requested to prevent the development of a chronic fistula which may occur after needle aspiration.

Diagnosis

The presentation of several small cervical lymph nodes that have been present for months in a well 4-year-old child is most likely to be due to reactive lymph nodes. This is confirmed by a clinical assessment shows that he is active, healthy, has no bruising or bleeding from mucous membranes and has freely mobile discrete nodes of up to 0.5–1 cm in size.

Management

Explain to the parents that these glands have increased in size in response to infection and may never completely disappear. Blood tests do not aid in management and are not routinely required. This is usually reassuring for the parents.

Follow up

None required.

Discussion

Four-year-old children often have several palpable glands (lymph nodes) in the neck. These might be pea-sized nodes which form part of the normal anatomy of a child and can persist for months if not years.

The overwhelming majority of children referred with this problem tend to have reactive lymph nodes which have enlarged in response to a focal infection/inflammation. They increase and decrease in size but may never completely disappear. A prolonged history of months in an otherwise well child makes it more likely to be a reactive cause.

Malignant lymph nodes steadily increase in size and usually present after a couple of weeks with painless enlargement of the gland and there may be associated systemic symptoms of tiredness, pallor or bruising.

Rapidly enlarging lymph nodes over 1 – 2 days are invariably due to infection/ inflammation and are often painful and tender, and are treated initially with antibiotics.

Further reading

Stutchfield CJ, Tyrell J. Evaluation of lymphadenopathy in children. Paediatr Child Health 2012; 22:98-102.

Patient information

Patient.co.uk

    www.patient.co.uk/doctor/Generalised-Lymphadenopathy

Macroglossia

Dear Paediatrician,

I would be grateful if you could see this 5-month-old baby who has presented with an enlarged tongue. The pregnancy was uneventful and her birth weight was 8 lb 9 oz. Her development is so far normal. She has some feeding difficulties. It takes up to 1 hour for her to take her feed and she is drooling a lot. She has also had two choking episodes and has received several courses of antibiotics for chest infections.

Dr Beverley Kenwright

Case analysis

An infant presenting with macroglossia should immediately raise the suspicion of an underlying genetic problem. The enlarged tongue would be one of the most obvious presenting features, as noticed by the parents and general practitioner. The most important condition to consider is Beckwith–Wiedemann syndrome (BWS), an overgrowth and cancer predisposition syndrome which most commonly presents with macroglossia, exomphalos and increased growth.

The general practitioner has commented on normal development, which would be expected in a child with BWS. However, there are other causes of macroglossia on the differential list that are associated with developmental delay such as chromosomal disorders. It is important to ascertain if the feeding issues described in the referral letter are related to the macroglossia or are related to a separate problem which may provide further clues to an underlying diagnosis. This would also apply to the increased number of infections reported.

Differential diagnosis

Macroglossia can be classified as true or relative macroglossia.

True macroglossia

This may be due to BWS, chromosomal disorders, e.g. Down's syndrome, 9q34 microdeletion syndrome, 17p11.2 microdeletion syndrome, hypothyroidism (isolated or syndromic), lysosomal storage disorders or disorders on the 'ras' pathway (rasopathies), such as neurofibromatosis type 1 (NF1), or cardiofaciocutaneous syndrome. It could also be an isolated finding.

Relative macroglossia

The tongue may be relatively enlarged due to adjacent structure size or an impingement upon the tongue, e.g. a vascular malformation or cystic hygroma.

Consultation essentials

History/examination

Developmental milestones including hearing, vision and growth

A detailed history ought to be taken focusing on developmental milestones, hearing and vision to indicate if there is an underlying syndromic diagnosis.

Congenital anomalies

Look for features of congenital anomalies, developmental delay, growth abnormalities and hearing or visual problems. Any of these features may indicate a chromosomal disorder or a rarer genetic diagnosis. Establish if the macroglossia was present from birth or developed postnatally. Consider whether it could be a mass such as a neoplasm or lymphangioma. If there are features of a storage disorder, consanguinity or family history of other problems, a mucopolysaccharidosis should be considered. Look for other features of hypothyroidism and perform thyroid function tests. Ask about a family history of problems related to NF1, especially if there are café au lait patches.

Dysmorphic features

Look for other features of BWS. These include prenatal overgrowth or macrosomia, abdominal wall defects, umbilical hernia or evidence of diastasis recti, anterior linear earlobe creases, posterior helical ear pits, visceromegaly, hemihypertrophy, renal abnormalities and embryonal tumours, particularly Wilms' tumour. Look for facial naevi or haemangiomas. Trisomy 21 is also a cause of macroglossia but is usually apparent on facial appearance. However, mosaic trisomy 21 may be more subtle but still result in macroglossia.

Pregnancy, neonatal and family history

When considering BWS, ask about a positive family history; 85% of cases are sporadic and 15% are inherited. There is an increased risk of BWS with assisted reproductive technology, e.g. intracytoplasmic sperm injection. Ask about a history of polyhydramnios or scan abnormalities such as exomphalos. Babies are usually large for gestational age (above 98th centile). The placenta and/or umbilical cord may have been noted to be large. There is often a history of neonatal hypoglycaemia.

If there are no other features and a positive family history of isolated macroglossia, this may suggest autosomal dominant macroglossia.

Tests/investigations

If any of the above features are present, molecular testing for BWS is important but since BWS is a common cause of macroglossia, even in the absence of other clinical findings, molecular testing could be considered. Request karyotyping and/or detailed array comparative genomic hybridisation (array-CGH) on bloods. Microdeletions or microduplications which may or may not be clinically significant can be identified on array-CGH and parental samples may be required to establish significance. The chromosomal imbalance may be associated with macroglossia. Karyotype searching for mosaicism will, for example, identify mosaic trisomy 21. Thyroid function tests should be done to exclude hypothyroidism. Consider urine for gylcosaminoglycans (GAGs) if there are other features suggestive of a mucopolysaccharidosis.

Diagnosis

The clinical diagnosis is BWS. The umbilical cord was noted to be very thick at birth. On examination, the patient's head circumference was above the 25th centile but her weight was on the 91st centile. She had a small capillary haemangioma on her forehead in the midline as well as on the back of her neck. Her ears were normal and there was no asymmetry of her upper or lower limbs. Systemic examination was also normal. Since this condition can be associated with Wilms' tumour, further genetic assessment is required to determine the risk. Regular abdominal scans are indicated depending on the genetic abnormality.

Management

Consider management for macroglossia and management of the underlying diagnosis. Common complications of macroglossia that are reported include speech problems, swallowing difficulties, drooling, recurrent upper respiratory tract infections and airway obstruction. Refer to a speech and language therapist for assessment and treatment for feeding, respiratory and/or speech problems. Consider input from the craniofacial and plastics team for possible tongue reduction surgery if the enlarged tongue is severe and significantly affecting the baby. However, if mild to moderate, this may improve with time as the mandible grows to accommodate the tongue.

Refer to clinical genetics for assessment if possibility of BWS, chromosomal disorder or any other genetic disorder. Molecular testing can be carried out but also individuals and families can be counselled for rare conditions and be counselled for future pregnancies.

Depending on the risk of abdominal neoplasm, renal and abdominal ultrasound scans should be organised according to local guidelines (described in text below).

Hemihypertrophy may require input from orthotics and orthopaedic surgery if severe.

Follow up

A paediatrician (possibly with an oncology interest) should follow up a child with BWS, unless the genetics favour low or no Wilms' risk. A referral back to the clinical geneticist for discussion of offspring risks when the child is older and thinking of having a family of their own may be appropriate at a later time.

Discussion

Beckwith–Wiedemann syndrome (BWS) is an imprinting disorder involving chromosome 11. The region of chromosome 11 contains many genes but *CDKN1C* (growth suppressing gene) and *IGF2* (growth promoting gene) have been strongly implicated in BWS.

CDKN1C is controlled by KvDMR1 and *IGF2* is controlled by H19 DMR. Methylation studies examine whether these genes are active or not. Children with KvDMR1 loss of methylation do not require Wilms' tumour screening, therefore establishing a molecular diagnosis can avoid unnecessary screening and anxiety. Children with uniparental disomy and those with a methylation error at H19 are at higher risk of developing a tumour than children with BWS with a different aetiology. The tumours in BWS are predominantly of embyonal origin, e.g. Wilms' tumour and hepatoblastoma. Because they are fast-growing tumours, it is recommended that all children with BWS should have an abdominal ultrasound scan every 3 months. Early identification of the tumours may lead to improved survival. The risk of Wilms' tumour declines significantly after the age of 7 or 8 years, and therefore abdominal ultrasound scans are not required after this age.

It is difficult to detect hepatoblastoma on abdominal ultrasound therefore 3 monthly α-fetoprotein, which is significantly raised in children with hepatoblastoma, is recommended until the age of 3 years, after which the risk declines.

Sometimes a clinical diagnosis may remain even in the absence of a positive molecular test if all the diagnostic clinical criteria are met **(Table 45.1)**.

Table 45.1 Clinical diagnostic criteria for Beckwith–Wiedemann syndrome	
Two or more of the major criteria	Macroglossia
	Prenatal overgrowth
	Anterior ear lobe creases
	Abdominal wall defect
	Hemihypertrophy/growth asymmetry
	Embryonal tumour
	Characteristic renal abnormalities
And one or more of the minor criteria	Polyhydramnios
	Neonatal hypoglycaemia
	Facial nevus flammeus
	Characteristic cardiac abnormalities
	Characteristic facial appearance

Further reading

Prada CE, Zarate YA, Hopkin RJ. Genetic causes of macroglossia: diagnostic approach. Pediatrics 2012; 129:e431–e437.

Bradley-Smith G, Hope S, Firth HV, Hurst JA. Oxford Handbook of Genetics, Ist edn. Oxford: Oxford University Press, 2009:278.

UK Genetic Testing Network: Gene Dossier for Beckwith–Wiedemann syndrome. http://www.ukgtn.nhs.uk

The Wilms' Tumour Surveillance Working Group. Surveillance for Wilms'Tumour In: At-Risk Individuals – Pragmatic Recommendations For Best Practice. The British Society for Human Genetics 2005. http://www.bshg.org.uk

Patient information

Beckwith–Wiedemann syndrome support group
www.bws-support.org.uk

MMR vaccination

Dear Paediatrician,

Please can you advise the parents of this 1-year-old girl. Even after extensive discussion with the health visitor they are reluctant to allow MMR immunisation. The child is healthy and developing normally. She already has a vocabulary of 10 clear words. She has had the first three doses of primary immunisation. However, the parents (both university graduates) are aware of concerns about MMR and are most worried because the mother's nephew (aged 10 years) has recently been diagnosed with Asperger's syndrome.

Dr Simon Kopelowitz

Case analysis

In February 1998, the Lancet published a paper by Andrew Wakefield et al, suggesting a link between the measles, mumps, rubella (MMR) immunisation and autism. Although this paper suggested a theory, it was seized upon by interested parties as making a definite statement. Subsequently, many other studies were conducted from a wide variety of angles, all of which refuted the theory and confirmed that the association between MMR and apparent onset of autism was temporal and not causal (i.e. the two events happened around the same time but were not cause and effect). One journalist suggested that it would also be possible to link wearing of shoes to apparent onset of autism since both those events tend to happen around age 1 year. Ultimately Andrew Wakefield was removed from the medical register because of concerns about his research, in particular, regarding MMR and autism.

At around the same time public interest in autism increased and the diagnosis rate has risen exponentially. It has been very hard to quash the concern about MMR vaccination, mostly centred around the individual vaccines, and the capacity of a baby to cope with three antigens simultaneously – hence the vogue for requesting single antigen vaccines. In reality the immune system is designed to cope with many thousands of antigens at once, and the MMR vaccine provokes a better response when the three vaccines are given together rather than separately.

Consultation essentials

If you are going to answer this type of query you need to be clear about the facts, and be able to show and explain some of the science behind the facts. You also need to be able to explain probability. As with all medical interventions, there are risks and benefits. There is a genuine risk of adverse reaction to the MMR vaccine, notably with modified forms of the illnesses manifesting as fever and possibly a mild measles rash at about 14 days, and potentially mild parotid swelling at about 21 days. The child is not infectious during these events, and usually requires no more than antipyretic treatment. There is some reassurance if this response occurs when the child has been protected from the illness. This risk needs to be set against the risks of problems should the child contract the wild-type illness.

In the case of measles as an illness, there is approximately a 1 in 10 chance of complications, including croup, pneumonia, conductive or sensorineural deafness, encephalopathy and subacute sclerosing panencephalitis (a degenerative disorder similar to Creutzfeldt–Jakob disease). The risk of encephalopathy is 1 in 500 and the risk of death was 1 in 5000 when measles was common in the UK. The risks are more severe for immunosuppressed children.

Mumps can cause sensorineural deafness, viral encephalitis and is well known as a cause of male, and female, infertility.

Rubella's main risk is to the fetus: variable congenital abnormalities can be caused depending on the time of gestation when the mother contracts the illness. The purpose of immunising the entire population (rather than just immunising women) is to improve herd immunity to rubella.

The difficulty in explaining relative risk is that the possibility of a complication depends not only on the risks outlined above, but also the risk of contracting the disease when some of the population is immunised. Current immunisation rates in the UK remain below target levels (currently around 90% with a target of 95%) and there continue to be outbreaks of all three diseases. During 2011 the incidence of measles rose significantly with a wide age range affected (mainly individuals who were unimmunised because of parental fears).

The scientific evidence is clear that the balance of risk is very strongly in favour of immunisation.

Suggested discussion points

- Cover the facts, as above, on the risks of the diseases and the relative lack of risk of the vaccine. This should include the fact that cases of measles are currently on the increase.
- Discuss the issue (if raised) of single vaccines. These are not licensed and not available on the NHS. The supplies are not reliable and they are not subject to the same level of quality control as the licensed vaccines. There may be questions about 'cold chain' reliability, i.e. appropriate storage from manufacture to delivery. Additionally, vaccines tend to be less effective when given separately because seroconversion rates are lower. Also, the child will require three separate injections (and ultimately six if the parents want separate vaccines for the second dose too). There is no reliable data about the timing of the separate vaccines and how to space them.
- Discuss issues related to the second immunisation, given around the time of pre-school boosters. This is not a true 'booster'. It gives a second chance for seroconversion for those who did not convert with the first dose (about 10% of children for each component). However, it is not recommended to use blood tests to check immunity because of the additional intervention required, and the cost. All three components would require testing because response to one component does not guarantee response to all. Most labs are set up to test for recent illness rather than the low levels of antibodies present after immunisation, and therefore a false negative result is possible.

Follow up and discussion

Some parents can be persuaded, if their fears are taken seriously and a clear explanation has been given. However, for those who are not swayed immediately, it is worth remembering that there is no upper age limit for MMR immunisation and it is better to immunise late than never. Some parents may be willing to reconsider immunisation when their child is a little older and language development is well established. This compromise should not be seen as a concession to the argument for a link between MMR and autism, but as a pragmatic solution towards increasing immunisation rates. Some parents will be reassured by offering to perform the vaccination in hospital but this cannot be a solution offered to everyone. The follow up can usually be left between the family and the family doctor.

Further reading

Salisbury et al. Department of Health. Immunisation against infectious disease (The Green Book). 2006. www.gov.uk

Wakefield AJ, Murch SH, Anthony A, et al. Ileal lymphoid nodular hyperplasia, non-specific colitis, and pervasive developmental disorder in children [retracted]. Lancet 1998; 351:637–641.

Patient information

NHS Choices website www.nhs.uk

Case 47

Multiple unexplained symptoms

Dear Paediatrician,

Thank you for seeing Theadora. She is 14 years old and complains of a number of perplexing symptoms which have been present for the last 18 months. These include worsening nausea with occasional difficulty swallowing, frequent headaches and numbness on either side of her body. At these times she says that her limbs feel 'too heavy to move.' Recently, she has also mentioned that her vision is abnormal and she sees things changing size.

I suspect that these symptoms have a psychological basis but Theadora says that she is very happy at home, and has good friends at school. Surprisingly, despite her symptoms she is only missing 1 or 2 days of school a week. Despite my frequent reassurances that these symptoms are unlikely to be organic, the family feel that they would like her to be fully investigated. Routine blood tests including full blood count, urea & electrolytes, liver function, thyroid function, antinuclear antibody, erythrocyte sedimentation rate, C-reactive protein and coeliac screen have all been normal.

Her family are very concerned, and mum has had to give up her job as an accountant because of Theadora's problems.

Dr Julian Large

Case analysis

This is a difficult presentation of multiple unexplained symptoms. There are a number of challenges, which need to be addressed.

- Are these all one presentation or could there be multiple problems? For example, some of her symptoms sound like migraines, but migraine would not explain everything.
- Which, if any, of the symptoms may have an 'organic' basis? This is always challenging. There is always one obscure organic condition which might present, atypically in this way, and it would be embarrassing to overlook this. This can lead to only considering anxiety or conversion disorder as a diagnosis of exclusion, rather than using the positive symptoms and signs which can eliminate or reduce the need for investigations.
- Understanding the child's and family's agenda. In some situations, they may expect a miracle cure; they might alternatively be seeking permission to remain in the sick role. Despite the general practitioner's suggestions and the normal blood tests, the family have not embraced the diagnosis of a conversion disorder. This could be that they do not understand it, or maybe they are worried that there is a sinister underlying diagnosis.
- The impact on the family can be great, but as in other chronic conditions in which the family may be 'fighting or fuelling' the condition. It is not clear why the mother has given up work, and what gains there may be from this.
- People who can psychologise don't need to somatise, or if you have to somatise you will respond less well to psychology.

Differential diagnosis

Conversion disorder

A conversion disorder is characterised by the occurrence of symptoms and/or signs which are inexplicable anatomically or pathophysiologically. They are different from fabrication in that the patient usually has no control over them. Conversion disorders most commonly start in adolescence, but can start much earlier. Although they are often triggered by anxiety, the patient's level of anxiety usually falls after the onset of physical symptoms, because the symptoms may act as a distraction, or permit removal from the anxiety-generating situation, e.g. school.

Many of the symptoms described could be part of an organic illness, and it can be hard to establish which symptoms may be organic. For example, Theadora's dysphagia maybe due to 'globus hystericus', or she may have syringobulbia or achalasia. Her neurological symptoms could be due to partial seizures or transient ischaemic attacks, and her insistence that she is not suffering from anxiety, and the only thing that would make her happier would be finding the medical treatment for her ailments (which she suspects are serious) can lead to multiple investigations and referrals to other teams.

It is best to make a positive diagnosis of conversion disorder as soon as possible, because the longer it goes unchecked the more established it becomes, and the more difficult it is to treat. There are many advantages to completing all necessary investigations quickly and moving on to the correct diagnosis. It is often difficult for families to make the transition to a diagnosis of conversion disorder. What investigations are necessary may have to be negotiated. Some families may feel that the examination and explanation is enough, or they may insist on further tests.

Think how to explain the symptoms. It is important to acknowledge them and not say they are 'made up' or 'false'. Describing conversion disorders is difficult. There are many helpful analogies. These include suggesting that it is a 'software' rather than 'hardware' problem, where a normal brain is overloaded and has difficulty reading and sending signals. Extending the analogy, in this situation, the person to mend the problem is a software engineer. In human terms this is usually a psychologist.

Alternatively, 'The best way to get you better is for you to see somebody who can help with the way that your body and brain work together, for example in athletics, the best athletes aren't necessarily the ones that can run the fastest – they are often the ones with the best psychologist.' Occasionally, it is worth suggesting that all of the symptoms can evaporate in the same way that they arrived.

Persuading families to engage with psychology help can be difficult. Often a more multidisciplinary approach is required, including physiotherapy and education. From the GP's letter it is easy to underplay the level of school absence, which is actually significant. This level of absence is likely to impact seriously on her educational and social achievement. It is also quite likely that things have become worse recently – hence the referral – and her school attendance may have dropped further.

In Theadora's situation any other diagnosis is unlikely, though sometimes there are some underlying organic symptoms which become amplified.

Other conditions

There is always a vast differential diagnosis. And this creates the dilemma as to how many investigations and referrals are necessary. It is almost unheard of for epilepsy or brain tumours to present in this way without there being other symptoms and signs. Rare metabolic conditions are rare – and although some may present in adolescence, they would usually present earlier. Her symptoms seem fairly specific and the fact that she reports normal social functioning with family and friends makes early onset psychosis unlikely.

Consultation essentials

History/examination

Documenting all the symptoms and their progression is often a complicated process. Examination should focus on trying to establish if there may be an organic cause for the symptoms. In some cases, this will be clear, e.g. neurological signs that have no anatomical basis; in other situations it may be less clear, for example, nausea may have some associated epigastric pain.

Tests/investigations

It is impossible to make progress until the family are happy that physical causes have been excluded. In extreme cases, this can be very challenging, and an unwillingness to acknowledge the psychological component to illness might need to be addressed by a joint meeting with the Child and Adolescent Mental Health Service (CAMHS), and occasionally will become a safeguarding issue. The longer it takes to complete physical investigations, the more ingrained the behaviour and symptoms become, so it is important to carry out any tests as soon as possible.

Ask the family what physical conditions they are worried about, and make sure the explanation or investigations address these.

Diagnosis

Theadora has classic features of a conversion disorder. She did have symptoms of oesophagitis and was given ranitidine. As this did not improve her symptoms, it was stopped after 6 weeks.

Management

Theadora should be referred to CAMHS and physiotherapy – the family may resist this and the ensuing discussion may be difficult. The use of medication should be resisted. Occasionally, it might seem sensible to engage in a therapeutic trial of medication, and in this instance set clear guidelines and goalposts and do not give unhelpful medication for too long.

Any medication may have a placebo effect, or more commonly a semi-placebo effect. This means that some symptoms will improve a bit. The implication from this is that the symptoms are organic and just finding the right medicine will make them all go away. A common suggestion is that if the 'physical symptoms' improve then the patient will return to normal functioning. Actually it is returning to normal functioning which is most likely to alleviate the symptoms.

Follow up

It is likely that the family will want medical follow up. This is a double-edged sword. Whilst the medical input may aid 'recovery with honour', it may discourage engagement with CAMHS.

Discussion

Working with families in this situation is often complicated. It is essential to use language which is supportive and does not belittle the family or the symptoms, which need to be fully acknowledged. For most families recovery is a hard process. This is because they may have to confront difficult issues at home or school. Many children who are abused may present with conversion disorders, but frequently only disclose the abuse many years later. This, however, does not mean that every child with a conversion disorder is being abused. Abuse usually presents with a disclosure. Whilst children should always be given the opportunity to disclose, if they deny any concerns this denial should be respected.

Further reading

Griffin A, Christie D. Taking the psycho out of psychosomatic: using systemic approaches in a paediatric setting for the treatment of adolescents with unexplained physical symptoms. Clin Child Psychol Psychiatry 2008; 13:531–542.

Hardwick P. Engaging families who hold strong medical beliefs in a psychosomatic approach. Clin Child Psychol Psychiatry 2005; 10:601–616.

Kozlowska K. The developmental origins of conversion disorders. Clin Child Psychology and Psychiatry 2007; 12(4):487–510.

Case 48

Neonatal follow up

Dear Paediatrician,

Please could you arrange local follow up for Clara who was born prematurely whilst the family were on holiday in Portugal. She was born at 26 weeks' gestation weighing just 540 g and was airlifted to the regional hospital in Lisbon. There is a full summary, in Portuguese, of her stay on the neonatal unit, of which the family have a copy.

The family have explained that she had a brain haemorrhage which was 'not very serious'. She was ventilated for 1 month and received oxygen for a further 2 months. She was discharged as soon as her condition allowed, so the family could get back home. They understand she needs an eye examination and she did not pass a hearing test but overall are relaxed as she seems to be feeding and growing well. They have also had one previous preterm infant who has done very well.

Yours sincerely,

Dr Ayokunle Ogungbemi

Case analysis

Clara is an extremely low birth weight, extremely preterm infant. She is likely to have had a difficult period soon after birth, including postnatal transfer. She had a prolonged period of ventilation and has chronic lung disease; all factors that put her into the highest risk group for later adverse neurodevelopmental outcome. The fact that she has not passed a hearing assessment raises the possibility of hearing loss, and retinopathy of prematurity has not been excluded. These are both significant co-morbid factors.

She needs a planned schedule for long-term monitoring as well as simultaneous referrals to the local audiology and ophthalmology services for early evaluation.

Although policies may vary between centres, most will have a plan for following up babies discharged from the neonatal intensive care unit (NICU), such as the one below. The main aims of neonatal follow up are to:
- Assess developmental outcome
- Identify and manage medical needs
- Offer support to families

Developmental outcome

Because this group of babies are at an increased risk of long-term developmental issues, neonatal follow up might be considered to be 'heightened surveillance'. Obviously, as soon as any problems are found then referrals to appropriate teams are required, e.g. community paediatricians, physiotherapists, etc.

Parents are generally poorly informed on the risks and outcomes for their premature child. There is a great reliance on the presence or absence of structural brain lesions in how parents are counselled – that reliance may be misplaced. There are increasing reports of cerebral palsy in children, particularly those born very prematurely, with normal ultrasound scans. There is also increasing evidence that even babies born a few weeks prematurely are at an increased risk of neurodevelopmental problems, compared to babies born at term.

Predicting long-term outcome is complicated by the fact that a proportion of infants will develop transient patterns of neurologic abnormality that may require intervention but resolve over the first few years of life.

It is also important to keep things in perspective, as the vast majority of neonatal graduates will be normal, or have such minor issues that they will function completely normally.

Discussing outcome is challenging and it can be hard to strike the right balance. Parents invariably want to be told the truth, and may struggle with the uncertainty inherent in trying to predict the future. Whilst it is wrong to give false hope, parents don't always want to be told the worst possible scenario. There are limits to medical prediction skills, and the most important measure is how the baby is actually doing. Parents should understand that the aim of surveillance is the early detection of any problems, and not to confirm normality. However, if problems are not detected, the more likely their baby will be normal. National data is now available for disability rates at 30 months of age in extremely premature infants and other regional and international data on disability rates exist which should help inform the discussion. In some centres, this will form part of a wider research programme into neonatal outcome.

Managing medical needs

Babies who have been admitted to NICU will have an increased number of medical issues and there can be long-term consequences of prematurity itself, such as chronic lung disease.

Support

The neonatal course is often a stormy one; parents may need additional reassurance in the first few years of life.

Follow-up programme

Not all babies need follow up from the neonatal unit. Each unit will have their own criteria. Babies listed in **Table 48.1** should receive some follow up. Their first appointment is usually about 6–12 weeks post discharge.

All infants born at < 30 weeks' gestation should be referred to the physiotherapist covering NICU as soon as their clinical condition allows. A separate physio follow up intervention programme may be set up for them post discharge.

Babies may need a number of appointments. The following tables provide a checklist for the timing and essential content of these appointments.

Table 48.1 Common reasons for follow up after admission to a neonatal unit
• All infants < 32 weeks' gestation at birth
• Twins < 34 weeks at birth
• Infants with abnormal cranial ultrasounds or MRI
• Term infants (to include the late preterm infant) who have had severe illness, e.g.
– Persistent pulmonary hypertension of the newborn
– Perinatal asphyxia + cooling therapy
– Severe haemolytic disease of the newborn
– Significant congenital anomalies
– Encephalopathy + abnormal scans

First clinic follow-up visit (Table 48.2)

- 8 weeks corrected gestation for infants discharged after 35 weeks' gestational age
- 3 months of age for 'term' infants
- Term corrected for those infants discharged before 35 weeks' gestational age

Table 48.2 First neonatal follow-up visit: what to do	
Issue	Action
Hearing	Ensure has been checked and decide on whether this needs on-going follow up or can be removed from the active problem list
Retinopathy of prematurity screen	Ensure complete (if applicable) and decide on whether this needs on-going follow up or can be removed from the active problem list
Immunisations	Have they started or are they continuing. Stress importance of completion plus advice on flu or respiratory syncytial virus vaccine if appropriate
Discharge medications	Advising on change in dosage, when to stop, etc. for example, iron supplements can be stopped when fully weaned
Feeding	Think about intolerance, constipation, reflux, colic, etc. and plot growth parameters looking for early signs of suboptimal growth
Physical examination	Examine hips for developmental dysplasia, check for hernias, assess tone and posture; both passive and active, record reproducible parameters – popliteal angles, adductor angles, stretch at achilles, scarf sign, shoulder retraction, etc.
Cot death prevention	Back to sleep/feet to feet/smoking/ co-sleeping
Explain neurodevelopmental follow-up schedule	Stress early detection of neurodisability as opposed to confirmation of normality
Parental concerns	Ensure any concerns are addressed
Referrals	Make these as and when necessary

Second clinic follow-up visit (Table 48.3)

- 16 weeks corrected gestation for preterm infant
- 6 months of age for 'term' infant

Table 48.3 Second neonatal follow-up visit: what to do	
Issue	**Action**
Feeding	Should make an easy transition to spoon feeding
Growth	Measure and plot growth parameters and consider stopping preterm formula – usually at the time of weaning
Development	Assess developmental progress, especially social , verbal /non-verbal interaction
Physical examination	Perform a clinical examination which should focus on neurodevelopment – limb/truncal tone and posture, sequencing/transitional movements to rolling, abolition of premature reflexes; recordings of reproducible parameters
Parental concerns	Ensure any concerns are addressed
Referrals	Make these as and when necessary

Third clinic follow-up visit (Table 48.4)

- At 8 months corrected for preterm infants
- Omit for 'term' infants

Table 48.4 Third neonatal follow-up visit: what to do	
Issue	**Action**
Growth	Measure and plot growth parameters
Development	Assess developmental progress to include social/language/exploratory skills
Physical examination	Perform a clinical examination which should focus on neurodevelopment – limb/truncal tone and posture, sequencing/transition movements: prone to sitting to all fours, commando moves, saving reflexes, etc.
Parental concerns	Ensure any concerns are addressed. Any developmental concerns at this stage should prompt a multidisciplinary assessment request

Fourth clinic follow-up visit (Table 48.5)

- at 12 months corrected

Table 48.5 Fourth neonatal follow-up consultant visit: what to do	
Issue	**Action**
Growth	Measure and plot growth parameters
Development	Assess developmental to include social/language/exploratory skills
Physical examination	Examination is largely observational looking at motor development/ function – gross and fine – best done on the floor with suitable variety of toys and stimulation. Any abnormalities e.g. toe walking should prompt careful physical examination and referral if any abnormalities detected
Parental concerns	Ensure any concerns are addressed. Any concerns at this stage should prompt a multidisciplinary assessment request

Optional visit at 16 months (if previous concerns have been raised)

Clinic essentials:
- review general progress

Fifth clinic follow-up visit

- At 21 months corrected

Clinic essentials:
- Review general progress
- Speech and language development – specific assessment

Six clinic follow-up visit

- 30 months of age

Clinic essentials:
- Perform developmental assessment using standard assessment tool, e.g. Bailey II.
- Discharge from clinic at this stage, ensuring community follow up if required.

Patient information

The March of Dimes
> www.marchofdimes.com

Tommy's campaign
> www.tommys.org.uk

Bliss
> www.bliss.org.uk

Nocturnal enuresis

Dear Paediatrician,

Thank you for seeing Harvey, who is now 9 years old. He has nocturnal enuresis and is wetting the bed every night. He has had the occasional dry night, the last one was about 3 months ago.

He is a very sensible boy from a good family, who have tried to be as helpful as possible. He tried some desmopressin a few years ago, but this did not really help. He is due to go to cub camp in a few months time and is keen to be dry for this.

Dr Simon Kopelowitz

Case analysis

This is a straightforward referral, the diagnosis of nocturnal enuresis (NE) has been made and the request is about management. As far as classification is concerned this is a primary nocturnal enuresis as he has not had a significant period of dryness. The presence of other symptoms, notably daytime symptoms, determines whether this is monosymptomatic (no other symptoms) or polysymptomatic.

Differential diagnosis

Nocturnal enuresis can be multifactorial. There may be specific contributory factors such as constipation and bladder overactivity, but there is some overlap and it is helpful to take a more holistic approach.

Primary nocturnal enuresis

Given the description, it is difficult to make any other diagnosis. In the absence of other symptoms no other diagnosis comes into question.

There are three cardinal messages for the patient:
1. It is not your fault
2. You are not alone
3. It will get better

Being dry at night is a developmental rather than a behavioural skill. That is, different people will attain dryness at different times (**Table 49.1**). The 'three systems approach' is a popular way of explaining what factors, which may coexist, determine being wet or dry overnight. These are:
1. Overnight urine production
2. Bladder volume and activity
3. Rousability – the bladder and the brain talking to each other

Table 49.1 Proportion of children with enuresis at different ages	
Age (years)	Number of children bedwetting
5	1 in 6
7	1 in 10
10	1 in 15
18	1 in 100
Caveat: enuresis is variably described from those who wet every night, to those who wet every few months.	

Constipation, partly because of its effect on bladder function, can be considered the fourth system, and it is hard to treat any urinary tract problem in the presence of constipation. It is essential to assess and address any constipation/stool withholding.

Aim to reduce overnight urine production as much as possible by avoiding caffeine, and stopping drinks for 1 or 2 hours before bedtime (there are some clinics that encourage later drinking but this seems counterintuitive at best). The bladder should be empty before sleeping, by making sure the child has passed urine before going to bed.

It is hard to change rousability, but some children may wake, and go back to sleep again.

Although some families want reassurance or a discussion of options, they may also want some treatment.

Lifting

This entails waking the child every night and taking them to the toilet. Clearly, this is not a cure for NE and will not speed up the time to natural dryness. However, neither does medication. Therefore, many families will opt for lifting if it works, rather than medication, as the interim measure. Ideally, the time of lifting should be gradually brought closer to the child's bed time.

Alarms

It is not clear how or why these work, but they certainly do have some success. They require perseverance and dedication, which can be hard for the families involved. The National Institute for Health and Care Excellence guidelines recommend alarms as first line treatment. Because in the UK they are not available on prescription, patients have to get these from enuresis clinics which are run by school nurses. Families may choose to purchase the alarms themselves as they are now available relatively cheaply - especially through internet sites. As a result, paediatricians will tend to see families who have either not responded to the alarm or not wanted to try it.

Medication

The two main medications are desmopressin (antidiuretic hormone) and antimuscarinics such as oxybutinin. It is usual to start with desmopressin. If desmopressin does not work at normal doses, then adding in oxybutinin is more likely to be successful than increasing the desmopressin. If there are prominent symptoms of overactive bladder, consider starting with oxybutinin alone.

Diabetes (insipidus or mellitius)

These present with polydipsia and polyuria, not just nocturnal enuresis. They are more likely to be a cause of secondary, rather than primary enuresis.

Spinal or urogential abnormalities

Underlying anatomical problems such as these are unlikely, especially in this case as he has had some, albeit only a few, dry nights. These problems would generally present with continuous dribbling of urine.

Consultation essentials

History/examination

In order to establish where the problem lies, and hence what the most effective treatment may be, there are a number of areas that need elucidation. This may be readily available from the history, although it is not unusual for patients not to know the answers. In which case, ask them to report back.

Primarily establish if there are other symptoms, notably daytime symptoms suggestive of bladder overactivity, namely frequency, urgency and wetting. Some children control this by severely restricting drinks, but when they drink freely they are noted to produce frequent, small wees.

Try to see if there is a pattern to the occasional dryness, what happens differently on dry and wet nights – most often families are unaware of any differences.

Take a drinking and urinating history of an average day focussing on when drinking occurs, what is being drunk and when, and how often the child needs to go to the toilet. Ask specifically about constipation.

Enquire about night-time routine, when the last drink is taken and when the child goes to the toilet.

Once asleep does the child ever rouse? This needs to be addressed specifically to the child, as parents are likely to be unaware of points during the night when their child rouses. If they do rouse what might prevent them going to the toilet? They may be scared of the dark. Providing a torch, night light (or light sabre) may help with this.

Establishing a family history of delayed dryness is of theoretical value, but also may offer some comfort to the child, that others in the family had the same problem.

It is easy to overplay the psychological factors in enuresis. Most anxious children do not wet the bed and children who wet the bed are no more anxious than those that don't. In a few children there will be a clear emotional factor to the bedwetting, but it is practically unheard of for bedwetting to be the presenting feature. Similarly, sexual abuse presents with disclosure. There is no evidence that bedwetting will reveal hidden abuse any more than asthma would.

There is little specific need in performing an examination. It often provides such limited information, that the need for genital and anal examination must be seriously questioned, particularly in those children that are reticent to be examined.

Tests/investigations

Measurements

The overactive bladder is often overlooked. Measuring urine volumes over a few days is instructive:

Expected bladder volume = $(Age+2) \times 30$ mL

Or $(Age+2) \times$ Fl oz

Volumes consistently below those predicted are highly suggestive of overactive bladder. Children may enjoy the challenge of measuring their urine in a jug.

Urine testing

Testing urine is of limited value. Many children have already had urine tested for infection. Diabetes mellitus or insipidus should be evident from the history.

Renal ultrasound scan

A urinary tract ultrasound can be useful if there is uncertainty. It can be used to assess bladder volume and emptying, but is probably less valuable than actually measuring the urine voided.

Diagnosis

Harvey had some daytime symptoms, and so has primary polysymptomatic nocturnal enuresis.

Management

The use of an alarm was offered but was felt to be inappropriate for the family circumstances. Simple measures were introduced which were ineffective, so Harvey started medication. He became essentially dry on a combination of oxybutinin and desmopressin. As regards the cub camp Harvey and his family found information on the Education and Resources for Improving Childhood Continence (ERIC) website such as pinning pull ups into 'disposable' pyjama trousers. He was wary of taking medication in front of his friends, so was advised that if asked he could say that he was on antibiotics.

If the medication is completely unsuccessful, it can be retried after 3–6 months – when the child's body has become a bit closer to being naturally dry. If it is partially effective, consider if the gain is worth the medication. If it is completely effective it can be continued for 3–6 months and then weaned to see if the child has become naturally dry. If the wetting resumes, so can the medication. Do not stop medication prior to an important event such as cub camp.

Follow up

Follow up largely depends on the treatment option chosen. Follow up after a few months is usually appreciated. Certainly some contact should be made before cub camp to ensure that he is prepared.

Discussion

Because bedwetting is developmental rather than behavioural, behavioural approaches are unlikely to work. There may be a small behavioural component so behavioural approaches may be worth trying for a few days, but should not be done for longer, as this may worsen the situation. This would include the use of star charts for dryness and removing the pull ups (star charts can be used to encourage appropriate behaviour such as proper drinking, weeing and taking medication). Needless to say, punishment for bedwetting is entirely unacceptable. Involving the child in changing wet sheets can be done to inculcate responsibility, but should not be seen as a consequence for wetting.

Similarly removing the pull-ups is a common suggestion, the idea being that the wetting would stop if the child felt the wet. Whilst this may work occasionally, it would do so in the first few nights. If it is not effective, then the increased in discomfort and washing is detrimental to both the child and the parents.

There are a number of considerations in treating NE. Clearly, the aim of treatment is dryness, but if this is achieved at the cost of frequent waking and consequent daytime drowsiness, there is little real benefit. Similarly if daytime symptoms are as disabling, or more so, than the night-time symptoms, then both need addressing.

Even with maximal treatment the child may not attain total dryness, but might be dry enough to 'make a difference', e.g. if the urine is contained within the 'pull up' as opposed to soaking the bed that may be an improvement worth having.

The investigation and management of secondary nocturnal enuresis is essentially similar to that for primary nocturnal enuresis.

Further reading

National Institute for Health and Care Excellence. Nocturnal enuresis – the management of bedwetting in children and young people. Clinical Guideline 111, 2010.
www.nice.org.uk/guidance/cg111

Patient information

Education and Resources for Improving Childhood Continence (ERIC)
www.eric.org.uk.

Noisy breathing

Dear Paediatrician,

Thank you for seeing this 3-week-old boy whose parents are worried because he makes a loud noise when breathing. This noise is getting louder over time and increasing in frequency.

He seems to be well in between episodes and is breastfeeding normally.

Dr Kenneth Rider

Case analysis

It is important to make clear what is meant when a patient is referred for noisy breathing. 'Stridor' is a high-pitched sound that in the early stages sounds like breathing-in whilst phonating (adducting the vocal cords), but in advanced stages the phonatory quality disappears to be replaced by a more whispery quality. It usually emanates from the larynx and is inspiratory but may also emanate from the trachea and be biphasic or expiratory. 'Stertor' is a low-pitched or throaty respiratory noise. It usually emanates from the oropharynx.

Noisy breathing in children can present both as urgent and as non-urgent referrals. Urgent referrals are usually for inflammatory (largely infective) conditions, or an inhaled foreign body. Nonurgent referrals can be due to a wide variety of conditions, depending on the nature of the noisy breathing. Referrals very early in life are, in the large majority, due to congenital pathologies.

Since the era of the haemophilus influenzae B vaccine the incidence of paediatric epiglottitis has plummeted. Acute laryngotracheobronchitis (croup) and throat infections (e.g. tonsillitis, quinsy and glandular fever) remain acute causes of upper respiratory noisy breathing, alongside conditions such as diphtheria and whooping cough. Non-urgent referrals early in life may be due to congenital pathologies. By far the commonest congenital pathology is laryngomalacia, but other diagnoses must not be missed. Later in childhood common causes of noisy breathing are enlarged tonsils or adenoids and nasal obstruction.

Differential diagnosis

Laryngomalacia

This is the commonest cause of stridor in neonates and infants. In-drawing of floppy supraglottic structures on inspiration causing intermittent stridor that presents within weeks of birth. The stridor is worse on feeding, crying and when lying supine. Cry and voice are otherwise normal. It is usually self-limiting by 2 years of age. It may, uncommonly, require surgical intervention.

Recurrent laryngeal nerve palsy

This is idiopathic, or due to birth trauma or Arnold–Chiari malformation. Bilateral palsies present with inspiratory stridor. Unilateral palsies present with a weak voice. It rarely requires tracheostomy and when no specific treatable cause is found, it usually recovers spontaneously by early childhood.

Subglottic stenosis

Congenital subglottic stenosis is quite a common cause of neonatal stridor due to incomplete recanalisation. It presents in neonates but often only after an upper respiratory tract infection (URTI). Often there is biphasic stridor. It may require surgical management. Acquired subglottic stenosis occurs post-intubation but is less common with modern endotracheal tubes.

Vascular rings

A vascular ring causes noisy breathing due to external compression of trachea due to a vascular anomaly, e.g. double aortic arch. It presents with biphasic stridor and may cause secondary tracheomalacia. It can require surgical intervention.

Laryngeal papillomatosis

Pailomatosis of the larynx is a common cause of hoarseness in children. It may cause inspiratory or biphasic stridor. It is caused by maternal genital HPV type 6 and 11 infections. It usually spontaneously regresses but can require surgical intervention.

Neoplasm

The commonest neoplastic cause of noisy breathing in children is haemangioma. Laryngeal haemangiomata are usually subglottic. They present within the first few months of life with inspiratory or biphasic stridor which is worse with crying. Associated cutaneous haemangiomata are common. They often spontaneously involute in early childhood.

Congenital laryngeal web

Laryngeal webs are usually anteriorly based and at the level of the glottis so cause an abnormal cry or voice. If symptoms are significant they may require surgical intervention.

Laryngeal cleft and fistula

Rarely, the posterior cricoid lamina does not fuse or tracheoesophageal septum does not develop. This presents with inspiratory stridor, cyanosis, coughing or aspiration.

Acute larynotracheobronchitis or croup

Croup is the commonest cause of stridor in children and is usually viral, e.g. parainfluenza. It presents in very small children during cold months. There is gradual onset, harsh or barking cough and hoarse voice, moderate fever, no drooling or dysphagia and inspiratory or biphasic stridor. It is self-limiting with supportive treatment. Oral steroids have been shown to be of benefit.

Epiglottitis

This is much less common since haemophilus influenzae B vaccine. It usually presents in young children between 2 and 7 years of age. It is characterised by rapid onset, absence of cough, normal voice, high fever, drooling and dysphagia with soft inspiratory stridor. It is a medical emergency and requires urgent intubation, antibiotics and steroids. An ENT senior doctor must be present when there is a risk of critical airway narrowing.

Foreign body

Most upper aerodigestive foreign bodies causing noisy breathing remain in the oropharynx and cause stertor. Only small foreign bodies can pass into the larynx to then cause inspiratory stridor if caught at laryngeal level or an expiratory wheeze, segmental collapse and pneumonia if inhaled into the bronchi.

Stertor

A variety of conditions and situations may cause stertor including tonsillar hypertrophy, macroglossia, craniofacial abnormalities and oropharyngeal infections.

Nasal causes

Narrowing of the nasal passages due to, e.g. rhinitis, polyps or foreign body, and adenoidal hypertrophy may be a cause of noisy breathing through the nose or constant mouth-breathing.

Consultation essentials

History/examination

Firstly, clarify what is meant by noisy breathing. Determine the quality of the sound and whether it occurs on inspiration, expiration or both. It is also most important to get a feel for the effect the cause of the noisy breathing may be having on the child. For example if it is associated with shortness of breath, poor feeding, failure-to-thrive or even cyanosis. Other features to look out for in the history are an abnormal cry, body position, coughing, recurrent chest infections, snoring and other sleep-related obstructive breathing symptoms. Asking the parents to do an impression of the noise or record an audio clip or video of it (most mobile phones can do this) can be very helpful.

It is not always possible to listen to the sound that the child is making but this can sometimes be heard if the child cries. Examination should be made, e.g. for any signs of increased respiratory effort, craniofacial abnormalities, masses in the head or neck and changes in thoracic shape. Auscultation to detect the quality or level of the noisy breathing can be helpful.

Tests/investigations

In the uncomplicated case these are not necessary. Where clinically indicated, plain neck and chest radiographs, contrast swallow, CT or MRI, angiography, pulse oximetry, allergy tests and sleep studies may be helpful. Where symptoms and signs raise concerns, microlaryngoscopy and bronchoscopy may be indicated.

Diagnosis

In view of the age of presentation, the presenting complaint and the lack of worrying associated features, the working diagnosis here would be laryngomalacia.

Management

The family were reassured that as the baby was quite well and not at all distressed during the episodes, or apparently suffering any more generalised ill-effects, a wait-and-watch policy should be adopted. It was also explained to them that the likelihood was that the symptoms would improve spontaneously in time. If there are any concerns, a referral to ENT should be made.

Follow up

Review should normally be arranged, e.g. in 8 weeks' time. This is partly to ensure that there has been no deterioration, so that the working diagnosis is still consistent with the clinical picture, and partly to reassure parents, who will naturally be anxious, that whilst there has been no improvement, the clinical course is as expected and stable.

Discussion

The causes of noisy breathing in children are many and varied. A careful history should be taken to define what is meant by noisy breathing and the effects the condition has on the child. The objective is to distinguish the many children with benign, self-limiting causes who can be reassured and observed, from those who may require more active intervention and onward referral.

Further reading

Friedman EM, Vastola AP, McGill TJ, Healy GB. Chronic pediatric stridor: etiology and outcome. Laryngoscope, 1990; 100(3):277–280.
Halpin LJL, Anderson CL, Corriette N. Stridor in children. BMJ 2010; 340:c2193.
Maloney E, Meakin G. Acute stridor in children. Contin Educ Anaesth Crit Care Pain 2007; 7(6):183–186.

Patient information

Patient.co.uk
   www.patient.co.uk

Case 51

Obesity

Dear Paediatrician,

Please could you see Eileen, she is 11 years old, and about to enter secondary school. She is concerned about her weight, which is well above the 99th centile, despite a healthy diet and regular exercise. She is also quite tall for her age.

Dr Rachel Mann

Case analysis

Obesity is due to excess energy intake which is largely behavioural, although there are many societal factors such as food manufacture and retail which can encourage it. In general, a child who is relatively short and obese is more likely to have an underlying medical problem, whilst for one that is tall and obese the cause is almost certainly nutritional.

Obesity in wealthy populations is a problem of critical proportion, which is unfortunately often highly resistant to medical intervention. In many cases of obesity within wealthy populations, effective treatment will be a variation of 'do more and eat less'. This is likely to be most successful in the self-motivated families, who would then not seek medical advice. This implies that those who seek medical advice may be expecting somebody to 'cure' them, which is is less likely to be successful.

There are rare medical causes of obesity, and some genetic conditions have associated obesity. There are normally fairly obvious dysmorphic features to suggest these conditions.

Differential diagnosis

Nutritional

The overwhelming number of children with obesity will simply be eating more than they burn off. As mentioned above, this is a problem for the individual, for which society should take a lot of the blame.

Endocrine

Occasional endocrine causes of obesity would normally result in a child being relatively short. This includes Cushing's syndrome and hypothyroidism.

Drugs

Some drugs can cause considerable weight gain. The commonest culprits being oral steroids, pizotifen, sodium valproate and atypical antipsychotics.

Consultation essentials

History/examination

Identifying the onset of obesity can be helpful, in that children with medical conditions may have previously been slim. Obesity due to energy imbalance is often familial, and looking at the relatives can often help make the diagnosis. Many families will deny over eating, and overestimate the amount of exercise that is undertaken.

Ask if there is any suggestion of sleep apnoea, notably snoring loudly, interrupted breathing whilst asleep and poor quality sleep. If there is any doubt, overnight sleep studies should be arranged.

Accurate measurement of height and weight should be recorded and plotted on appropriate centile charts, along with a calculation of the body mass index (BMI). Blood pressure should be measured with an appropriate-sized cuff and plotted on blood pressure centile charts. The pattern of obesity should be noted. Marked central adiposity is associated with more cardiovascular co-morbidity. Upper body fat, or looking like a 'lemon on matchsticks' may suggest Cushing's syndrome.

Examine the skin. In any form of obesity, stretch marks (striae) are common and of no significance. The thickened velvety darkened skin of acanthosis nigricans is indicative of, but not particularly sensitive for, significant insulin resistance. It is usually seen first around the neck and in the axillae, but in severe cases may occur in all flexures. In hypothyroidism, the skin may be thickened and yellow, whilst in Cushing's syndrome there may be striae hirsutism and telangiectasia.

In the presence of any other problems such as dysmorphism, learning difficulty or deafness, genetic causes of obesity need to be considered.

Tests/investigations

In simple obesity, these are rarely required. If there is concern about an underlying cause, then appropriate tests should be performed, such as cortisol and thyroid function. The Obesity Services for Children and Adolescents Network Group have given suggested guidance on investigations.

There is no clear guidance as to which children should be routinely investigated for co-morbidity. Almost certainly a child whose BMI falls above three standard deviations from the mean would merit investigation. In this situation tests should include a fasting blood glucose and insulin test, with consideration for a glucose tolerance test. A full lipid profile should be organised and liver function tests carried out. If the alanine transaminase (ALT) is above 70 U/L then further investigations looking for non-alcoholic fatty liver disease, should be undertaken.

Diagnosis

Eileen's height is on the 75th centile which gives her a very high BMI, in the obese category. She does not exercise much, apart from PE at school, and eats many unhealthy snacks through the day.

Management

The theory of managing obesity is incredibly simple; yet implementing it is very hard.

The first challenge is for the child and family to recognise that there is a problem. There then follows a need to want to change and the determination to implement this. Trying to promote change in patients is always a challenge, and techniques of motivational interviewing are worth learning, as these have been known in many settings to improve the likelihood of change. The principles are simple, and involve using a guiding rather than directing style, developing strategies that elicit patients' motivation, and encouraging them to talk about change.

In some families there are simple misunderstandings and dietetic input may be useful. For example, many people believe that fruit drinks are healthy, whereas they actually are high in calories. You should be able to provide some motivation, but obviously it is the individual and family that need to carry on with this.

There are some, but too few, groups which focus on childhood weight loss and approach this from a multidisciplinary angle involving input from dieticians, psychologists and personal trainers.

Depending on the level of obesity, co-morbidities need to be assessed and managed. The most significant of these are:

- Hypertension: systolic or diastolic blood pressure ≥98th centile for age – remember to use an appropriate sized cuff
- Obstructive sleep apnoea
- Significant mobility or joint problems
- Abnormal glucose or insulin metabolism
- Acanthosis nigricans
- Dyslipidaemia
- Nonalcoholic fatty liver disease – if ALT >70 U/L
- Features suggestive of polycystic ovarian syndrome

It is rare in children to require medication or bariatric surgery, and these would only be undertaken in specialist centres.

Follow up

For simple obesity, no follow up is required, although offering appointments may act as a motivator. Any capability needs to be appropriately managed, and if the child continues to gain weight they may need to be reassessed for the development of co-morbidities.

Discussion

Unfortunately, the referral rate for obesity is increasing. Perhaps even more alarming are the number of obese children who do little or nothing to address the issue. Many obese patients fail to acknowledge the problem, either in denial or as a variant of body dysmorphism. On a population level, this has serious implications, but is also important in clinic, as many children presenting with medical problems will also be obese. It is important to be able to discuss this openly and compassionately.

Many parents will avoid the subject, perhaps hoping that it will go away. The children will usually be sensitive to it, and will often have suffered stigmatisation and bullying. Effective treatment is hard, and involves decreasing intake and increasing energy expenditure. Undertaking this in a group or as a family is most likely to be effective, although significant success remains elusive for many, and there is an urgent need for an effective weight loss programme for children.

Further reading

Rollnick S, Butler CC, et al. Motivational Interviewing. BMJ 2010; 340:c1900.
OSCA consensus statement on the assessment of obese children and adolescents for paediatricians. Obesity
    Services for Children and Adolescents (OSCA) Network Group, 2009.
www.rcpch.ac.uk

Patient information

Kids Health
    www.kidshealth.org
Healthier Generation
    www.healthiergeneration.org

Palpitations

Dear Paediatrician,

I would value your opinion on this 12-year-old boy who presented with short-lived episodes of palpitations lasting about 10 seconds. Some of these are associated with physical exertion, but he experienced some at rest while watching television. He has had these symptoms for about 4 years but only recently told his parents as they are now occurring monthly. His palpitations are not accompanied by any other symptoms apart from feeling slightly light-headed. He is an active sportsman involved in various sports, football in particular. I have suggested he avoid sports until you have seen him.

Dr Stella Verberne

Case analysis

Older children start to become aware of their own body and heart beat and may interpret this as worrying. In the overwhelming majority of cases there is no significant dysrhythmia. The prevailing benign nature of palpitations in older children does not mean that they do not represent a significant problem for the patients and their family.

Differential diagnosis

Normal

As children become aware of their bodies, they may feel their heart beating, especially after exercise, or when excited or stressed. Often when asked how fast their hearts are going the rate will be fast, but within the normal range.

Stress/anxiety

Psychological pressure and stress at home or at school can lead to a perception of an unusually fast heart beat, sometimes described as short-lived palpitations. It may also be a 'cry for help' from a stressed or anxious child, particularly in situations where there appears to be health anxiety.

Supraventricular tachycardia

This is the most common dysrhythmia present in older, otherwise healthy, children. In supraventricular tachycardia (SVT) the heart rate should be above 180 beats per minute in children over 1 year old (> 220 beats per minute in < 1 year old). The rate is similar in each episode, and asking patients to measure this during an episode is helpful. The recurrent and sometimes relatively frequent nature of palpitations associated with this diagnosis does not mean that they represent a threat to health or life in older children. There is often a family history, and this may reinforce the likelihood of SVT, but can also offer reassurance to the relatively benign nature.

SVTs are commonly short-lived and self-limiting in older children without any preceding symptoms. Given this, they usually cause little or limited cardiac compromise and so have few, if any, associated symptoms. Pallor, dizziness, loss of appetite or nausea, increased sweatiness, irritability are mostly associated with tachycardia lasting more than a few minutes, although their absence even in palpitations lasting longer than 30 minutes does not exclude the diagnosis, as severe compromise of cardiac output may not be present here. In younger children and neonates SVT may precipitate heart failure with all its accompanying signs and symptoms.

Whilst most patients with an SVT appear to have a structurally normal heart, they can also have associated congenital (e.g. atrioventricular septal defect, Ebstein's malformation of tricuspid valve) or acquired (e.g. hypertrophic cardiomyopathy, myocarditis) heart disease in childhood.

Ventricular tachycardia

This is very rare but highly significant. Even short-lived ventricular tachycardia may reduce cardiac output and blood supply to the brain causing light-headedness, blurred vision, headache, nausea, and loss of consciousness; alternatively the slower heart rate associated with ventricular tachycardia may be very well tolerated if short-lived and self-limiting.

Family history is often an important lead with early, unexpected or premature death in otherwise healthy family members raising the level of suspicion. The circumstances of such deaths are important, e.g. physical exertion, particularly swimming, immediately preceding death point at a significant risk for the referred child. Family history of long or short QT syndrome, Brugada syndrome, hypertrophic or dilated cardiomyopathy will guide further investigation, assessment, and referral. Patients with suspected ventricular tachycardia need immediate discussion with a paediatric cardiologist or paediatric electrophysiologist.

Metabolic causes

Thyrotoxicosis, hypoglycaemia or a sudden increase in circulating level of endogenous catecholamines (e.g. phaeochromocytoma) can cause palpitations which are more prolonged and are invariably a sinus tachycardia. The presence of other signs and symptoms should point to the diagnosis, which can then be appropriately managed.

Medication and substance overdose

Common culprits in this category include β-agonists taken for asthma, theophyllines, stimulants used to treat attention deficit hyperactivity disorder (e.g. methylphenidate) and caffeine-containing drinks consumed in large quantity. In older children alcohol and recreational drugs need to be considered. This list is not exhaustive and a drug history is essential. The pharmacopeia (e.g. BNF-C) or pharmacist can advise on whether particular drugs are associated with arrhythmias. If there is a link to a drug, then it may need to be withdrawn from the patient.

Consultation essentials

History/examination

Obviously, it is imperative to establish what is meant by palpitations – is this awareness of a normal or abnormal heart beat. Parents may feel that their child's heart is beating very fast, being unaware that this may be normal. If they have felt their child's heart beating previously, ask them to do this in clinic, to confirm that the presenting heart beat was different. Children or parents may be able to reproduce what the heart beat sounds like and they may be able to tap its rate on a desk. It is important to establish if there are any triggers to the onset of palpitations, any associated symptoms and how long they last for.

Ask about systemic features and about any medication or drugs taken, including dosage and the time interval between doses. Caffeine consumption should be established with a specific dietary history.

The family history should focus on the presence of any early onset of heart disease, sudden, early or unexpected death and the circumstances surrounding any such death if known. Often there will be a family member with a history of fast heart beat (supraventricular tachycardia and/or pre-excitation, long or short QT syndrome, Brugada syndrome, hypertrophic or dilated cardiomyopathy). Although families may not know specific details, ask about the treatment delivered or expected in close relatives. With the relatives' permission they may bring their information to subsequent appointments. If one family member has a significant arrhythmia it is important that any family member at risk is offered appropriate screening. This may require the affected person to discuss hereditability with their own cardiologist. Generally, each family member with abnormal cardiovascular signs may need to go to their general practitioner for a referral. Sometimes, the web spreads across not only generation, but also continents.

In the examination pay special attention to the cardiovascular system looking for any abnormal cardiovascular signs related to presence, quality, rate and regularity of pulse (auscultation of heart sounds with concomitant palpation of the pulse will test for a peripheral pulse deficit), peripheral perfusion, skin changes and oedema, the size of the liver, heart sounds and presence, or absence, of a murmur. This will be complemented by blood pressure measurement – right upper and one lower limb – and assessment of oxygen saturation.

Investigation

A 12-lead ECG is mandatory, although of limited benefit. Any abnormalities are clearly significant, but a normal one certainly does not exclude pathology. Remember to look at the P wave morphology, P wave and QRS complex axes, and PR interval (a short PR interval requires further investigation). Look specifically for the presence of delta waves, ventricular depolarisation (ST segment elevation in leads V1-3 in Brugada syndrome), and QT interval prolongation.

Recording of an ECG trace at the time of symptoms will be diagnostic. If the child has presented to hospital or the emergency services whilst symptomatic, obtaining any ECGs taken at this time is invaluable. If palpitations are happening frequently, asking the child or family to have an ECG at the time of palpitations may be practical, especially if the general practitioner surgery has an ECG machine.

If there is uncertainty, the child should be referred to a paediatric cardiologist who can consider the need for prolonged ECG monitoring with a symptom diary for 1–7 days. Given the relatively infrequent nature of palpitations mentioned in the above referral letter, a cardiac event recorder is more likely to provide an ECG trace at the time of symptoms. In selected cases implantation of a loop ECG recorder may be indicated following assessment, and extensive testing by a paediatric electrophysiologist. The symptoms and risk of the arrhythmia would need to be significant to merit this level of investigation. Formal exercise test is mandatory where symptoms are triggered by physical exertion and the patient is involved in competitive sporting activities.

An echocardiogram to assess cardiovascular anatomy and function and to exclude ventricular hypertrophy or dilatation may be helpful, particularly when there are symptoms of cardiac dysfunction, or audible murmurs. The decision to do an echocardiogram and the examination itself would usually be reserved for the paediatric cardiologist.

Diagnosis

This child's mother had Wolff–Parkinson–White syndrome and underwent radiofrequency ablation of an accessory pathway at the time of cardiac catheterisation 5 years ago. A 12-lead ECG of the patient revealed short PR interval with delta wave in lead V1. Subsequent cardiac event recorder showed short-lived (10–15 seconds) spells of SVT and Wolff–Parkinson–White syndrome.

Management

Short-lived and self-limiting episodes of supraventricular tachycardia without significant symptoms do not usually require a change of life style or treatment. When medication or caffeine-rich drinks exposure is suspected as the cause of palpitations, reducing or stopping medication (following consultation with the specialist overseeing its administration) and abstinence from caffeine are indicated, should symptoms cause considerable anxiety or discomfort. In cases where anxiety is a major factor, input from psychological services is helpful.

Follow up

Regular follow up in a paediatric cardiology outpatient clinic is advised to monitor the frequency and duration of symptoms and to exclude adverse effect of protracted and clinically silent episodes on myocardial function.

Discussion

The majority of short lived palpitations need little more than reassurance. If the ECG is normal and there are no associated symptoms, then watchful waiting, with an annual review is appropriate. In the unlikely event of a change of symptoms some safety netting is required, to allow referral to a paediatric electrophysiologist or cardiologist. Further cardiac investigations are best performed by the cardiologist, or after discussion with them.

Further reading

PACES/HRS expert consensus statement on the management of the asymptomatic young patient with a Wolff-Parkinson-White (WPW, ventricular pre-excitation) electrocardiographic pattern. Heart Rhythm 2012; 9(6):1006–10024.

Patient information

Wolff–Parkinson–White syndrome
    www.nhs.uk
KidsHealth
    www.kidshealth.org

Partial epilepsies

Dear Paediatrician,

This 5-year-old girl, Emily, who had pneumococcal meningitis as a toddler and subsequently some 'absence' attacks, has recently started a new type of attack. She looks shocked, she trembles, her pupils become uneven, she flushes red under her neck and around her jaw, then her tongue deviates, her head turns and her jaw deviates always to the left 'as if someone had a fishhook in her mouth'. This attack lasts from 10 seconds to 1 minute. She is drowsy or sleeps afterwards. She has also had a number of episodes of similar flushing and thumb sucking.

Dr Daniel Okuonghae

Case analysis

This seizure has features of a simple partial seizure with versive features which involve conjugate deviation of the head and eyes, often but not always away from the discharging hemisphere. However, it also has features of a complex partial seizure with possible aura suggesting some cognitive change and the autonomic phenomena of unequal pupils and flushing. It also seems she may have auras which do not progress to a motor seizure. Her 'absences' may also have a focal origin. Bacterial meningitis and other types of brain injury can cause diffuse cerebral injury leading to multifocal epilepsy.

Differential diagnosis

Partial seizures

These can present in a myriad of different ways, depending on where the focus of the seizure is. This makes them very difficult to diagnose, as they range from olfactory changes to more dramatic features as typified by Emily. There can be secondary generalisation. Awareness of the fits is variable. Most fits appear to be stereotypical, so they all look the same. Most parents should be able to provide a video of the fit. It is extremely rare for them to cause a significant deterioration in social behaviour, although parents may want a child whose behaviour is challenging to be tested for partial seizures. EEG is usually crucial in confirming the diagnosis, but in the presence of a normal EEG a trial of therapy may be indicated if the clinical picture merits it.

Nonepileptic or behavioural attacks

These might present with more complex motor and psychological phenomena or even flashbacks in children subject to psychological trauma. Nonepileptic seizures (pseudoseizures) are unlikely at 5 years old, usually developing from 9 years. In these episodes, the nature of the seizure often changes, and they are usually very frequent, often more than 20 times a day, and 'resistant' to treatment. The strong motor component coupled with the past medical history in Emily's case is strongly suggestive of organic epilepsy.

Migraine or migraine equivalents (e.g. benign positional torticollis of infancy)

Migraine can present in various ways. As some migraine equivalents respond to antiepileptic drugs, there is debate as to whether there is overlap between migraine and seizures. Usually in migraine there will be some family history.

Other seizure types

Other types of seizure disorder may present in this way, especially benign epilepsy of childhood with rolandic spikes, which involve one side of the face, are strongly associated with sleep, have an onset at around 5 years but do not have features of complex partial seizures.

Consultation essentials

It is important to establish the medical background. In this case, the meningitis was associated with some regression and then slow developmental catch-up. Other types of epilepsy are associated with a family history particularly of febrile convulsions in the case of rolandic epilepsy. In temporal lobe epilepsy, characterised by automatisms, there may be a history of a prolonged febrile convulsion (FC) in infancy, with the possibility of mesial temporal sclerosis, and of short FCs in siblings suggesting a genetic predisposition to FCs.

History/examination

The eye witness history of the attack is the key to the diagnosis of all seizure and episodic phenomena. Additionally, it is very important to look for focal neurology, especially signs of a hemiplegia which may be relatively subtle and, if congenital, may also manifest as slight differences in the size of the hand and/or feet.

Tests/investigations

The two main investigations would be an EEG and brain imaging. The EEG may show a discharge over the area causing the epilepsy and slow waves are common where there is a brain lesion. Rolandic epilepsy is characterised by a centrotemporal sharp wave focus.

Brain imaging is essential to exclude a focus which may need treatment in its own right, e.g. a brain tumour. Most brain tumours would be detected on CT scanning but an MRI is preferable being better at detecting some gliomas. It does require a cooperative or sedated/anaesthetised child. This may be difficult to arrange, in which case a CT scan may be easier. CT is also better at detecting calcification. It is best to discuss which scan would be most appropriate with a radiologist.

Depending on the results of these investigations, or other features in the history, further tests may be required.

Diagnosis

In this case, the diagnosis is complex partial seizures on a background of brain injury following bacterial meningitis.

Management

The family should be given information about the epilepsy. Epilepsy action provides excellent advice. Ideally every child should have access to an epilepsy nurse specialist, but this is unfortunately the exception rather than the rule. They need information about any lifestyle adaptations – for instance avoiding bathing alone and to be careful when climbing trees. They should also be told about managing epileptic emergencies. There is some debate about which, if any, families should be told about sudden unexplained death in epilepsy. Many paediatricians feel that raising this incredibly rare complication merely generates unnecessary anxiety.

Carbamazepine or lamotrigine are recommended by the National Institute of Health and Care Excellence as first-line therapy for partial seizures. Make sure that families are aware of side effects, particularly haematological problems with carbamazepine.

Follow up

Patients started on anticonvulsants need close follow up until settled on an anticonvulsant. A referral to a paediatric neurologist is indicated in all children under 2 years old, those with epilepsy not responding to first-line agents and any suggestion of continuous partial seizures.

In this case, the epilepsy progressed to a more complex refractory myoclonic type and the complex partial seizures subsided. A ketogenic diet was initially successful but this could not be sustained and after many different medications she eventually settled on lamotrigine monotherapy.

Discussion

There is always a debate about starting medication. Essentially, medication does not alter the course of epilepsy, its aim is to reduce or better still, eliminate the fits, to improve quality of life. For a child with only occasional fits, or where the fits occur in a 'safe' manner, e.g. in many cases of benign rolandic epilepsy, it is entirely reasonable not to start medication. In some cases a balance is struck between controlling fit frequency and avoiding too much medication.

Families often worry about the educational and developmental problems associated with epilepsy. It seems that epilepsy does not itself cause problems, but that there may be a common 'lesion' causing both epilepsy and other problems. This means that other than the rare regressive diseases, a child that starts having fits would not be expected to show any change in their developmental trajectory. Similarly, in a child with epilepsy and developmental issues it is unusual that treating the former will have any major impact on the latter, unless the epilepsy is stopping participation in school. Some antiepileptic drugs may impair intellectual performance, with sodium valproate being the most notorious.

Further reading

Guerrini R. Epilepsy in children. Lancet 2006; 367:499–524.
National Institute of Health and Care Excellence (NICE). The epilepsies: the diagnosis and management of the epilepsies in adults and children in primary and secondary care, Clinical Guidance 137. London: NICE, 2012.

Patient information

Epilepsy action
www.epilepsy.org.uk
Epilepsy Research UK
www.epilepsyresearch.org.uk

Case 54

Plagiocephaly

Dear Paediatrician,

I would be grateful if you would see this 4-month-old girl who has a very asymmetrical head shape. She is preferentially looking to the right when lying supine because of her flattened occiput. Her parents have read about helmets and are keen to discuss this.

Thank you for your assessment,

Dr Malcolm Taylor

Case analysis

The key here is to differentiate positional plagiocephaly from abnormal sutures or prematurely fused/close sutures.

Differential diagnosis

Positional plagiocephaly

Babies commonly have an unusual head shape after birth. This can be caused by the in-utero position of the baby during pregnancy. Some 'moulding' occurs during birth. Often the head will return to a more normal shape in about 6 weeks after birth. Sometimes a baby's head does not return to a normal shape and the baby may have developed a flattened area at the back or side of the head. Usually, the baby has normal development. The head looks asymmetrical with flattening on one side posteriorly. This facilitates the child lying preferentially on that side and looking towards it. It is probably a direct consequence of the introduction of the back to sleep campaign in the early 1990s, encouraging parents to lie their babies on their back to sleep in order to reduce the risk of cot death. The skull does not completely ossify until after infancy and is therefore vulnerable to moulding and external pressure. Positional plagiocephaly manifests as left or right posterior skulls flattening, usually associated with prominence of the frontal area creating a parallelogram shape to skull when viewed from above.

Craniosynostosis (syndromic or nonsyndromic)

This condition causes plagiocephaly, or asymmetrical skull, but there may be a more symmetrical but abnormal shape. It may be present from birth or develop later in childhood. Craniosynostosis is due to fusion of one of the sutures joining the skull bones together. These results in specific skull shapes described (**Table 54.1**). It requires further investigation and referral to a craniofacial surgeon.

Table 54.1 Types of cranial synostosis			
Synostosis	%	Sutures involved	Skull shape
Sagittal synostosis	Most common 50%	Fusion of sagittal suture down the midline top of the skull	Lack of growth in width and compensatory growth in length, resulting in a long, narrow skull (scaphocephaly)
Coronal craniosynostosis	Second most common 25%	Fusion in one or both of the coronal sutures that run from the top of the ear to the top of the skull	If only one coronal suture is fused, a flattened forehead on the affected side is seen. They may also have a raised eye socket and a crooked nose
			If both coronal sutures are fused, the infant will develop a flat and elevated (prominent) forehead and brow. The head is small (brachycephalic)
Metopic synostosis	4–10%	Fusion occurs in the metopic suture, which runs from the nose to the top of the skull	Develop a pointed scalp that looks triangular (trigonocephaly)
Lambdoid synostosis	2–4%	Fusion occurs in the lambdoid suture which runs along the back of the head	Develop a flattened head at the back, like positional plagiocephaly. Not all children with a flattened head at the back have lambdoid synostosis, they are more likely to have positional plagiocephaly Differentiating lamboid stenosis from plagiocephaly is therefore a challenge; however lamboid stenosis is the rarest of the craniosynostoses. Also, the parallelogram-shaped head is characteristic of positional plagiocephaly compared to the trapezoid-shaped head typical of the lambdoid craniosynostosis

Consultation essentials

History/examination

Look at the general features noting any dysmorphisms. Note any head tilt; it is quite common in plagiocephaly and may have an associated toticollis which would need a referral to a physiotherapist. View the head from all sides, and particularly from above. Note the position of the ears and forehead if the ears are asymmetrical this is more likely a cause for concern. Occipital flattening will be identifiable. In positional plagiocephaly a parallelogram appearance will be seen.

According to age, test degree of ease of active movement of the head by encouraging the infant to fix and follow a suitable object. Check passive movements for muscular spasm and general tone.

Measure head circumference and plot on centile chart. Check against height and weight. Describe the asymmetry, flattening, ridges. Assess whether child is making appropriate developmental progress.

Tests/investigations

Positional plagiocephaly is diagnosed on history and clinical findings, it is not usually necessary to do imaging. However, a skull radiograph may help to rule out craniosynostosis or identify obliteration of the lambdoid suture. There is some promise for ultrasound sonography of the lambdoid sutures as a screening test for lambdoid craniosynostosis, avoiding radiation. A computed tomography scan would confirm craniosynostosis, and this would warrant a referral to a neurosurgeon or a craniofacial team if found.

Diagnosis

This is most likely to be positional plagiocephaly in this baby.

Management

There are some simple noninterventional measure that parents can do:
- Early recognition of the condition can help prevent progression
- Tummy time – while all babies should sleep on their backs, there is active encouragement for them to spend some time of their fronts during the day and during play when old enough to begin to hold their head up. This can aid natural re-moulding that will occur
- Positioning – making the opposite side of the cot interesting than the side preferentially looked towards and gently repositioning (counter positioning) the head while asleep can prevent progression. Ensure the car seat is adjusted to discourage the same side being looked towards
- Physiotherapy – this may be helpful if the is an associated torticollis, and to help the baby begin to look in the other direction
- Helmets and bands – the use of helmets remains controversial. There seems to be no added advantage over conventional treatment and therefore their use is not funded by the National Health Service.
- They cost several thousand pounds and the condition is likely to improve naturally. They have to be worn for 23 of 24 hours each day, which is a significant undertaking

Follow up

Essentially there is no real need to follow-up unless one of the more abnormal head shapes evolves over time prompting concern and reassessment. However infrequent reviews until the parents are happy that the child's head shape is looking better (which usually coincides with a better covering of hair) is reassuring for everyone.

Discussion

The head shape is normal in plagiocephaly, it is the pressure from positioning on repeated occasions that 'moulds' the head shape. Once these pressure effects are no longer as influential, as the child is able to move their head independently and change their sleeping position in sleep, the shape starts to normalise. This is usually by the age of 1 year but may be take longer. Growth or hair can cover minor abnormalities as a child grow up, but there are many adults out there who would have asymmetrical skull shapes which would be obvious if they chose to shave their head. Recent studies suggest that there may be a link between plagiocephaly and developmental delay. This is likely to be of little clinical significance. If further studies support this, it is more likely that the developmental issue causes plagiocephaly rather than vice versa. The helmet companies are likely to use this research to insinuate that aggressive treatment of plagiocephaly might have long term benefits, and not treating it might be deleterious – families should be warned about this.

Further reading

Bialocerkowski AE, Vladusic SL, Howell SM. Conservative interventions for positional plagiocephaly: a systematic review. Developmental Medicine and Child Neurology 2005; 47(8):563–570.
Singh A, Wacogne I. What is the role of helmet therapy in Positional plagiocephaly? Arch Dis Child 2008; 93:807–809.
Collett BR, Gray KE, Starr JR et al. Development at age 36 months in children with deformational plagiocephaly. Pediatrics. 2013; 131(1):109-15

Patient information

Great Ormond Street Hospital
   www.gosh.nhs.uk

Case 55

Polydipsia

Dear Paediatrician,

Thank you for seeing this 2 and a half-year-old who drinks a lot of juice. He constantly requests the bottle, even at night. I wonder if he has diabetes insipidus.

Dr Christopher Pryke

Case analysis

Parents of toddlers will often report that their child drinks a lot, usually as information volunteered during the consultation than the main reason for referral. Young children, who are reportedly drinking a lot, are not in sole control of the amount they drink. Who is filling up their bottle or beaker? It is often the parents who are fuelling the habit by constantly having the bottle topped up. A 2-year-old child should be drinking from a beaker or cup and not the bottle, especially not juice or sugary drinks as that will erode their primary dentition. Investigation is often not necessary and the simplest management would be to encourage the parents to reduce the number of 'free refills' being offered. However if there is a real concern about the amount a child is drinking there are some important conditions to consider. The volumes of water a child should drink have been described (**Table 55.1**).

Differential diagnosis

Diabetes insipidus

Water balance is essential for homeostasis and intracellular and extracellular water needs to be balanced for normal cell functions. Three mechanisms do this in humans: antidiuretic hormone (ADH), regulation of thirst and renal function. In diabetes insipidus (DI) there is a polyuric state which is due to an absence of ADH from the posterior pituitary (central) or resistance of the kidneys to its effects (nephrogenic). There are long lists of central and nephrogenic causes and a separate group, polydipsic DI, which could be acquired

Table 55.1 Differentiating organic/true polydipsia from habit/psychogenic polydipsia

Organic cause (e.g. DI)	Habit/psychogenic
Water seeking behaviour	Always has bottle/beaker with them
Drinks anything	Prefers sweetened juices in preference to water
Wakes in the night for drinks	May take a bottle to bed but does not wake in the night
Constantly saturated nappies	Thriving
Poor weight gain	
Adapted from Carr and Gill, 2007	

(following chronic meningitis, granulomatous disease, or other diffuse cerebral pathology), or due to a psychiatric illness. It can also be idiopathic.

Another separate group is dipsogenic DI or primary polysdipsia (see below). There is a link to polyuria and excessive drinking, defined as volumes in excess of 2 L/m^2/day or approximately 50 mL/kg/day in older children.

Primary polydipsia (dipsogenic DI)

Excessive fluid intake will suppress ADH secretion and contribute to increased urine output. Mostly serum sodium remains normal. However, serum osmolality will be low to normal. This situation is usually caused by excessive fluid intake, which is commonly habitual but there are rare hypothalamic abnormalities which lead to excessive thirst. This situation is usually a diagnosis of exclusion. It may be that there should be further assessment for DI, e.g. by a water depravation test before deciding there is excessive/habitual drinking in the presence of a normal ADH-renal axis.

Diabetes mellitus

The possibility of type 1 diabetes mellitus should of course not be ignored. Other signs such as polyuria and polyphagia may be present. Weight loss should be checked for. In a more chronic presentation with very high sugars and a long history, Kussmaul breathing and ketoacidosis will necessitate urgent resuscitation and treatment according to national diabetic ketoacidosis protocols. A more insidious course with polydipsia is less common.

Consultation essentials

The key is to differentiate abnormal drinking behaviour from normal or habit. It is also important to differentiate between frequency of urine and true polyuria. Polyuria results from excessive fluid intake, DI (due to an absence of central release of ADH, a renal tubular insensitivity to ADH), or an osmotic diuresis. It is nearly always associated with polydipsia and an increased frequency of passing urine.

History/examination

The history is key and will likely yield enough information to distinguish organic from habit. The obvious question is 'how much does your child drink in a day?' Charting frequency and volume of intake and urine volume voided may help to determine accurate amounts of urine produced over 24 hours. The type of fluids is also important. Just like the 'milkaholic' who drinks milk through the day and at night, children with DI usually wake in the night with thirst. Other aspects of the child's drinking behaviour should be assessed. Normal drinking behaviour is very variable and largely dependent on carers in young children as indicated above. Children with DI exhibit extreme thirst and water-seeking behaviour. They may drink from the bath, toilet or puddles. Toddlers may not sleep very well in the day because they are looking for water. Their dehydration state can cause irritability, constipation and vomiting.

Tests/investigations

In cases of habit drinking no investigations are required. If there is any doubt the first assessment should be a 24-hour urine collection to confirm the polyuria as indicated above. A urine dipstick for glucose is obligatory. Baseline blood levels of blood glucose and renal function as well as serum calcium and potassium should be checked. The best in vivo assessment of the kidneys' concentrating ability is to check an early morning urine specimen. The specific gravity of an early morning urine sample will help assess the renal concentrating ability, so will a measurement of urine osmolality in an early morning sample. This can be conclusive if the urine is very concentrated. If there is any doubt then it can be compared with a paired plasma osmolality level. This may then direct the need for a more formal evaluation of the pituitary-renal system. The standard test is a water deprivation test. This should only be performed by experienced professionals as there is a real risk of significant dehydration.

Children who drink a lot will produce more urine. They often have low serum sodium. In DI, the polyuria is inappropriate compared to the input and they are thirsty. Sodium is usually normal, except where there is imbalance with excess loss compared to intake, such as in vomiting or excessive sweating.

Diagnosis

This child was habitually drinking juice from a toddler beaker.

Management

He was reported to have a poor appetite and had loose, frequent stool. He was taking in excess of 2.5 L/day. He was still in nappies at night. He was waking in the night and was given more juice to settle off back to sleep. He was otherwise well. His weight was on the 2nd centile and height on the 50th centile. An early morning paired serum and urine osmolality were 285 mOsmol and 750 mOsmol respectively, suggesting a good concentrating ability of the kidney with a slightly low serum osmolality. A much lower serum osmolality would be expected in DI with more dilute urine. His parents were encouraged to reduce the amount of juice he was being given. This was successfully done and his loose stool improved too.

Follow up

Concern about underlying DI necessitates endocrine referral unless there is a facility to carry out the required water deprivation test safely on the ward.

Discussion

Many children do not drink water, but prefer juice. In excessive volumes, this causes its own problems, including loose stool or a label of 'toddler's diarrhoea'. Hourihane and Rolles coined the term 'squash drinking syndrome' for children with poor appetite (or reluctance to eat) at mealtimes, who consume > 30% of the recommended daily intake of energy from drinks other than milk, and have loose stools which resolve or improve with the reduction of energy taken in drinks, either by replacement with water or drinks of lower energy content.

Carr and Gill used the term 'polypopsia' to describe toddlers and pre-school children ingesting excessive amounts of carbonated drinks. The ingestion of these fluids results in the passage of dilute watery urine where the kidney partially loses its ability to concentrate, known as 'medullary washout syndrome'. The long-term excessive water intake will partially suppress ADH, causing a similar pattern to central DI. The high osmolality of carbonated drink and juices can also cause an osmotic diuresis which will make the situation worse.

Further reading

Baylis P, Cheetham T. Diabetes insipidus. Arch Dis Child 1998; 79:84–89.

Carr M, Gill D. Polyuria, polydipsia, polypopsia: "Mummy I want a drink". Arch Dis Child Educ Pract Ed 2007; 92:ep139–ep143.

Hourihane JO, Rolles CJ. Morbidity from excessive intake of high energy fluids: the 'squash drinking syndrome'. Arch of Dis Child 1995; 72:141–143.

Petter LPM, Hourihane JO, Rolles CJ. Is water out of vogue? A survey of the drinking habits of 2–7 years old. Arch Dis Child 1995; 72:137–140.

Patient information

The Infant & Toddler Forum
    www.infantandtoddlerforum.org
Childsmile
    http://www.child-smile.org.uk/

Poor feeding in a baby

Dear Paediatrician,

Please could you see Emily who is now 4 months old and is struggling to feed, and often takes over an hour to finish a bottle. Mum had to abandon breastfeeding. The family has tried a variety of different milks, but none seems to be to her taste. She also has not gained weight as expected.

She was born at full term, and has no other obvious problems.

Thank you,

Dr Jameel Mushtaq

Case analysis

Many referrals like this are for a baby who is normal but has parents with unrealistic expectations. Here, with faltering growth, the situation is more urgent. Observing the baby feed is highly instructive. Parents often receive little practical advice on feeding either in relation to expected intake or technique. If Emily is struggling to feed adequately then she may need urgent feeding intervention, even admission and assisted feeding, e.g. via a nasogastric tube.

Differential diagnosis

Unrealistic expectations

Parents are often unaware of what is normal for babies. By about a week of age, most babies will drink approximately 120–150 mL/kg/day of milk at each feed (or 2–2.5 floz/lb/day), feeding every 3–5 hours. Each feed may take 30–40 minutes. Identifying how, and how much, a baby feeds is essential.

Common problems include overfeeding, because when a teat is placed in the baby's mouth it will initiate a sucking reflex, even if the baby is full. This overfilling can lead to vomiting, an exacerbation of reflux symptoms and a presumption of feeding issues. Babies who are overfed will be thriving. Most feeding advice can be provided by health visitors.

Normal development/'catch down' growth

Co-ordination of sucking and swallowing is established between 34 and 37 weeks of gestation. Some large babies born prematurely may be erroneously said to be term babies, and their feeding reflexes may not be properly established. This is often exacerbated in infants of diabetic mothers.

Some babies just seem to be a little slow, and do pick up in time.

Some babies who are large for gestational age will exhibit 'catch down' growth. They may be within the normal range, but large for themselves. For example, a baby who should have been on the 9th centile, but was born on the 91st may slowly return to their destined centile. They will appear to be losing weight, and will not be taking the volume expected of a 91st centile baby.

Neuromuscular

Feeding requires neuromuscular integrity. A history of a difficult birth might suggest hypoxic-ischaemic encephalopathy (HIE). Babies with altered tone should obviously cause concern, cerebral palsy can present with initial hypotonia. There is a host of rare neurological causes, many with an underlying metabolic abnormality. Specific investigations, following specialist advice are often required.

Missed diagnoses: cleft palate/Down's syndrome/congenital abnormalities

Although these should be identified at birth, a few cases slip through the net. The cleft soft palate is a classic example. Ideally palatal examination requires two people and the palate should be clearly visualised with the aid of a tongue depressor and torch. Down's syndrome can also have a delayed diagnosis, especially in certain ethnic groups. The fact that others may have missed the diagnosis should not be a reason to delay making it now.

Hypothyroidism

This should have been picked up in the Guthrie test in the first week of life, but if the baby is generally sluggish is worth testing for.

Sepsis

Infection is usually a cause of short-term feeding difficulty. If the symptoms are short lived, this would always be the first diagnosis to exclude.

Congenital infection

A congenital infection should be evidenced by other features, including organomegaly, cataracts, etc. If there is a suspicion, then a discussion with the microbiologists may be helpful.

Oral aversion

This is slightly unusual at this age, unless the baby has had a protracted time on a ventilator, or a long time without feeding. The baby will often object to anything being put near the mouth and will gag and vomit easily. 'Desensitisation' with the input of the speech and language team can take some time. Alternative feeding via nasogastric tube or gastrostomy may be necessary.

Gastro-oesophageal reflux/Cow's milk protein allergy

Babies who have severe oesophagitis, due to gastro-oesophageal reflux disease or cow's milk protein allergy, may be reluctant to feed because of the pain. Most babies will have other symptoms of reflux, but in some it may be silent. Often the only way to diagnose it is with a trial of medication. Babies with reflux often suck a lot to generate alkali saliva, this is often misinterpreted as hunger or early teething. Stool withholding can present with symptoms very similar to gastro-oesophageal reflux disease. To exclude cow's milk protein allergy, a 2-6 week trial of hypoallergenic formula milk can be tried to see if the symptoms improve or the baby gains weight.

Cardiac

Babies in cardiac failure would normally present with breathlessness and sweating during feeds. The failure should be easy to diagnose on clinical examination.

Toxic

Most drugs, prescribed and recreational, including alcohol pass through breast milk. Very occasionally, there may be deliberate poisoning such as with salt. There is usually an associated social history of concern.

Trauma

Without a history, any head trauma at this age is likely to be abusive. The most useful test is measuring the head circumference and comparing with previous readings. An increasing head circumference should trigger immediate investigations.

Consultation essentials

History

A full feeding history should determine whether the symptom is recent or has been present since birth. Establish how and how much the baby feeds, and what their behaviour is like during a feed. Reflux is painful, in cardiac failure there will be sweating and breathlessness, and in neuromuscular conditions passivity. With a cleft palate there may be spluttering and nasal regurgitation.

A detailed history of the pregnancy and delivery is required. If the child was conceived through in vitro fertilisation, the reason for needing treatment may be relevant. For example, myotonic dystrophy is associated with fertility problems and can cause problems in children. Unfortunately, sometimes a mother's myotonic dystrophy is only diagnosed after her child's.

During the pregnancy, decreased fetal movements and polyhydramnios both indicate possible neuromuscular problems and a history of maternal infection raises the possibility of a congenital infection. If there were any delivery issues, then HIE and cerebral palsy may be factors.

Examination

This must include a weight and head circumference, which should be plotted and compared to previous values. General examination should look for physical abnormalities suggestive of a genetic problem and assess muscle tone. The eyes need to be examined for cataracts and the abdomen for organomegaly.

Specifically, the palate should be fully inspected, which may need assistance. One person should depress the tongue allowing visual examination of the entire palate with a torch. The suck reflex should be checked.

Investigations

Clearly, these depend on the differential diagnosis and vary from none to a vast array. Try to target investigations.

Diagnosis

On examination Emily looked dysmorphic and had poor tone. She was only drinking half of her expected feeds.

Management

She was admitted to the children's ward to teach the parents nasogastric (NG) tube feeding. She was referred to geneticists, neurologists, the feeding team and community paediatricians. The NG tube was replaced with a gastrostomy button. At 9 months she still did not have a diagnosis, but showed features of significant developmental delay.

Follow up

This should be with the individual teams. The family will have so many hospital appointments that they do not need any extra ones. However, with everybody seeing one bit of Emily, the community paediatrician should have overall charge.

Discussion

In many babies no firm diagnosis is made and they recover spontaneously. However, malnutrition in the first year of life can have serious long-term consequences, and should be prevented as much as possible. Babies who feed poorly may be especially vulnerable. It is important to 'draw a line in the sand' as regards intervention. It is too easy to think that the situation is just about alright and to wait and see. This cannot go on indefinitely. It is best to have a clear target, which if not met will trigger intervention.

Further reading

Galler JR, Bryce C, Waber DP et al. Socioeconomic outcomes in adults malnourished in the first year of life: a 40-year study. Pediatrics 2012; 130(1):e1–e7.

Patient information

Family lives
www.familylives.org.uk

Case 57

Poor feeding in a toddler

Dear Paediatrician,

Please can you see Archie who is 22 months old. His mother is worried because he will not eat properly. He is growing well along the 25th centile, but is only eating first food baby jars and drinking formula. He gags or vomits if given any other foods. Please advise.

Dr Daphne Manning

Case analysis

Feeding is such an intrinsic part of nurturing, that a child refusing to feed can challenge the entire essence of motherhood. Physical or mechanical causes are rare but it is essential to ensure, and reassure, that the child is getting an adequate diet. Most feeding problems are dealt with very capably in the community by health visitors. If they are being referred it is likely that the problem is more 'resistant'. In theory a combination of speech and language therapy and psychology can be helpful in treating these issues. Unfortunately, these services are so overstretched that few cases reach the threshold for treatment.

Differential diagnosis

Gastro-oesophageal reflux

Babies, who have had oesophagitis, particularly if it has been untreated, can develop feeding problems. Because feeding has been painful in the past, there is little pleasure associated with feeding. They often have an exaggerated gag reflex. If there has been 'silent reflux' ('he was never sick') the diagnosis of oesophagitis may not have been made previously. Sometimes secondary symptoms persist even if the reflux has resolved. A trial of anti-reflux treatment may be worthwhile.

Iron-deficiency

There is a vicious cycle with iron-deficiency and poor appetite 'feeding' into each other. A blood test is diagnostic, but in practice it may be easier prescribing a short course of iron.

Behavioural food avoidance/aversion/phobia

A few analogies may be helpful, although each has its limitations. The first is that food refusal arises if children are not exposed to different foods at a young age. This is akin to animals in the forest. A mother will identify to her children which plants are edible. By a certain age, any plant that the young animal has not been shown will be considered poisonous. Self-preservation will prevent him from eating it. Similarly, a child will not eat foods that seem threatening. These children seem to have a real fear of either trying new tastes or textures or of swallowing often starting from an early age. Their food repertoire is limited and constant, eating a few foods which need to be prepared in particular ways, e.g. a specific brand of baked beans. Sometimes the aversion starts later, after a specific 'trauma' such as severe tonsillitis or emergency intubation. Children with autism will often have similar limited dietary repertoires and be very sensitive to any changes.

The next analogy perhaps as an extension of the first is that the child really thinks that the food being offered is obnoxious. Everyone else may be licking their lips, but it does not help. Common advice suggests that if a child is hungry enough they will eat the food that is offered to them. This does not work because in their eyes, however hungry they still see a plate of undesirable food in front of them. In some cases, introducing new foods gradually can work, but this requires patience and perseverance; often with little rewards. It is wise to not build up parental expectations unduly. Ultimately, what is important is that the child is ingesting a balanced diet. It is remarkable how often seemingly very limited diets actually contain everything that a child needs. A dietary assessment is essential, and is best done by a dietician. If the child is ingesting a balanced diet then this allows everybody to relax a little, which often in itself helps the situation. If there is anything missing, the dietician can advise about supplements.

It is crucial to address parental anxiety. Remind the mother that her primary obligation is to give her child a balanced diet. If she is doing this, she is fulfilling her role. If the child decides that he is not going to eat different foods that is up to him. If a feeding clinic or speech and language therapy team are accessible they may be able to work with the family.

Playing up

Although on the surface children who play up at mealtimes behave like the group above, their food repertoire, whilst narrow, does change over time. The ritual of parents presenting children with numerous choices at each meal is quickly established. Various games are devised in order to encourage each mouthful (choo choo train, one for mummy, etc.). Consequently each meal takes forever. In this group of children the parents will get excited when the child eats baked beans for 2 days in a row, but will then become disappointed when the child refuses to eat them on day 3. There are parenting groups and courses to help parents deal with these issues.

Mechanical problems (cleft palate, tongue problems, etc.)

These will present as general rather than specific feeding difficulties. A soft palatal cleft can remain undiagnosed for years. Whether tongue tie can cause feeding problems in much younger babies is a matter of debate. The practice of releasing tongue tie – which is a simple procedure – moves in and out of favour. Similarly macroglossia is a rare cause of feeding difficulty. If there are neuromuscular problems they are likely to be evident by other signs and symptoms.

Consultation essentials

History/examination

Identify if the problem is with different tastes, textures or both. If the repertoire is narrow, does it vary with setting or over time? If it varies, it is less likely to be phobia/aversion. A feeding history should start from birth. Ask about how settled Archie was as a baby – reflux may be diagnosed retrospectively. Measure and plot Archie, whilst this may reassure everybody that calorie intake is adequate, it does not fully assess the diet. Be supportive and realistic.

Tests/investigations

Investigations are not usually required unless specific indications are found in the history and examination.

Diagnosis

Archie's food refusal seems to have started young. He had many symptoms of gastro-oesophageal reflux disease which were untreated.

Management

A trial of reflux treatment caused some improvement and a dietetic review established that he was receiving a balanced diet.

Follow up

Medical follow up is not really needed, dietetic follow up may be. On-going reflux could be managed by the general practitioner. As in many situations one follow up to 'close the loop' may be indicated.

Discussion

A child that does not feed well is a major challenge to the parents, especially mothers who often feel very sensitive about this. It is important that they feel supported and not undermined. Often the best result that can be achieved is the reassurance that the child's diet, although restricted, is at least adequate.

Patient information

Infant and toddler forum
    www.infantandtoddlerforum.org
Phelan T. 1-2-3 Magic: effective discipline for children 2-12. Child management incorporated, 2010.

Case 58

Precocious puberty in girls

Dear Paediatrician,

Thank you for seeing Matilda who is now 6 years old. Mum has noticed some early breast development which she is concerned about. Matilda has been noted to be taller than her peers but is otherwise well.

Yours,

Dr Richard Tiley

Case analysis

Early puberty requires a systematic approach so that investigations are kept to a rational level and an accurate diagnosis is made, ensuring that the appropriate management plan can be instituted. The first challenge is distinguishing true precocious puberty from normal development.

The staging system utilised to assess pubertal development is that published by Marshall and Tanner and the sequence of changes is commonly referred to as 'Tanner stages'. Precocious puberty in a girl can be defined as stage 2 breast development on the Tanner scales, before the age of 7 years. Many parents are surprised that pubertal changes can start normally from the age of 7 years, and need reassurance that this is within the expected range. Some younger children may have isolated changes such as the presence of pubic or axillary hair (premature adrenarche) which would not be considered true puberty.

True precocious puberty

This is gonadotrophin-dependent (central) with early activation of the hypothalamic-pituitary-ovarian axis.

It follows a normal concordant pattern: breast development first, followed by pubic and axillary hair, a growth spurt and finally menarche. Most cases in girls are idiopathic, but may occasionally be secondary to CNS pathology.

Discordant puberty includes

- Gonadotrophin-independent development due to peripheral ovarian activation such as in McCune-Albright syndrome causing breast enlargement and vaginal bleeds, but no pubic or axillary hair
- Adrenal pathology – congenital adrenal hyperplasia, adrenal tumour or Cushing's syndrome causing virilisation with development of pubic or axillary hair, body odour, rapid growth, clitoromegaly and acne but no breast development.

Differential diagnosis

Normal development

The age of onset of normal puberty in girls varies greatly. The external physical changes can start appearing from between 7 and 13 years of age, although hormonal changes can precede these by a year or so. The first change is normally the formation of a breast bud, followed by the development of pubic and axillary hair, a growth spurt and the onset of menses. In about 15% of girls pubic hair develops before breast budding. There is significant ethnic variation. Premature adrenarche and thelarche are variants of normal.

Adrenarche

The development of pubic and/or axillary hair is called adrenache, with body odour and acne, but with no breast development. Premature adrenarche is usually benign and can start from about 5 years of age. It is particularly common in girls of Afro-Caribbean origin. If the girl is growing normally and does not have any other signs of virilisation, such as clitoromegaly, this may be a benign variant of normal. Investigations may be required to exclude congenital adrenal hyperplasia (CAH) or an androgen secreting tumour, especially in girls who have a rapid growth spurt or virilisation.

Thelarche

This is isolated breast development before 7 years of age with no signs of androgenisation. This is a normal physiological variant in girls under the age of 3 years. If there are no other signs of puberty, and growth and development are normal, no further investigation or intervention is required. In girls between the ages of 3 and 7 years, the onset of breast development may need to be investigated. A luteinising hormone releasing hormone (LHRH) test will identify any significant abnormalities.

True precocious puberty

This is the presence of early breast development, with or without androgenic changes, with an abnormal LHRH test and raised oestrogen. In the young girl under 5 years, further investigations are recommended, such as an MRI of the brain to rule out intracranial pathology such as a hypothalamic hamartoma or pituitary tumour. In the majority of girls no cause is found and this is then deemed to be idiopathic precocious puberty.

Congenital adrenal hyperplasia /adrenal tumours

These conditions are androgen producing and cause discordant changes of adrenarche with no breast development. Although severe forms of CAH would be expected to present in the neonatal period, milder forms can present later. A urinary steroid profile will confirm, or refute the diagnosis. Blood androgens can do the same for an androgen secreting tumour.

Other endocrine causes: Cushing's syndrome, hypothyroidism

Cushing's disease and hypothyroidism are rare causes of early puberty and need to be considered and investigated.

Consultation essentials

History/examination

The purpose of the consultation is to try to distinguish whether there is a problem at all, and if there is, to narrow down the possible causes. Determine what pubertal changes have occurred at what age, and how they have progressed. Androgenisation without breast development needs different management.

Although the patient's ethnicity is usually obvious, this needs to specifically be considered, as accelerated development is more common in Afro-Carribean girls. Check parental heights.

There may be a history of brain injury or neurosurgery in some children with central precocious puberty.

Some conditions may have cutaneous manifestations, such as café au lait spots in McCune–Albright syndrome.

Plot the child's height and weight. Size is a trigger for normal puberty and taller children go into puberty earlier. The shorter, overweight girl who has signs of early puberty is more likely to have underlying pathology.

The child should be examined fully, and puberty staged according to the Tanner scale. This should be done sensitively, ideally with a chaperone present. Girls of any age should be able to ask for a female doctor to examine them, and if they do so, this wish should be respected.

Investigations

A bone age is useful as it is usually advanced in a child with precocious puberty – whether gonadotrophin-dependent or independent.

In true precocious puberty the following baseline blood tests should be performed:
- Thyroid function
- Luteinising hormone/follicle-stimulating hormone
- Oestradiol
- Prolactin

If the examination and/or baseline investigations are suggestive of true precocious puberty then an LHRH stimulation test can be arranged. This usually requires admission to a day unit, and should only be undertaken by an expert.

If a central cause is suspected, an MRI of the brain may be required.

If there is only androgenisation/virilisation, the basic investigations would include:
- Blood androgens – testosterone, 17 hydroxy progesterone, dehydroepiandrosterone (DHEAS) and androstenodione
- Cortisol
- Urine steroid profile

If these are normal, then no further action is required.

If the investigations suggest congenital adrenal hyperplasia, then a Synacthen (ACTH stimulation) test should be performed in a specialist unit.

Diagnosis

As this girl is 6 years old, tall for her age, and has breast development she needs further investigation. The most likely diagnosis in this clinical situation would be idiopathic, central (gonadotrophin-dependent) precocious puberty.

Management

All cases of early puberty need sensitive management. Clearly any underlying pathology needs to be treated, but even when it is said to be 'normal' it is often socially and psychologically difficult for a child in primary school to deal with the physical changes of puberty, let alone the practical challenges of menstruation.

Follow up

The findings will determine what follow up is required. If any investigations are required the family will need a method of getting the results promptly and starting any necessary treatment. Regardless of the cause of any early puberty, the girl and family are likely to need support managing this. It is likely that regular follow up will be required until the family feel comfortable with the situation.

Discussion

The management of early puberty focuses on a number of issues.

Treating any underlying problem

Underlying causes, e.g. endocrine diseases, should be treated.

Delaying puberty

In girls who are very young and have gonadotrophin-dependent precocious puberty, delaying the progression of puberty may be achieved by using a depot preparation of a gonadotrophin-releasing hormone analogue such as leuprorelin or triptorelin.

Growth

As the growth spurt occurs early, girls with early puberty may have a short final height. This may be moderated by using growth hormone in addition to delaying puberty, but again needs expert management.

Emotional/social

This can be the most difficult aspect to deal with. For most girls, the early onset of puberty is difficult to deal with and will need sympathetic support from doctors, home and school. Some children might need formal psychological support.

Cycle control

If puberty is allowed to progress early and menarche is attained at a very young age, the child may need treatment to reduce the frequency of menstruation, or at least make it manageable.

Pregnancy

Children with precocious puberty will need to be given patient appropriate advice about the risks of pregnancy. This is especially true if they have associated learning difficulties and are therefore increasingly vulnerable. Contraceptive medication or implants may need to be considered.

Patient information

Child Growth Foundation
    www.childgrowthfoundation.org

Proteinuria

Dear Paediatrician,

Please could you see this 15-year-old boy, who was found to have significant proteinuria (3+ on dipstick testing), when he had a medical for 'scuba diving' lessons. He seems fit and well and has no oedema or haematuria. I repeated the urine test after 1 week and it continues to show 3+ protein.

   The urine protein: creatinine ratio is very high at 180 mg/mmol.

   I wonder if he has nephrotic syndrome?

Dr Nav Su

Case analysis

In view of the heavy proteinuria, nephrotic syndrome is the most serious diagnosis to consider. The age group would make minimal change nephrotic syndrome unlikely. At this age with an insidious onset the rarer types, membranous or membranoproliferative glomerulonephritis is more likely. Unfortunately, there is no mention of blood being present on urine dipstick or a blood pressure measurement being done. Haematuria and hypertension would suggest nephritis, associated with, or independent of, nephrotic syndrome, e.g. recovering post-infectious or Henoch–Schönlein purpuric (HSP) nephritis.

   A simple exercise-induced proteinuria is possible, although the proteinuria has persisted on repeat testing, this and the high protein:creatinine ratio, effectively exclude a spurious cause. Orthostatic proteinuria needs to be considered as the child seems well.

Differential diagnosis

Nephrotic syndrome

In this age group, an insidious onset of puffiness around the eyes or ankles over a period of several weeks is the usual presentation. A urine dipstick would show 3+ to 4+ protein. Urine must be sent for microalbumin:creatinine ratio and protein:creatinine ratio to confirm the diagnosis. In nephrotic syndrome, urine albumin:creatinine is > 30 mg/mmol and urine protein:creatinine is > 200 mg/mmol. Single 'spot' urine is adequate; there is no need for a 24-hour urine collection.

   If the urine dipstick is positive for blood or if macroscopic haematuria is present, the urine must be sent for microscopy to check for red blood cells or casts. This would suggest an associated nephritis.

   Blood pressure must be checked manually with the correct sized cuff. Check the 95th centile for age and sex on the standardised blood pressure centile charts. If the blood pressure is persistently above the 95th centile (at least three separate readings in the same clinic, after allowing the child to relax if necessary), discuss the patient with a renal team.

   Blood levels must be urgently checked for urea, creatinine, serum electrolytes, protein and albumin to confirm the diagnosis, which would be suggested by hypoalbuminaemia. Other tests such as antinuclear antibody, double-stranded DNA (dsDNA), antineutrophil cytoplasmic antibody), complement (C3 and C4) and varicella IgG can be requested at the same time.

Presence of heavy proteinuria, oedema and low serum albumin would confirm the diagnosis of nephrotic syndrome. The age group and insidious onset would suggest the rare types that would need a referral to a paediatric nephrologist for a renal biopsy before definitive treatment. In addition, hypertension and/or haematuria would point towards a nonminimal change type.

Nephritis

The possibility of nephritis should be considered if there is a history of HSP or sore throat in the preceding weeks or months, which may have resulted in nephritis with blood and protein in the urine. There may be a history of cola coloured or reddish urine with reduced urine output. Blood pressure must be measured and a urine dipstick test performed. If blood is present on stick testing the urine should be sent for urgent microscopy. If proteinuria is present, the urinary albumin:creatinine ratio must be checked – this can be on a single sample. Arrange the same blood tests as above and in addition an antistreptolycin titre, immunoglobulins and anti-DNAse B titres. If C_3 is low over the course of 8 weeks after the onset of nephritis, or if the proteinuria is ongoing or increasing and significant (urinary albumin:creatinine ratio > 2.5 mg/mmol), this will require discussion with a paediatric nephrologist to consider whether a renal biopsy is necessary.

Exercise induced proteinuria

Proteinuria can be present after vigorous exercise. Hence repeat urine protein:creatinine ratio is essential to exclude this possibility in a very active sporty child.

Orthostatic proteinuria

Some individuals have proteinuria when they are up and about, dependent on posture and after standing for a while. This is evident on checking paired urine protein:creatinine ratios on first morning urine and on a random daytime sample. If the first morning sample has no protein on dipstick testing and this is further confirmed on urine protein:creatinine ratio <20 mg/mmol, while the random sample has significant proteinuria (urine protein:creatinine >20 mg/mmol) it would confirm this diagnosis.

Consultation essentials

History

Ask for a history of puffiness around the eyes especially on waking up, oedema of the feet and ankles and increase in abdominal girth, which would suggest ascites. Also an increase in weight or clothes getting tight may indirectly suggest oedema.

A history of viral upper respiratory infection or gastroenteritis in the few weeks preceding the proteinuria may indicate the possibility of nephrotic syndrome.

A history of sore throat, impetigo or vasculitic rash in the preceding weeks or months may indicate a nephritis (post-streptococcal or HSP), which has progressed to a nephrotic stage. The nephritis may have been obvious in the acute stage with dark or reddish urine or may have been missed if haematuria had been microscopic or urine had not been tested. If blood and protein are present on dipstick testing, urine should be sent for urgent microscopy and urine protein:creatinine and microalbumin:creatinine ratio checked.

If there is no history of oedema or illness and the proteinuria has been detected incidentally, the likelihood of orthostatic or exercise-induced proteinuria is high. Sometimes protein is detected on the dipstick in highly concentrated specimens and needs to be substantiated by the urine protein:creatinine ratio.

Examination

It is essential to record the weight, manual blood pressure (with the correct-sized cuff) and the urine dipstick in clinic.

Investigations

Urine must be sent so that protein:creatinine and microalbumin:creatinine ratio can be checked. In addition urine should be sent for urgent microscopy for red blood cells and red cell casts if blood positive on dipstick test. Further blood tests should be done as listed above.

Diagnosis

Orthostatic proteinuria was diagnosed as the child was clinically well and the first morning urine was negative for protein. The blood pressure was normal. This was confirmed on the first morning urine protein:creatinine ratio being < 20 mg/mmol with a normal serum protein and albumin.

Management

Parents were reassured and the child discharged.

Follow up

No follow up is required for this condition. If proteinuria was also present on the first morning specimen of urine and blood tests were normal, repeat urine testing after 1 week to check if it resolves. In case of persistent proteinuria, a specialist opinion must be sought.

Discussion

Orthostatic or postural proteinuria is a benign condition and usually resolves with time.

Further reading

Webb NJA, Postlethwaite RJ. Clinical paediatric nephrology, 3rd edn. Oxford: Oxford University Press, 2003.
Leung AKC, Wong AHC. Proteinuria in Children. Am Fam Physician. 2010; 82(6):645–651.
    www.aafp.org
The National Heart, Lung and Blood institute. Blood Pressure Tables for Children and Adolescents.
    www.nhlbi.nih.gov

Patient information

HealthyChildren.org
    www.healthychildren.org
Great Ormond Street Hospital (GOSH)
    www.gosh.nhs.uk

Case 60

Pyelonephritis

Dear Paediatrician,

Thank you for seeing Jenny. She is 4 years old and has been having recurrent episodes of fever and loin pain. She has been diagnosed with recurrent urinary tract infection. Recently, she was treated with intravenous antibiotics for a urinary infection while on holiday. She was unwell for 3 days. She is otherwise well. Her mother has had recurrent urinary tract infections as a child. I enclose the notes from her admission.

Many thanks,

Dr Lesley Quigley

Case analysis

Differentiating upper from lower urinary tracty infection is of significance because of the need for urgent antibiotic treatment to reduce the possibility of renal parenchymal damage in pyelonephritis. Upper urinary tract infections (UTIs) usually make children more unwell and usually prompt a need for further investigation depending on age and clinical course. Of primary importance are the method of diagnosis and a reliable urine collection method. Bag urine samples are generally avoided and clean catch specimens are required. The National Institute for Health and Care Excellence (NICE) guideline 53 (UTI in children – urinary tract infection in children: diagnosis, treatment and long-term management) is used to guide further assessment.

Differential diagnosis

Pyelonephritis

Since the presentation of pyelonephritis can be nonspecific, particularly in younger children, considering the diagnosis in all children with feverish illness is important (see NICE guidelines for Feverish illness). The classic collection of symptoms of loin pain, abdominal pain, vomiting with high fever and cloudy/offensive urine are supportive of upper tract symptoms and renal infection.

Lower urinary tract infection or irritation
Other infection

The possibility of another infection needs to be considered. Localising signs for infections which might not be apparent (suggested by earache or sore throat), as well as more obvious disctractors pointing to another cause (such as diarrhoea) should be considered. In the outpatient setting, a history of a prior event and the memory of the specific detail may have diminished with time, so any documentation of presentation assessment during the acute episode can be helpful.

Consultation essentials

History

Asking about the symptoms during an episode will help assess the likelihood of pyelonephritis being a diagnosis. However, the focus will likely be on the urine sample and the associated results. Asking how the urine was collected and processed can help determine whether the sample can be believed. For example, a sample may have been collected without washing the external genitalia – sterile water is adequate, without soap or antiseptic. A clean catch is exactly that, obtaining a sample of urine from the bladder directly into a sterile pot, via washed genitalia. In younger infants this is challenging, but with perseverance, following a good feed (if the baby is able to) and sometimes a cold hand on the lower abdomen, a sample can be obtained. Ask what the sample was collected in, particularly if collected at home – tin foil trays, carrier bags, a potty or the change mat are some of the non-sterile, inappropriate methods used to collect urine in which then cause contamination. If afore-mentioned methods have been used, a true assessment of the result cannot be made. Commercial pads have been researched and found to be an acceptable alternative, but not cotton wool or absorbant pads. A catheter specimen sample or suprapubic aspiration could be considered in the emergency department.

A dipstick can be helpful to assess for urea-splitting organisms. Nitrate is converted to nitrite by *Escherichia coli* and this is the positive dipstick finding supportive of urinary infection. It is a time-limited conversion, so in infants passing urine frequently, there may not be time for nitrite formation, despite the presence of bacteria. The presence of leucocytes is also reported on the dipstick. Presence of nitrites and leucocytes are very suggestive of a UTI.

Once a cleanly caught sample is obtained it needs to be processed urgently. If this is not possible, the sample should be stored in the fridge. The lab should be asked to do microscopy – to assess white cells, red cells and other cells, e.g. epithelial cells which, if present, imply skin contamination. A sample containing greater than 50 white cells per cc, and no epithelial cells is suggestive of infection. The lab will process the sample for culture and the gold standard will be a pure growth, in presence of pyuria, of $>10^5$ colony forming units per millilitre per high powered field. So, making the diagnosis of UTI is not a simple matter of reporting a positive culture.

Good practice suggests that two clean catches are obtained.

Examination

A general exmination to assess for palpable kidneys and other stigmata of chronic renal disease can be performed. Examination of the external genitalia is more important in lower urinary tract infection.

Investigations

Further urine samples are not usually necessary unless chronic infection is suspected in a child with urogenital anatomical abnormailites. This is unlikely to be the case for Jenny.

Tests and investigations are discussed in the management section below. Inflammatory markers will be high in pyelonephritis, and a presentation with septicaemia is a possibility.

Diagnosis

Jenny has a good history for pyelonephritis based on the report from the illness on holiday. There were episodes of previous infection reported. On close review (and having obtained all the sample results from the lab, including microscopy), none of these previous samples were confirmatory of UTI with pure growth and pyuria, in the presence of typical symptoms. As such these previous episodes were 'undiagnosed' as UTIs. However, the episode on holiday is more suggestive and review of the notes confirms a fully sensitive *E. coli* infection with pyuria of 200 white cells per high powered field obtained by clean catch.

Management

There is specific guidance in the NICE UTI guideline on further investigation based on age. Children who respond well within 48 hours of starting treatment require no imaging. Otherwise, imaging is required. For Jenny, a child with a one-off infection and no recurrent or atypical features, an ultrasound is recommended and no further tests.

The history of Jenny's mother having had renal problems when younger needs to be explored. Since vesicoureteric reflux runs in families, this may make the possibility of reflux in Jenny more likely, although it should improve over time and is unlikely to still be present. If she had reflux, the possibility of renal scars should be considered. However in the presence of a normal ultrasound at this age, and according to the NICE guidelines (which do not reference a positive family history as being relevant), no further tests are required.

Follow up

This may not be necessary if the ultrasound is normal. It is important to safety net with advice to collect a clean catch urine sample if Jenny is unwell with a fever and there is no obvious cause. That sample needs to be processed urgently. Treating with antibiotics while waiting for the culture result is a reasonable plan.

Discussion

While obtaining a sample is important, nothing should delay the prompt treatment if the child is acutely unwell with signs of sepsis in an acute presentation.

There is some controversy about the NICE guidelines. They would reduce the number of tests done compared to previous consensus guidelines and suggest the renal community should advocate a more cautious approach. Following this approach, a small number of significant lesions may be missed and the debate hinges on the risk of missing these versus the risks inherent in investigating many children needlessly. An approach reducing the number of radioisotope tests will reduce the radiation exposure to the kidneys and, conversely, there is a real, if small, risk in such investigations. Ultrasound, in good hands, can be good at determining peripheral scarring. Dimercaptosuccinic acid (DMSA) scan would be the gold standard for excluding scars. The NICE guidelines do not routinely advise prophylaxis. A review of tertiary unit practice in Australia following the introduction of the guidelines found no change in the proportion of patients undergoing renal ultrasound, a decrease in the proportion undergoing micturating cystourethrogram (MCUG) scan and receiving antibiotic prophylaxis, and an increase in the proportion undergoing DMSA.

Further reading

National Institute for Health and Care Excellence. Urinary tract infection in children: quick reference guide. Clinical Guideline 54, 2007.
http://guidance.nice.org.uk
Judkins A, Pascoe E, Payne D Management of urinary tract infection in a tertiary children's hospital before and after publication of the NICE guidelines. Arch Dis Child doi:10.1136/archdischild-2012-303032

Patient information

National Institute for Health and Care Excellence. Urinary tract infection in children. Clinical Guideline 54, 2007.

Case 61

Raynaud's phenomenon

Dear Paediatrician,

Alice is now 12 years old. She has episodes of finger swelling and redness, especially in the cold. This has been present for some time. Her aunt has scleroderma.

Please advise on appropriate management.

Many thanks,

Dr Lionel White

Case analysis

This letter strongly suggests a diagnosis of Raynaud's phenomenon/syndrome, which can happen from any age. It is important to determine if this is an isolated condition or part of a generalised connective tissue disease, and then determine what level of treatment is required.

Differential diagnosis

Raynaud's phenomenon

Raynaud's phenomenon (RP) is very common. There are a number of formal definitions, and clearly the more rigidly these are applied, the lower is the incidence of RP. A recent UK study suggested a prevalence of up to 20% in secondary school children, whereas most international studies suggest a prevalence of 3–5%.

There remains uncertainty about the pathophysiology of Raynaud's, and it is divided into primary RP, where there are no associated conditions, or secondary RP. The most common association with secondary RP is connective tissue disorders which occurs in about 20% of sufferers. Other associations are rare in childhood but include drugs (including methylphenidate), endocrine problems, infections such as mycoplasma and, extremely rarely, malignancy. Most cases do not have an obvious autoimmune cause, and girls are affected four times as often as boys.

To clinch the diagnosis there need to be three colour changes to the affected area:

1. Pallor – caused by initial artery and arteriole spasm
2. Cyanosis – due to capillary dilatation and venous stasis
3. Rubor – caused by reactive hyperaemia

These are accompanied by varying degrees of swelling and pain. It is usually the pain that spurs the family to seeking help. RP affects exposed areas, of which the hands are the most vulnerable. It should affect both sides equally. If the symptoms are unilateral, then another cause must be sought. The commonest trigger for an episode is exposure to cold, but there can be other triggers, including psychological ones.

Management depends upon the severity of symptoms. Avoiding triggers is obviously important. This might need school involvement, e.g. staying inside at break-times, wearing gloves in school and not doing cross-country runs in the snow.

Keeping warm is essential: the warmest gloves (and socks) available should be worn to try and avoid symptoms. Specialised products (including silver gloves) are available.

In severe cases, medication may be required. The commonest medication used is nifedipine. Usually, a low starting dose is increased slowly, with the aim of finding the lowest effective dose. Blood pressure should be monitored, checking for hypotension. Nifedipine is often taken during the winter months only.

Secondary RP

It is important to ascertain if there are any other symptoms, particularly involving skin, muscles and joints, as the RP may be part of a connective tissue disease (CTD). Clinically, in CTD the nail bed capillaries may be abnormal, but most units will not have the necessary equipment to check this.

In some instances the cause of secondary RP will be obvious. A major distinguishing factor between primary and secondary RP is that in the former there should be no raised inflammatory markers and normal autoantibodies. An erythrocyte sedimentation rate (ESR) and antinuclear antibody (ANA) may be helpful in distinguishing between them, although beware of the slightly positive ANA which is more often than not a coincidental finding.

Juvenile idiopathic arthritis

This can present with finger swelling, and is normally more protracted and less obviously triggered by exposure to cold. It can be a cause of secondary RP.

Chronic regional pain syndrome (reflex sympathetic dystrophy)

This is a poorly understood conversion disorder. Normally, there is significant continuous coldness of the affected limb, and severe pain. The limb seems ischaemic, and may look pale and feel cold, but should not have the characteristic colour changes of RP. Usually, only a single limb is affected. Treatment is with physiotherapy and psychology input.

Sickle cell disease

Bony sickle crises often affect the hands causing dactylitis. This should be evident from the history, and by this age it would be unusual to make a first diagnosis of sickle cell disease.

Consultation essentials

History/examination

After getting a clear history, try to ascertain if there are any features of CTDs. Make sure that the patient is not on medication which may trigger RP. Many patients will have a family history positive for autoimmune disorders.

Tests/investigations

If there are no other signs, an ANA and ESR seem reasonable to at least reassure if this is primary RP.

Diagnosis

Alice appeared to have primary RP. An ANA was weakly positive, but this was felt to be coincidental.

Management

A letter to the school explaining her problems and the acquisition of silver gloves seemed to suffice initially. However, as the weather worsened so did her discomfort. She was started on nifedipine, and the community nurses checked her blood pressure until she was on a stable dose.

Follow up

Depends on severity of symptoms and treatment instituted. Because RP can be the first symptom of other conditions, safety netting should ensure that the family represent if symptomatology changes.

Discussion

Raynaud's phenomenon is common, especially in children of secondary school age. Because symptoms cover a wide spectrum, the management varies between cases. The longer the symptoms have been present, and in the absence of anything more worrying and a normal ANA and ESR, the more likely it is that this is primary RP, and the family can be appropriately reassured.

Further reading

Nigrovic PA, Fuhlbrigge RC, Sundel RP. Raynaud's phenomenon in children: a retrospective review of 123 patients. Paediatrics 2003; 111(4):715–721.

Patient information

Raynaud's and Scleroderma Association
www.raynauds.org.uk.

Case 62

Reaction to first vaccine

Dear Paediatrician,

Please can you advise on the future management of this 3-month-old baby?

He presented for immunisation at 2 months. When he was examined, he was healthy and the first of his primary immunisations was given. The following day he was very unsettled and didn't feed as well as usual. His parents think he was a little feverish and he had some reddening and swelling of the left leg, which was the site of the DTaP/IPV/Hib immunisation. The site of the pneumococcal vaccine was slightly red but not swollen.

He recovered within 2 days and is now back to normal and doing well.

The parents are aware of the benefits of immunisation and would like the course to continue but they are worried that there will be a worse reaction next time. He is due to be immunised next week.

Dr Enrique Alvarez

Case analysis

The reaction described is quite common and is definitely a significant local reaction – possibly an adverse systemic reaction because of the fever and loss of appetite.

Consultation essentials

The reaction may be due to an active vaccine component but could also be caused by any one of many other ingredients in the vaccine or equipment used to administer. The main message is that these are mild, self-limiting reactions which do not escalate to anaphylaxis or a more severe reaction. In practice a child who has reacted this way to a first vaccine is probably no more likely to have an adverse event with subsequent vaccines than any other. The clear message to the family is to go ahead with the remainder of the vaccine schedule as normal. They should be advised, however, to have suitable paracetamol available for the baby.

Because it is not known which component of the vaccine would have triggered the reaction there is no logic to giving vaccines separately and in practice it is not possible to obtain the vaccines separately. In the past the pertussis component was blamed for many of the reactions but changeover to the acellular vaccine reduced adverse reactions noticeably and this is no longer seen as the main suspect component.

In this situation it is important that the person responsible for immunising the child satisfies himself that the child is fit and healthy for each immunisation. If the general practitioner is clear that this is the case and the parents are reassured it is probably not necessary to delay immunisation in order for the child to be seen by a paediatrician.

However, if there is doubt, or the child appears to be unwell, then a thorough assessment of the child would be helpful.

True contraindications

The only general true contraindication to immunisation is an anaphylactic reaction to the same vaccine previously, or an anaphylactic reaction to one of the antibiotics used as preservatives within the vaccine (neomycin, streptomycin and polymyxin B). There are other special considerations regarding vaccines, e.g. for patients with significant immunosuppression and those with HIV, but these should be discussed and explored individually, with advice from any specialist treating the child. There are also special considerations for some vaccines in patients who are severely egg allergic or who have latex allergy, but these are unlikely to be factors for a young baby. All the contraindications are related to personal history. Family history of any potential problem is not a contraindication.

Further reading

Salisbury, et al. Immunisation against infectious disease (The Green Book), 3rd edn. Department of Health, 2006.

Patient information

The Department of Health
   www.nhs.uk

Case 63

Rectal bleeding

Dear Paediatrician,

Please could you see Jemima? She is 3 months old, and has started passing blood in her stool. She seems very uncomfortable. She was a normal delivery – an elective home birth – and mum is breastfeeding exclusively.

Dr Hugh Mayor

Case analysis

Any bleeding in a baby this age needs to be taken seriously. The greatest concern would be whether the child has a bleeding disorder, either inherited or as a result of a vitamin K deficiency. In the latter situation there may be a herald bleed, before a more catastrophic one. Similarly, if the child has a surgical cause of bleeding, e.g. a Meckel's diverticulum, there can be quite severe blood loss. On receiving this letter it is wise to contact the family immediately. Unless the story is highly suggestive of a fissure, i.e. a small amount of blood associated with a constipated stool, the child should be seen as soon as possible, and preferably immediately.

Differential diagnosis

Haemorrhagic disease of the newborn, vitamin K deficiency

Haemorrhagic disease of the newborn (HDN) can present with any degree of bleeding or bruising, often with minor symptoms preceding catastrophic ones. Babies who have received intramuscular vitamin K seem to be completely protected from HDN. Those that have received oral vitamin K are likely to be protected but they may have low levels due to the presence of liver failure. Babies who have not received any vitamin K will be vulnerable to HDN. Breast milk contains very little vitamin K. A controversial health scare in the late 1990s led to a drop in the uptake of vitamin K, and a predictable rise in cases of HDN. Some parents are still wary of administering vitamin K especially intramuscularly.

It is essential to ask about vitamin K administration. Check clotting and if there is a prolonged prothrombin time, vitamin K should be given. The baby should be monitored until clotting has normalised.

Bleeding diathesis

Other bleeding diatheses may present this way occasionally. They are more likely to present with bruising and oral bleeding. A clotting screen will identify most abnormalities, although there can be rare abnormalities, e.g. platelet dysfunction, where the numbers are normal but the function is not.

Cow's milk protein allergy

There is some debate about whether this is an allergy or intolerance, or indeed whether there are two separate entities; it is probably a form of non-IgE-mediated immunity. Cow's milk protein allergy (CMPA) causes many symptoms including colitis – other symptoms include eczema, reflux and change in bowel habit. The colitis will cause the baby to be unsettled and pass blood mixed with loose stool. Even though Jemima's mother is breastfeeding, if she is consuming dairy produce the cow's milk protein can be passed through breast milk.

Generally, the diagnosis is made by excluding dairy. If a mother is breastfeeding, she should go dairy-free and if this is prolonged she may need dietary supplements, especially calcium. If the baby is having formula this can be changed. Babies less than 6 months can first be tried on an extensively hydrolysed feed (eHF) and the majority will respond to this. In those that do not, an elemental/amino-acid feed (aaF) can be tried. It is important to recognise that eHFs are quite expensive and aaFs very expensive. Prescribing the latter unnecessarily is a poor use of either the patient's or the health system's resources. Although there is some crossover with CMPA and soya allergy, most babies with CMPA can tolerate soya. It is reasonable to suggest a soya formula to babies over 6 months.

If the baby improves with a change of milk, it is hard to know whether this is causal or coincidental. The only way to prove this would be with a challenge. After 2 to 6 weeks, the baby can be exposed to small but increasing quantities of the presumed offending agent in the form of cow's milk infant formula. If the symptoms recur, then it supports the idea that it was to blame. In general CMPA improves with age. Therefore, over time the baby can be challenged intermittently. For example, at 6 months of age a baby on an eHF may be tried with soya, and one on an aaF tried with an eHF or soya. If this is tolerated then at some stage in the future, usually by 1 year of age, they may be challenged with dairy.

Unless there is a history of anaphylaxis, theses challenges can take place at home, usually by introducing a small amount, e.g. a small yoghurt, or mixing 30 mL of the old milk in a bottle of the new one, and seeing if this causes symptoms over the next few days, if everything is well, the amount offered can be increased slightly until symptoms recur or the previous feed is fully reintroduced.

Anal fissure

This is rare in children this young, unless there has been significant constipation/stool withholding. Usually, there will be a small quantity of fresh blood associated with a hard stool. Treatment is with fluid, fibre and laxatives, finding the right combination to allow the passage of a soft, easy, regular stool.

Meckel's diverticulum

Meckel's diverticulum presents with profuse rectal bleeding, often with very little pain. There is often much blood and little stool. Because the bleeding can continue and proceed to shock, it is important to diagnose this early. A radioisotope – a Meckel's scan – is required. Treatment is with resuscitation and surgery.

Intussusception

An intussusception would be rare in this age group. If in doubt speak to the radiologists and surgeons.

Artefact

It is always worth checking that the red component of the stool is actually blood. Urate crystals can look like blood in a nappy, although this would be at the front of the nappy from urine.

Extremely rarely, parents will put their own blood or other blood like substances in the nappy, in fabrication. This diagnosis should only be considered after organic causes have been excluded.

Consultation essentials

History/examination

The nature of the blood and the stool can help distinguish between colitis, fresh brisk bleeding, such as from a Meckel's diverticulum, or a small bleed from a fissure. It is important to know how long the symptom has been present and how the baby has been. A feeding history, including what a breastfeeding mother is eating can identify if there has been any change in the diet. A stooling history is as important, checking for any constipation.

Ask about vitamin K administration and whether there is any bleeding diathesis in the child, e.g. prolonged bleeding after vaccinations – or in the family.

Examination must include an assessment of circulation (ABC), and in some cases resuscitation will be required.

Tests/investigations

It is hard to argue against arranging a full blood count and clotting screen as minimal investigations. If there has been only small blood loss with a clear explanation, these may not be strictly necessary. Other investigations will depend on clues from the history, and often none are required. Stool culture to exclude a dysenteric infection might be helpful.

Diagnosis

Jemima was passing blood mixed in with her stool and was increasingly uncomfortable – all features of colitis, secondary to CMPA.

Management

Jemima's mother was advised to go on a dairy-free diet, and over a few weeks Jemima's symptoms resolved. She was challenged a few weeks later when her mother took a trial of dairy again and Jemima's old symptoms showed signs of returning.

Jemima's mother remained dairy-free, and received calcium supplements from her general practitioner. She exclusively breast fed till Jemima was 8 months of age, following which Jemima was successfully weaned on to a dairy-free diet using soya milk instead of cow's milk in her feeds.

Follow up

This depends on other services available. After making a change, some review will be required after a few weeks to check if this has been effective, or if something else needs to be done. If the child or mother is on an exclusion diet, they may need dietetic follow up.

Further management could be with the general practitioner, dietician or paediatrician but rarely needs all three together. In children with diagnosed CMPA, challenges with dairy are usually commenced at about 1 year of age. If dairy is not tolerated then subsequent challenges can take place every 4–6 months.

Discussion

Most CMPA is of the non-IgE-mediated type. Onset can be insidious and an elimination diet may need to continue for at least 2 weeks. Rarely children present with more acute IgE-mediated symptoms. In this situation, they should be managed as any other child at risk of a serious allergic reaction/anaphylaxis.

Further reading

Koletzko S, Niggemann B, Arato A et al. Diagnostic approach and management of cow's milk protein allergy in infants and children: ESPGHAN GI Committee practical guidelines. J Pediatr Gastroenterol Nutr 2012; 55:221–229.

Vandenplas Y, Brueton M, Dupont C et al. Guidelines for the diagnosis and management of cow's milk protein allergy in infants. Arch Dis Child 2007; 92 (10):902-908.

Ludma S, Shah N, Fox AT. Managing cows' milk allergy in children. Br Med J 2013; 347:5424.

Patient information

NHS Choices
   www.nhs.uk

Case 64

Recurrent fever

Dear Paediatrician,

This 5-year-old boy has recurrent fevers every few weeks with recurrent tonsillitis. During one illness he did seem to have a swollen ankle and limped for a week but then got better. He gets a non-specific rash with the fevers. There are reports of occasional mouth ulcers. His mother says she can predict when the the fever will occur within a day or two. She is worried that there may be an underlying condition.

Thanks for seeing him,

Dr Angela Power

Case analysis

Many children, particularly pre-school, are referred to outpatients with recurrent fevers. The differential here is wide and an analytical approach is essential to be able to distinguish what is normal or not. In the latter case, is there an underlying immune deficiency causing recurrent infection, or a systemic condition with recurrent fever as a presenting feature?

There are many different definitions of recurrent fever. One commonly used is three or more episodes of fever in a 6-month period, with no obvious medical cause for the fevers, and at least 7 days interval between each fever episode. Fever is usually defined as a temperature of over 38.0°C. A distinction between fever of unknown origin (FUO)/pyrexia of unknown origin (PUO) needs to be made. The differential in PUO is more diverse than for recurrent fevers, so the distinction is important.

The distinction between whether fever is recurrent at regular or irregular intervals can help determine aetiology.

Differential diagnosis

Recurrent viral infections of childhood

Children can have around 8–10 viral illnesses in a year. The fever from a viral illness can last for up to 10 days. The majority of children cope with these and are unwell for a short-period of time. Occasionally, a run of infections can seem like the illness and the fever is never ending, but there are usually a few discrete days of wellness in between. There are usually signs that indicate the cause of the fever: tonsillitis, coryza, cough, etc.

Bacterial infection

As for viral infections, children can have bacterial infection in recurrent fever. They are more usually occult so consider urinary tract infection (UTI), bacterial endocarditis, sinusitis or abscess. Although there may be repeated episodes of pyelonephritis, bacterial infections are less likely to occur with this frequency, e.g. a child with frequent bacterial infections needs investigating for underlying immunodeficiency.

Immunodeficiency

It would be unusual for a significant immunodeficiency to present this late. IgA deficiency is associated with an increased number of respiratory infections, commonly in the first few years of life. There is also an association with coeliac disease. Most immunodeficiencies are associated with the triad of failure to thrive, respiratory infections and diarrhoea. If an immunodeficiency is suspected, targeted investigations should be arranged, usually after discussion with an immunologist.

Other infections

Consider parasitic infections, such as malaria. Fungi should not cause invasive infection in immunocompetent children. Epstein–Barr virus (EBV) is said to cause recurrent fevers, but it is unusual to have this periodicity.

Fever (or pyrexia) of unknown origin

This is a vague condition which could be described as a discrete illness of at least 3 weeks' duration during which there is fever of over 38.3°C (100.9°F) present on most days and without a clear diagnosis despite investigation over 1 week, usually in hospital. Viral infections would have resolved in this time and bacterial infections are likely to have made the child more unwell, therefore this situation requires closer investigation. The causes are commonly infectious, inflammatory, vasculitic disorders and malignancies.

Inflammatory conditions

Chronic illnesses can present with recurrent fever in children. Consider inflammatory bowel disease, juvenile idiopathic arthritis, Bechet's disease, and hereditary periodic fevers (see below).

Marshall's syndrome (periodic fever, aphthous stomatitis, pharyngitis, adenitis syndrome)

The periodic episodes of high fever last 3–6 days and recur every 21–28 days. There is aphthous stomatitis, pharyngitis and cervical lymphadenopathy. It usually occurs in children under 5 years of age. The family usually know when the episodes are about to occur and parents will often explain that the fever comes on very regularly like clockwork. The presentation of the non-fever signs is variable, although lymphadenopathy is commonest; only around 70% will have pharyngitis and stomatitis. The episodes are formulaic, with every episode appearing the same as all of the others. Other nonspecific features may be present. The condition can last many months or years. Over time the episodes reduce. There are no long-term complications. Treatment is not usually required although use of a one-off dose of prednisolone, and tonsillectomy have been reported as being beneficial.

Cyclical neutropenia

This is a rare benign condition which affects humans and grey collie dogs. Neutropenia occurs every 21 days. There is an associated fever, malaise cervical lymphadenopathy, stomatitis or gingivitis. Neutropenia at the time of fever should raise the possibility of this diagnosis, which will need input from the haematologists.

Hereditary periodic fever syndromes

These are rare and distinct inherited conditions characterised by short and recurrent attacks of fever and inflammation that occur periodically. They cannot be explained by the usual childhood infections or illnesses. Each episode is usually self limiting and the children recover completely and are normal between episodes.. The episodes are usually associated with haematological signs of inflammation such as raised erythrocyte sedimentation rate (ESR) and leucocytosis.

Recent genetic advances have identified six periodic fever diseases:
- Familial mediterranean fever
- Hyperimmunoglobulinaemia D with periodic fever syndrome
- Tumor necrosis factor receptor-associated periodic syndrome
- Muckle–Wells syndrome
- Familial cold auto-inflammatory syndrome
- Chronic infantile neurologic cutaneous articular syndrome, also known as neonatal-onset multisystem inflammatory disease

The last three in the list are known as cryopyrin-associated periodic syndromes or cryopyrinopathies.

These conditions are normally definitively diagnosed and managed in tertiary centres.

Neoplasia

This is included in the differential as a malignancy and can rarely present with recurrent, unexplained fever. Lymphoma is the most likely cause.

Others

Drug induced (should be clear from the history), factitious (admit the child and document the fevers) and central nervous abnormalities (especially of the hypothalamus) are described as other rarer causes.

Consultation essentials

History/examination

Clarify the extent of the fever. How high is it? Is it consistent – every night, every week or every month? Do the family know when the next episode is due? How is the temperature measured? Ask about specific symptoms during an episode, especially arthralgia/arthritis and abdominal pain. Look for lymphadenopathy, oral ulcers, and rashes on examination.

Tests/investigations

Keep a dairy or log of the child's temperature. For an initial work up check:

- Blood count and film
- Inflammatory markers (ESR and C-reactive protein) – if raised initially, worth repeating in-between fevers
- Blood cultures
- Urine culture

Further tests can be carried out as directed and include serology for Epstein-Barr virus (EBV) the most common viral cause, saving serology for a convalescent sample, chest X-ray, tuberculin test if there is a possibilty of tuberculosis, serum protein electrophoresis, rheumatoid factor, antinuclear antibodies and anti-streptolysin O antibodies. A metabolic profile including uric acid and lactate dehydrogenase and quantitative serum immunoglobulins might be the next step, and consider bone marrow examination if no diagnosis had been made.

Diagnosis

Based on the story, a periodic fever, aphthous stomatitis, pharyngitis, adenitis (PFAPA) syndrome was diagnosed. There were no features of other diagnoses. The initial blood tests were all normal. In a subsequent episode the second line tests were done. Inflammatory markers were mildly elevated but returned to normal on recovery. The symptoms remitted over a period of months.

Management

There is no specific treatment for PFAPA. The fever does not always respond completely to antipyretics. They are not indicated if the child is not unwell. Over some years, the symptoms reduce, and resolves by later childhood. One treatment is to give a single dose of steroids (usually prednisolone) at the start of the symptoms in an episode. They have been shown to shorten or prevent the episode, and reduce the frequency of episodes. Tonsillectomy may be considered for very frequent, repeated attacks.

Follow up

Routine follow up could be done in primary care if the family know what to do and how to manage the episodes. It would be more usual for a paediatrician to monitor the child over time to ensure there are no new or different symptoms, prompting review of revision of diagnosis.

Discussion

Management of recurrent fevers often takes patience. If there are no worrying symptoms, and initial investigations are normal, a wait-and-see approach is appropriate. If the symptoms persist they should be investigated further and referred as necessary.

Further reading

Berlucchi M, Nicolai P. Marshall's syndrome or PFAPA (periodic fever, aphthous stomatitis, pharyngitis, cervical adenitis) syndrome. Orphanet encyclopedia, 2004.

John C, Gilsdorf JR. Recurrent fever in children. The Pediatric Infectious Disease, 2002; 21(11):1071–1077.

Marshall GS, Edwards KM, Butler J, Lawton AR. Syndrome of periodic fever, pharyngitis and aphthous stomatitis. J Pediatr 1987; 110:43–46.

Patient information

The American College of Rheumatology
www.rheumatology.org

Recurrent tonsillitis

Dear Paediatrician,

Thank you for seeing 15-year-old Toby. He has a 3-year history of recurring bouts of sore throats. This has been affecting his school performance for a while now and both teachers and parents are concerned regarding the number of weeks he has to miss school with his general certificate of secondary education approaching. He has missed 6 weeks of school this year.

When he attends the surgery, he has large inflamed tonsils with exudates and often a high fever. Previous throat swabs have grown group A β-haemolytic *Streptococcus* (GABHS).

Antibiotics have provided temporary relief only, and appear only to be effective for the next episode.

He is asthmatic, which is often exacerbated by these attacks. There are no significant developmental issues or relevant family history.

Dr Saleh Aljearah

Case analysis

Sore throat is one of the commonest presentations to a UK general practitioner: UK frequency 0.1 per capita per annum. Currently, there are no robust criteria for the diagnosis of tonsillitis. Important questions to ask are:

- Have the diagnoses been clinical or patient/parent-based?
- Has the patient had associated episodes of pyrexia, odynophagia, pharyngeal erythema with/out tonsillar exudates and painful cervical adenopathy?
- Have these episodes been documented by the general practitioner on a number of occasions?
- Has there been at least 12 months of symptoms that are not resolving?
- Have there been clear quality of life and educational issues?

Differential diagnosis

Recurrent tonsillitis

A large subgroup of children develops recurring infections of the tonsils and pharynx. The exact cause and prognostic factors in individuals are unknown. GABHS, viruses and anaerobes are common causative organisms.

A significant proportion of patients' symptoms resolve spontaneously if the duration history is under 12 months. With longer durations a large proportion will continue to suffer recurrent throat infections with significant adverse influence on quality of life, and reduced number of weeks of school and work attendance. Subcategories include subacute and chronic tonsillitis. Patients often suffer chronic low grade ill health affecting quality of life. They can develop tonsillar crypts, debris, tonsilloliths, halitosis, sometimes associated with abdominal pain, failure to thrive and low weight.

Infectious mononucleosis

Acute pharyngotonsillitis is a frequent manifestation of infectious mononucleosis (IM) and is caused by Epstein–Barr virus (EBV) infection. The clinical course is often longer than acute tonsillitis, typically lasting several weeks. Generalised lymphadenopathy is common and hepatosplenomegaly sometimes occurs. In these cases, it is important to advise avoidance of abdominal trauma/contact sports for 6 weeks. The diagnosis can often be made by measuring EBV antibodies, but this is not 100% reliable. Secondary infection occurs in up to 30% with GABHS, the commonest micro-organism implicated. It is important to avoid ampicillin as it can result in a severe allergic rash. If swallow is severely compromised consider systemic antibiotics and steroids.

Peritonsillar abscess (quinsy)

This is pus in the peritonsillar space (between the tonsil and its bed). It is often preceded by peritonsillar cellulitis.

Common causative organisms include GABHS, *S. viridans*, *S. aureus*, *H. influenzae*, anaerobes. Typical symptoms are severe unilateral/asymmetrical pharyngitis and marked adenopathy. The patient will often have severe trismus, making examination difficult. The uvula may be displaced to the contralateral side. Treatment includes adequate hydration, analgesia, antibiotics (a penicillin or a cephalosporin and metronidazole are good first line treatments), and often a short course of steroids to improve painful swallowing. An ENT specialist opinion is recommended as aspiration or incision and drainage under local anaesthesia often dramatically and immediately reduces symptoms. Rarely, airway obstruction can occur and requires careful examination by appropriately trained personnel and an experienced paediatric anaesthetist (as with acute epiglottitis), with availability of immediate resuscitation and airway support.

Most otolaryngologists recommend surgery for two quinsies in a lifetime. Some recommend concurrent tonsillectomy, although interval tonsillectomy is practiced by most.

Retropharyngeal and parapharyngeal abscess

These are rare but can be serious. They are more common in infants and young children under 5 years of age. Infection occurs in lymphoid tissue neck spaces. Clinical features include systemic upset with or without airway compromise, and untreated may progress to mediastinitis and be life-threatening. Initial investigations include plain films and CT with contrast which shows widening of soft tissue spaces of the neck. Recommended treatment is high dose antibiotics, urgent incision and drainage under general anaesthetic, and with airway protection. Tracheostomy may be necessary in extreme situations.

Lemierre's syndrome

This is a rare condition causing septic thrombophlebitis of the internal jugular vein +/- intracranial venous sinuses +/- metastatic abscesses. The causative organism is often fusiform bacillae. Clinical features include severe neck pain, torticollis, septicaemia, and typically runs a rapidly fulminant course. Investigations include CT/MRI with skilled imaging of neck veins and venous sinuses.

Immune complex disorders

Acute rheumatic fever and acute glomerulonephritis can cause tonsillitis. It is more common in certain ethnicities, e.g. Aborigines and Maoris in Australia.

Tonsillitis and psoriasis

Association between GABHS tonsillitis and guttate psoriasis. Some recommend tonsillectomy with uncontrolled trials showing benefit.

Consultation essentials

History

It is important to ask about age, the number and duration of episodes, effect on quality of life and education. Ask about similar history in siblings and the child's general health.

Examination

Examine the oropharynx using a small tongue depressor. A young child is best placed in the parent's lap with the child facing the examiner and the parent holding the child's head still against their chest. Older children may be asked to open their mouths and roar like a lion. In older children fibreoptic evaluation of the nasopharynx can be very useful in identifying the degree of adenoidal hypertrophy, especially if nasal obstruction or sleep disordered breathing is suggested in the history. The neck and abdomen are palpated for masses.

Diagnosis

Toby has recurrent acute tonsillitis.

Management

It is important to have a thorough and non-rushed discussion of the condition and management options with parents, as every child's management is very individual. It is important to discuss the likely natural history (about 50% recurring bouts resolve if the history is shorter than 12 months' duration though much less likely if longer). Audiovisual material is useful to show how the anatomy of the upper airway in a child can be affected.

All management options and treatment implications should be discussed, including the importance of active watchful waiting with symptom and video diaries in appropriate situations.

It is important to admit to any uncertainties without embarrassment, and therefore come to a consensual decision with the parents.

The Scottish Intercollegiate Guidelines Network (SIGN) criteria, quality of life and effects on education are the key factors to ascertain.

Further reading

McKerrow W. Diseases of the tonsil. In: Scott-Brown's Otolaryngology, Gleeson S, (Ed). Head and Neck Surgery, 7th edn. London: Hodder Arnold; 2008:1219–1228.
Paradise JL. Indications for tonsillectomy: setting the bar high enough. Arch Otolaryngol Head Neck Surg 2008; 134(6):673. doi: 10.1001/archotol.134.6.673-a.
SIGN
   www.sign.ac.uk

Patient information

ENT UK
   www.entuk.org

Scoliosis

Dear Paediatrician,

I would be very grateful if you could see this 12-year-old girl and advise on further management. She presents with a short history of chest asymmetry, noted by her family and friends, examination revealed an abnormal lateral curvature of spine. She is generally healthy and active, keen in sporting activities, particularly gymnastics. This is of a significant concern to the child and her parents because of the uneven appearance of her back when she puts on her gym gear. She also occasionally complains of back ache which resolves with rest. I have made a request for X-rays of thoracolumbar spine in anticipation.

Yours sincerely

Dr Humphrey Levine

Case analysis

The referral letter points to scoliosis as a possible diagnosis, and therefore it would be more appropriate if she presented directly to the orthopaedic team. There have been instances of patients being referred to the wrong clinic and the paediatrician should make an appropriate referral speedily.

The important aspects of this consultation would be to confirm scoliosis by examination, look for secondary causes and establish the need for further imaging/referral to orthopaedic surgeons.

Differential diagnosis

Scoliosis can be divided into two categories:

Functional scoliosis

This is where the spine itself is normal but curvature appears because of an underlying condition such as a difference in leg length or muscle spasms.

Structural scoliosis

There is fixed lateral curve to spine in the form of a 'C' or an 'S'. Idiopathic scoliosis is the most common, with girls affected more than boys. It often starts towards the end of primary school, and becomes more marked over time. Other causes are: cerebral palsy – especially when severe, spinal trauma, neuromuscular diseases, congenital vertebral anomalies and tumours. Historically tuberculosis (Potts disease) was a common cause, and remains so in countries where tuberculosis is rife and treatment limited.

Consultation essentials

History/examination

Focus firstly on the onset and severity of symptoms and the impact on life style such as the ability to perform day-to-day physical activities. Then determine any other presenting features such as a history of trauma, the presence of neurological symptoms in lower extremities, pain, and family history of spinal problems or neurofibromatosis.

A good examination does require that the back can be seen well. The old textbooks show people naked when being examined for scoliosis. This is probably a little overwhelming for most patients at a first consultation. Most young people will be prepared to take off their tops for a medical examination, girls can keep their bras on, and if very self conscious could wear a tight vest. They should be bare footed. It can be helpful to have a chaperone present. View the patient from the front looking for:

- Uneven shoulders
- Upper limb length discrepancy – one upper limb may seem longer because of shoulder tilt
- Prominence of rib cage on one side
- Prominent hip on one side
- Leg length deformity

Then view the patient from behind, looking for features as shown in **Figure 66.1**.

Next, perform the forward bending test – stand behind the standing patient and ask them to bend over and place their hands on their knees. In scoliosis, one side of the rib cage or lower back will appear prominent compared to other side (**Figure 66.2**).

Systemic features of illness, clinically significant pain, neurocutaneous markers, abnormal neurology, foot deformity and associated lordosis or kyphosis should be considered red flag signals and precipitate more urgent action.

Tests/investigations

The most useful initial tests are X-rays of the thoracolumbar spine – anteroposterior (AP) and lateral. Spinal curvature is measured using the Cobb method on an AP radiograph. Parallel lines are drawn along the plane of intervertebral discs at the beginning and end of the curve. A second line is drawn perpendicular to each of these lines and the angle of intersection of these second set of lines make the Cobb angle. Cobb angle >10° is indicative of scoliosis (**Figure 66.3**). The Cobb angle and how rapidly it changes determine the appropriate action.

- Cobb angle 10– 20°: usually managed by regular observation (3–6 monthly). A significant increase in Cobb angle (> 5° in 3 months would prompt further action)
- Cobb angle 20–45°: usually requires spinal bracing to prevent worsening
- Cobb angle >45° degrees: usually requires spinal fusion

MRI is becoming the investigation of choice, especially in severe cases or when a neurological abnormality is detected on examination. MRI is being used increasingly in the assessment of idiopathic adolescent scoliosis to look for occult intraspinal abnormalities.

Diagnosis

This girl had mild idiopathic scoliosis.

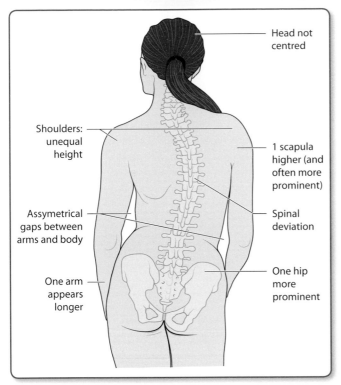

Figures 66.1 Features evident on examination of a child with scoliosis when standing with her back to the examiner.

Head not centred

Shoulders: unequal height

1 scapula higher (and often more prominent)

Assymetrical gaps between arms and body

Spinal deviation

One arm appears longer

One hip more prominent

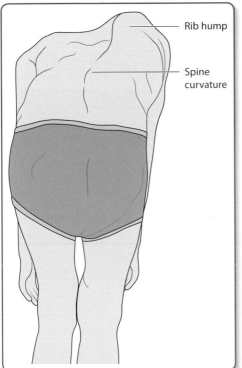

Figure 66.2 When the child bends over spine curvature may become more evident and a rib hump may form.

Rib hump

Spine curvature

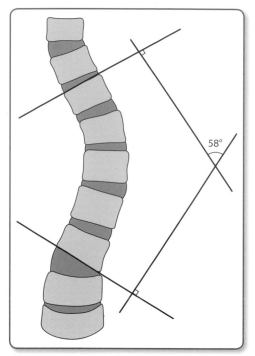

Figure 66.3 Measuring the Cobb angle in scoliosis – from an AP X-ray.

58°

Management

When a diagnosis of scoliosis is confirmed, most children are referred for an orthopaedic assessment. In cases of functional scoliosis, the correction of an underlying cause will result in resolution of scoliosis. This girl was referred to the orthopaedic surgeons who suggest watchful waiting. After 3 years the scoliosis had not markedly deteriorated.

Follow up

After referral to the orthopaedic surgeons, no paediatric follow up is required.

Discussion

Idiopathic scoliosis is the most common type of scoliosis seen in paediatric outpatient practice. Most patients have a mild form and just need reassurance and 3–6 monthly follow up until skeletal maturity is complete. Causes other than idiopathic scoliosis need to be considered.

Further reading

Altaf F, Gibson A, Dannawi Z, Noordeen H. Adolescent idiopathic scoliosis. Br Med J 2013; 346:f2508.
Hesko MT. Clinical practice; idiopathic scoliosis in adolescents. N Engl J Med 2013; 368:834–841.
Musson RE, Warren DJ, Bickle I, et al. Imaging in childhood scoliosis. Postgrad Med J 2010; 86:419–27.

Patient information

Patient.co.uk
www.patient.co.uk
The Scoliosis Association UK
www.sauk.org.uk

Case 67

Shared care of children with cancer

Dear Paediatrician,

Please can you help with the shared care of the 8-year-old boy who has recently completed a 3-year treatment for acute lymphoblastic leukaemia. He had normal treatment and has been essentially well since completing it.

Dr Sandeep Singh

Case analysis

Children with leukaemia are managed by shared care between a tertiary hospital primary treatment centre (PTC) and the local district general hospital (DGH) which is known as a paediatric oncology shared care unit. Treatment usually lasts approximately 2 years in girls and 3 years in boys. Following end of treatment children are seen regularly either at one of the two hospitals, or jointly for several years. The initial reviews are related to ensuring that the leukaemia has not relapsed, and long-term follow up is usually to assess any sequelae of treatment.

Consultation essentials

History/examination

At every out-patient assessment children should have their height and weight measured and plotted. There is a recognised association with children becoming overweight or even obese following treatment for leukaemia and several factors have been considered responsible, including the long duration of steroid use, the abnormal eating habits picked up during the period of chemotherapy and illness, and other possible contributing factors. Older children and adolescents should have pubertal assessment performed.

Examination during the first 5 years after the end of treatment should include assessment for anaemia, abnormal bruising, enlarged lymph nodes, liver or spleen and, very importantly, unilateral testicular enlargement which may indicate a relapse of disease.

After 5 years from end of treatment it is important to continue to monitor these children although they may now be considered 'cured' of the leukaemia. Modern chemotherapy regimens have a much lower profile of late effects and most survivors of acute lymphoblastic leukaemia do not have any significant long-term sequelae. It is important to assess cardiac function by echocardiogram.

Tests/investigations

Routine full blood counts are no longer recommended after the end of treatment and clinical surveillance is considered more useful and practical. In any child with symptoms/

signs of a possible relapse as listed above, a full blood count and film should be performed immediately and if abnormal they should be referred to the PTC for bone marrow and other investigations. Boys with testicular enlargement may have an isolated testicular relapse and may have a normal full blood count. They should always be referred back to the PTC for biopsy of the testis and bone marrow aspiration to check for relapse.

Myocardial abnormalities are a relatively rare but significant consequence of anthracycline drugs which are still routinely used for the treatment of leukaemia. Screening for cardiac damage is by assessing ventricular function on echocardiogram, specifically looking at contractility and shortening fraction.

Follow up

The schedule for follow up is often monthly for the first few months after end of treatment, then stretching through 2- and 3-monthly appointments to 6-monthly appointments from 2–5 years from end of treatment. At 5 years the child should be seen at the long-term follow-up clinic at the PTC where the focus of the consultation moves from looking for relapse to monitoring for sequale of treatment and any long-term problems such as cardiac damage, delayed puberty or fertility issues.

Further reading

Scottish Intercollegiate Guidelines Network. Long term follow up of survivors of childhood cancer. SIGN
	guideline 132, 2013.
	www.sign.ac.uk
Cancer Research UK. Childhood cancer statistics.
	www.cancerresearchuk.org

Patient information

Great Ormond Street Hospital
	http://www.gosh.nhs.uk
The Children's Cancer and Leukaemia Group
	http://www.cclg.org.uk

Case 68

Short stature

Dear Paediatrician,

I will be grateful for your assessment of this fourteen and a half-year-old boy with short stature. He has always been one of the smallest in his class. Currently, his height lies just below the 2nd centile with the mid-parental height on the 50th centile. His recent cause for distress is the fact that his 12-year-old sister has almost caught up with him in terms of height. He is also concerned about the appearances of his genitalia – he has not started developing yet. Of note, his father was a late developer and had a late growth spurt.

　　He was reluctant to be examined but does not report any secondary sexual characteristics. Please could you advise further.

Yours sincerely,

Dr David Thomson

Case analysis

Short stature is defined as height below the 2nd centile (minus two standard deviations for age and gender). The key to assessment in this case is whether the short stature is pathological or a normal variant.

Differential diagnosis

Normal variant short stature

Constitutional delay of growth and puberty

Children with constitutional delay in growth are healthy children with delayed skeletal maturation. The bone age lags behind the chronological age. Puberty is delayed compared with their peers and these children continue to grow later than their peers, leading to an adult height within the genetic potential. It is more common in males and there is often a family history of delayed growth and puberty.

Familial/genetic short stature

This refers to healthy short children who have short parents/family members. They grow at a normal velocity for age and track within their target centile range. In contrast to constitutional delay, the bone age is not delayed compared with the chronological age.

Pathological short stature

Pathological causes must be considered in all children who present with short stature. The major causes are discussed below. Broadly, short stature can be classified into disproportionate or proportionate. Plotting of sitting height and leg length (standing height minus sitting height) on appropriate growth charts helps to identify body disproportion.

Proportionate short stature
Small for gestational age
Nearly 90% of children who are born small for their gestational age show catch up growth in early childhood. Those who do not catch up to their genetic potential can benefit from growth hormone therapy.

Genetic syndromes
Short stature may occur in association with a genetic syndrome. It is essential that condition-specific growth charts are used to plot the growth of these children. Specific syndromes associated with short stature include:
- Turner's syndrome
- Down's syndrome
- Prader–Willi syndrome

Chronic disease
Virtually any chronic illness such as cardiac disorders, cystic fibrosis, coeliac disease, inflammatory bowel disease, etc. can cause growth failure.

Psychosocial deprivation
Neglect and emotional deprivation are known to cause psychosocial dwarfism that usually shows dramatic improvement in a safe, nurturing environment.

Endocrine disorders
Dysfunction of any endocrine system can lead to short stature, including:
- Hypothyroidism
- Growth hormone deficiency
- Cushing's syndrome
- Precocious puberty (an early growth spurt causes reduced final height)
- Poorly controlled diabetes mellitus

Disproportionate short stature
Short limbs
Conditions of skeletal dysplasia such as achondroplasia and hypochondroplasia will be evident as short limbs as well as short stature. The penotype also includes macrocrania.

Short trunk
Bone dysplasias primarily involving the spine, such as Morquio's disease or following spinal irradiation, for example in treatment for medulloblastoma.

Consultation essentials
History/examination
The following need to be considered in the assessment of the child with short stature:

- Detailed birth history, including birth weight for gestational age, history of hypoglycaemia/jaundice – which is rarely associated with hypopituatrism.
- Symptoms of any chronic disease process
- The psychosocial environment
- Thorough clinical examination; any dysmorphism (watch out for Turner syndrome in short girls)
- Pubertal assessment: delayed pubertal status in an otherwise short adolescent may indicate constitutional delay of growth and puberty (CDGP) with good potential for final height. Conversely, advanced pubertal status in a short child gives poor prognosis for final height.
- Accurate growth measurements, plotted on appropriate charts. A single height measurement has its value in screening for short stature. However, a more useful measure of growth is height velocity which requires serial measurements of height over a period of time (ideally 6 monthly intervals). It is expressed in centimetres per year after calculating the growth increment between two time points. Growth charts provide a benchmark reference based on measurements performed on thousands of normal healthy children. A normal growth curve is one that tracks along or is parallel to one of the printed centile lines in the child's target centile range (TCR). The TCR is derived from calculating the mid-parental height (MPH) +/– 8 cm and provides information about genetic height potential. The MPH is calculated by using the formula shown below:

For boys:

$$\frac{\text{Mother's height (cm)} + \text{father's height (cm)}}{2} + 7 \text{ cm}$$

For girls:

$$\frac{\text{Mother's height (cm)} + \text{father's height (cm)}}{2} - 7 \text{ cm}$$

Referral to a specialist/investigation should be considered in the following scenarios:
- Height below 0.4th centile
- Height falling through centiles
- Height centile lower than the target familial centile range
- Height velocity < 4–5 cm/year in childhood

Tests/investigations

First line investigations should generally include the following:
- Full blood count, erythrocyte sedimentation rate, urea and electrolytes, liver function tests – to screen for chronic illnesses
- Coeliac screen – as undetected coeliac disease is a cause of growth failure
- Thyroid function – to rule out hypothyroidism, an easily treatable condition
- Karyotype in girls – to exclude Turner syndrome
- Radiograph of left hand for bone age
- Serum insulin-like growth factor type 1 (IGF-1) concentration – as a screening test for growth hormone deficiency (beware nutritional causes for low IGF-1)

There are inherent difficulties in the diagnosis of growth hormone deficiency and hence referral to a specialist centre should be considered after nonendocrine causes have been excluded. The most important piece of information to forward is previous growth measurements/copy of the growth chart, along with the results of the first line investigations.

Assessment of growth hormone axis requires dynamic testing following administration of growth hormone secretagogues. The gold standard is growth hormone assessment following insulin-induced hypoglycaemia (insulin tolerance test). The test is dangerous in young children and avoided in most centres in the UK. The other commonly used alternatives are glucagon, arginine and clonidine. All children diagnosed with growth hormones deficiency should undergo MRI of the pituitary gland looking for any anatomical malformation or acquired mass lesion affecting the pituitary gland.

Based on the growth measurements and parental heights, the first analysis to be undertaken is whether the presenting child is short or not. The second step, based on history and careful examination is to exclude those who are healthy but short (familial short stature, constitutional delay, small for gestational age). The next step would be to exclude a nonendocrine cause of growth failure with the help of clinical evaluation and the first line investigations. Finally, endocrinopathies should be considered and advice from a paediatric endocrinologist should be sought.

Diagnosis

This young boy referred by the general practitioner is concerned about delayed puberty in association with short stature. This raises suspicion of CDGP. A family history of delayed puberty is in keeping with the diagnosis.

The young boy referred was healthy with no stigmata of chronic disease. He was short for his parental heights but previous measurements indicated that his growth had always tracked along a lower centile. The recent cause of concern was that his 12-year-old sister, who was in puberty had nearly caught up with his height (as she was experiencing her growth spurt). In contrast, on clinical examination it was evident that his puberty was delayed with testicular volumes of 4 mL bilaterally (Tanner stage II, onset of puberty). The bone age was delayed (12.5 years at a chronological age of 14.5 years); confirming the suspicion of CDGP.

Management

Specific treatment depends on the underlying cause. Support and education may be all that is required in some cases (familial short stature and CDGP). In the case of babies born small for gestational age where catch up growth is not achieved by 4 years of age, referral to a specialist for consideration of growth hormone therapy is indicated (Table 68.1). In this case of constitutional delay, supplemental treatment with sex steroids can be offered. Testosterone (or oestrogen in girls) will induce secondary sexual characteristics and alleviate anxiety.

Follow up

Regular review is essential if commencing therapy. Clear explanations are required and the input of a specialist team including nurse specialist is important. Such therapies and follow up will be in a tertiary endocrine clinic.

Discussion

Nutritional, psychosocial and systemic causes of short stature require correction of underlying problem. Endocrine causes of short stature are uncommon but important to recognise early as appropriate treatment can induce catch-up growth and a final height

Table 68.1 Growth hormone therapy indications
Growth hormone treatment is licensed in the UK for the treatment of short stature due to:
1. Growth hormone deficiency
2. Prader–Willi syndrome
3. Turner syndrome
4. Chronic renal insufficiency
5. Children born small for gestational age, who do not show catch-up growth by 4 years of age
6. Short stature homeobox (SHOX) gene deficiency

within the parental target range. For example, thyroxine replacement for the hypothyroid child is particularly effective in correcting short stature.

Further reading

Allen DB, Cuttler L. Clinical practice. Short stature in childhood--challenges and choices. N Engl J Med 2013; 368(13):1220–1228.
Brook CGD, Dattani MT. Handbook of Clinical Pediatric Endocrinology.Wiley-Blackwell, 2012.
Hindmarsh PC, Dattani MT. Use of growth hormone in children. Nat Clin Pract Endocrinol Metab 2006; 2(5):260–268.

Patient information

Child Growth Foundation
    www.childgrowthfoundation.org
Patient.co.uk
    www.patient.co.uk

Sickle cell disease

Dear Paediatrician,

I would be grateful if you could see this 12-year-old girl who has recently moved into the area. She was diagnosed as having sickle cell disease at the age of 3 years following a hospital admission. As she has not had a paediatric assessment for over a year we would like you to review her.

Yours sincerely,

Dr Charlotte Agnew

Case analysis

Sickle cell disease is becoming more common in the UK with the changes in ethnic mix. The UK antenatal and neonatal screening programme for sickle cell disease was set up in 2001 and uses the newborn blood spot to screen for the presence of the abnormal haemoglobin. The diagnosis of sickle cell disease might have been missed in the neonatal period in children born prior to 2004 when the programme became well established.

Consultation essentials

History

Sickle cell disease (SCD) is seen primarily in the Afro-Caribbean population. A history of sickle cell disease in other members of the immediate or extended family and in particular in the siblings needs to be established. The parents may be aware that they are carriers. Ask about:

- Painful crises including
  - Frequency of episodes
  - Whether requiring hospital admission or not
  - Sites of pain, e.g. limbs, chest, abdomen
  - Management of episodes – simple analgesia such as paracetamol or ibuprofen, or whether opiates have been administered in hospital
- Nocturnal enuresis – children with SCD are encouraged to drink large volumes of fluid to remain well hydrated. They also may develop renal impairment due to recurrent sickling. These factors increase the incidence of enuresis
- Snoring – children with SCD often have tonsillar and adenoidal hypertrophy and may have nocturnal hypoxia and sleep apnoea
- School attendance – children with SCD often have reduced school attendance for a variety of reasons and need to be monitored and addressed

- CNS symptoms of stroke/transient ischaemia – this is a less common, but devastating complication of SCD. All children should now be monitored regularly by transcranial doppler (TCD) scanning so that preventative measures can be instituted in those at risk.
- Immunisation history - children should receive pneumococcal vaccinations as part of the normal infant immunisation programme at age 2 years, followed by a booster every 5 years. Hepatitis B vaccination is recommended for all children as they may be exposed to hepatitis B if they receive a blood transfusion in a country where there is a less rigorous blood donor screening programme. Annual influenza vaccination is also recommended.

Examination

- Height and weight need to be measured and plotted at each visit. Pubertal status needs to be assessed. Children with severe SCD may have slow growth and delayed puberty
- Measure blood pressure and oxygen saturation
- Look for pallor of the mucous membranes and conjunctival icterus
- There may be a flow murmur due to chronic anaemia
- Palpate the abdomen looking for hepatomegaly and splenomegaly (in homozygous SCD, there is usually auto-infarction of the spleen by the age of 5 years and therefore the spleen is not usually palpable). Tenderness in the right hypochondrium may indicate the presence of gall stones and needs to be investigated

Investigations

A full blood count and reticulocyte count are checked on a 6-monthly basis unless the clinical situation necessitates more frequent checks.

- Liver function tests need to be checked, and children with more severe haemolysis may have a persistently raised bilirubin
- Some children may need measurement of their Hb F levels in monitoring response to treatment
- Sleep study may be indicated in children who snore at night, have tonsillar/adenoidal hypertrophy or low oxygen saturations
- Abdominal ultrasound scan may be indicated in children with abdominal pain or tenderness, especially in the right hypochondrium, to look for gall stones
- TCDs should be performed by a specialist trained technician on an annual basis in all children with homozygous SCD above the age of 2 years

Management

Medication

All children should be on prophylactic penicillin twice daily as they are at a high risk of pneumococcal infections.

Daily folic acid helps as this is a chronic haemolytic disorder.

Transfusions

Children with SCD do not need to be transfused routinely. Indications for a top-up transfusion include an acute severe haemolytic crisis, an aplastic crisis or pre-surgery. Some children may need an exchange transfusion, e.g. for chest crisis, severe priapism, acute stroke. Children who have abnormal TCD may be at increased risk of stroke and benefit from a regular transfusion programme.

- Families should be provided with 'open access' to the paediatric department or emergency department for urgent evaluation and treatment
- Management of an acute crisis includes intravenous hydration, analgesia, antibiotics and possible blood transfusion according to local or specialist guidelines
- Hydroxyurea (hydroxycarbamide) has been shown to be beneficial in children with severe SCD who have recurrent episodes of crisis. This should only be prescribed and monitored by trained clinicians

Follow up

Children with sickle cell disease need to have regular assessment with a paediatrician trained in the management of the condition. All children should have an annual review by a specialist paediatric haematology multidisciplinary team.

Further reading

NHS Sickle Cell & Thalassaemia Screening Programme
    www.sct.screening.nhs.uk

Patient information

The Sickle Cell Society
    www.sicklecellsociety.org

Case 70

Sleep problems

Dear Paediatrician,

Please can you help this family who are in a desperate situation? Reginald is 21 months old and has never slept through the night. He wakes a few times every night, and starts crying. Dad has a very challenging job, so Mum goes to Reginald to ensure that Dad gets his sleep.

They have tried controlled crying for a few nights but it was unsuccessful. He was unsettled during the day, but now seems happy, and whenever I have seen him he has been in good health. The only other relevant history is that Mum suffered from mild postnatal depression.

Many thanks,

Dr Andrew Bolton

Case analysis

It is difficult, if not impossible, to underestimate the exhaustion that accompanies being a parent of a child that does not sleep. Sleep deprivation is a method of torture and affects functioning on all levels. Parents consulting for sleep issues usually have little residual resilience and it is essential that any action plan acknowledges this. For example, although behavioural techniques may be indicated, they may be difficult to implement due to parental fatigue.

Sleep patterns are essentially habits and the longer bad ones are established the more difficult they are to break. So, by this age Reginald will have learnt to be awake at night. Whilst day time naps may provide him with an adequate amount of sleep in total, it is unlikely his mother will have the same opportunity to catch up on her sleep during the day.

Distinguishing cause from effect is complex, but poor sleep is associated with increased mental health problems, especially anxiety and decreased daytime effectiveness, reflected in poor school work in children, and an increased risk of accidents and reduced effectiveness in parents.

Although the child appears healthy and well, the impact that his poor sleep is having on his mother is not good for her well being, and not good for Reginald as her exhaustion will mean she is a less effective mother.

Parents are often reluctant to start treatment, so explaining that keeping his parents awake impacts adversely on him as well, is often helpful.

The postnatal depression may be relevant in many ways, as the condition may make her view her child negatively, and the exhaustion exacerbated by the poor sleep may make the depression worse.

Differential diagnosis

Individual factors/sleep behaviour

How long babies sleep obviously varies from baby to baby. Everybody has different thresholds for waking and falling back to sleep again. Environmental factors such as light, noise, heat/cold may have an impact. At this age he may have separation anxiety, affecting his ability to get to sleep, this leads to prolonged 'curtain calls' or his parents lying in bed with him till he gets to sleep (with separation anxiety it is often not clear which party is most disturbed at the thought of separation). In older children, poor sleep can be a manifestation of mental health issues, especially anxiety and depression.

When considering a sleep routine, the following factors should come into account. Each will be considered.

1. Daytime activity/sleeping
2. Getting ready for sleep
3. Getting to sleep
4. Staying asleep

1. **Daytime activity/sleeping:** If Reginald is completely happy and playful during the day, then the issue may be one of parental expectation. Some parents expect their children to sleep for a fixed amount of time, whereas in reality this is widely variable. If a child is sleepy or grumpy during the day, then it is likely that they are not getting enough sleep. Daytime naps are common at this age, and indeed aid sleeping at night. Late evening naps will not be helpful and keeping children awake till they collapse is not a way of guaranteeing good sleep.

2. **Getting ready for sleep:** It helps to have a bed-time regime. This can involve a bath and bedtime story, but should avoid too much excitement. Grandmothers visiting and expecting to play should be discouraged. Televisions/computer screens should be avoided while getting ready for sleep. The sleep environment should be appropriate, and ideally he should be in a place where he will neither be disturbed nor disturb others.

3. **Getting to sleep:** This can be difficult, and often the child will act in a way that delays the parents leaving the room. An exhausted mother will have battled through a challenging day. As she leaves, the child will say, 'Mummy I love you, can I have a cuddle?' and this can be hard to refuse. Similarly, the child may ask for one more song, story, etc.

   For parents who tend to stay with their children till they fall asleep, there will have to be some physical separation. This can be either gradual or sudden, depending on the level of crying/upset. In the first method, instead of lying with the child they may start sitting next to them and over time sit further and further away until they are outside the room. It may help to leave a reminder of the parent with the child such as an item of clothing. This is 'gradual withdrawal'.

   If the child starts crying then 'extinction' techniques can be employed. These again can be gradual or sudden. The best known example is 'controlled crying' where the child is left to cry for increasing amounts of time, starting at a few minutes, but stretching to 30–60 minutes if it proceeds for as long. At the end of each period the parent will go in, settle the child and leave. This may work less effectively than just letting him scream but the parents may feel they are being kinder to the child.

4. **Staying asleep:** Rousing during sleep is normal, and can happen many times a night. Normally, the baby should be able to get themselves back to sleep. Sometimes parents interpret stirring for waking and don't give the baby enough time to get back to sleep. Children will often take bottles if offered them in the middle of the night, but it should be possible to drop the night feed by 3 months of age. Assuming that the child is waking in the middle of the night to play, and will scream if ignored, then extinction techniques as highlighted above can be employed.

Pain/physical causes

Although treatment to encourage sleeping by controlled crying is often advised, if his waking is due to pain, this would be not only ineffective but also cruel. Frequent painful waking may be the predominant feature of reflux oesophagitis. If there is any doubt a trial of treatment, e.g. ranitidine for a few months, may be helpful. Other common causes of pain include muscle spasm in cerebral palsy, stool withholding, worm infections and eczema. Treatment usually brings about improvement in sleep, but sometimes the bad sleep habits may persist.

Obstructive sleep apnoea

This is rare in this age group, but more common in older children who usually give a history of loud snoring and fitful sleep. In these cases an ENT opinion is required.

Nocturnal fits

Fits during the night or sleep may cause daytime drowsiness but should not occur nightly.

Medication

Any medication can impact on sleep, such as salbutamol causing agitation preventing sleep or beta-blockers causing nightmares. In older children consider caffeine in drinks, alcohol and recreational drugs.

Night terrors

These tend to occur a few hours after onset of sleep, with the child waking, looking terrified. There can be semipurposeful activity such as sleep walking. Although frightening to observe, the child is unaware of them. Children usually outgrow them, but they can respond to anticipatory waking where for a few weeks the child is woken about 12 minutes before the night terrors are due to occur, although it is unclear, as yet, why this is effective.

Nightmares

Almost certainly occur in children of this age. They are often linked to anxiety or fear. If they are occurring this frequently, then questions need to be asked about what is triggering them. For example, is the child being exposed to inappropriate movies?

Consultation essentials

History/examination

This should identify any factors that might interfere with sleep (pain, drugs, and environmental factors) as highlighted above. Determine how long the problem has been present for; what part of sleep is involved, i.e. the getting to sleep or staying asleep, and what has been tried so far. Establish what support the parents may need to embark on a behavioural programme.

Tests/investigations

Unless anything specific is raised in the history these are rarely required. Polysomnography is generally reserved for more complex cases.

Diagnosis

Reginald was thought to have a behavioural sleep disturbance.

Management

He was given a short course of alimemazine which allowed his parents a few nights of sleep before embarking on a programme of extinction (controlled crying).

Follow up

As most parents often feel at their wits end, any form of advice will be appreciated. They may value the support of having a follow up appointment. If they are not engaged with their health visitor then a referral would be helpful.

Discussion

Behaviour and medication

Behavioural techniques are great in theory, but require energy which may be lacking in exhausted parents. In this situation, the parents need to find a way to gather strength before attempting their chosen technique. This might be accomplished by asking relatives to help look after Reginald for a few nights. A behavioural programme should start at a time when they have as much energy and support as possible, e.g. over a holiday. Sometimes parents might need to do 'tag parenting' taking time away from home to catch up on sleep. It is vital that everybody participates.

Medication can serve two purposes:

1. In very rare circumstances, a short course over a few weeks may help to break a habit.
2. If it does not change the habit it can at least provide some respite, making the behavioural battle easier.

Commonly used and effective medications include alimemazine and melatonin.

Prevention

'Prevention is better than cure'. Prospective parents may take note of three simple things which double the chances of a newborn baby sleeping through the night by a few months of age.

1. Don't let the baby sleep in your arms. If they do, wake them so they can go back to sleep by themselves.
2. Keep their bedroom dark and use minimal lighting at night time.
3. Don't feed the baby on waking, change or calm them first.

These should allow the baby to establish a day/night cycle and learn to go to sleep themselves, even if they have woken up.

Further reading

Matricciani LA, Olds TS, Blunden S, et al Never Enough Sleep: A brief history of sleep recommendations for children. Pediatrics 2012; 129(3):548–556.

Patient information

Sleep for Kids
    www.sleepforkids.org
Family lives
    www.family lives.org.uk
Crysis
    http://www.cry-sis.org.uk
Millpond
    http://www.mill-pond.co.uk

Soiling

Dear Paediatrician,

Please could you see Robert urgently; he is now 7 years old and has been soiling for over 2 years. He has just started school, however they have threatened him with exclusion if he is unable to remain clean.

Best wishes,

Dr Serena Martin

Case analysis

Soiling means different things to different people. The first goal is to find out what it means to this family. Establish when, where and how often it happens. Determining whether the soiling is with normal faeces, and the quantity of soiling is also essential.

Differential diagnosis

Developmental – not yet toilet trained

Although most children are fully toilet trained before they are 4 years old – there is some variation. Children with developmental delay or physical problems are likely to have delayed toilet training. However, it is important to encourage good toilet habits, as this is life changing for the child and family.

Toilet phobia

Toilet phobia is common. Many children will only use the toilet at home, or go in the presence of a parent. Up to 80% of children will not use the toilets at school. Factors such as privacy, hygiene and a fear of bullying have an impact, which can be very difficult to overcome. Often in practical terms this is best overcome by encouraging the child to go to the toilet before going to school.

Poor wiping

There are some children – including teenagers – who either do not wipe themselves, or do not check that they are clean. A reasonable way of asking is 'this may seem a silly question, but do you wipe your bottom after you have been to the toilet – I am asking this because I know lots of people don't' and then 'if you do wipe, do you look at the paper?' and 'how do you know when you are clean?' If the soiling is due to poor wiping this should be easy to address.

In some cultures, especially Islamic ones, people wash their bottoms as well as, or instead of, wiping. The lack of proper washing facilities may make it hard for these children to clean themselves at school, and make them even more reluctant to use the school toilet.

Retentive soiling – associated with constipation/ stool withholding

Most soiling falls within this category, although the constipation/stool withholding (C/SW) may not have been acknowledged. Essentially, if the child is trying to withhold, but failing then they will soil. In this type of soiling there is often the passage of frequent small amounts of abnormal stool, either small hard bits or softer overflow, which may be mistaken for diarrhoea. Often, the soiling happens when the child believes they are only going to pass wind. Usually treatment of the C/SW facilitates full continence although sometimes there is a progression to nonretentive soiling.

Nonretentive soiling – usually due to 'postponement'

Children who are used to soiling often seem to lack some self awareness and seem oblivious to sitting in their own stool. Sometimes this can be linked with other difficult behaviour, but more often it is an isolated problem. For these children the benefits of cleanliness do not outweigh the inconvenience of going to the toilet. They invariably absolve themselves with the comments 'I did not feel it coming,' or 'I did not know that it was there.' But if they have been to the toilet albeit only once then they have awareness of a need to go, and if they do not have bed sores, then they have demonstrated intact sensation. Management entails:

- Ensuring there is no C/SW
- Considering underlying issues, e.g. family issues, especially around siblings, attention fear of growing up
- Providing suitable motivation

If it is entirely clear that the soiling is due to postponement, then motivation techniques need to take this into account. So, whilst positive reinforcement can work, it seems to have limitations, and often consequences for soiling will need to be introduced. These can include the child being involved in clearing up the mess, missing special activities, etc. The aim is that when the child feels a need to go to the toilet, they will decide that they would rather go than face the consequences. The family are advised to stop describing soiling as an 'accident'.

For children who fail this programme, Child and Adolescent Mental Health Services (CAMHS) input may be required, but this often has limited success. Most children will outgrow the problem due to social pressure at school, but the aim is to get them clean before they get a bad reputation with their peers.

Intentional soiling – very rare, usually with significant underlying issues

Occasionally, children will soil intentionally, and this can, even more rarely, be in spiteful places such as their parent's shoes, the washing up bowl, etc. These children are often very disturbed and usually need multiagency input.

Organic (neuropathic) soiling

It is unusual for soiling to unmask a neurological condition. Many children with neurodevelopmental problems will have soiling, but this is more likely to be due to stool withholding and overflow.

Smearing of faeces

Smearing can occur in any of the above conditions. Sometimes children, particularly those with learning difficulties, may soil and explore what is in their pants. As they get their hands dirty, they try to 'clean' them on the wall, clothes, the carpet, etc. In these cases once the soiling is treated, the smearing usually stops.

Rapid gut transit

If the child is producing too much stool every single day, then they may have rapid gut transit, usually due to 'toddler diarrhoea' but this may also be seen in malabsorption or inflammatory bowel disease, and occasionally in autistic children. The history will identify this as a problem, which can then be treated accordingly.

Consultation essentials

History/examination

This is crucial. Questions to ask can include:
- Where does it happen? – If only at school it may be due to school toilets, if only at home it is more likely to be postponement/behavioural
- How often does it happen? If many times a day it is more likely to be overflow
- How much stool is in the pants? Small or variable amounts suggest overflow
- What does it look like? Normal stool (postponement) or abnormal stool (overflow or diarrhoea)
- In general, are there issues with opening bowels? When you feel them moving do you let the stool come out or try to keep it in?
- School toilets – are they clean? Does the child use them?
- Wiping
- Other issues in the family

Examination rarely provides much useful information if the history is conclusive, but most patients expect some form of examination.

Tests/investigations

Tests are rarely required. Soiling and stool diaries kept by the family can be useful.

Diagnosis

Robert had a long history of C/SW – his soiling was secondary to this.

Management

As the C/SW was properly treated, his soiling reduced. He did still have some issues of postponement, and was only fully clean after he missed a few sessions of cubs because he had to help clean his soiled pants.

Follow up

Some follow up is usually necessary. Often the input of children's community nurses can be helpful as there are day-to-day management issues.

Discussion

A possible analogy to offer the child for soiling is:
"Imagine playing football by the windows, and your mother asks you to go to the end of the garden because she thinks the window might smash. You don't listen to her repeated requests, but carrying on playing. You then do a big kick and smash the window. Would you consider that to be an accident?"

Further reading

Cohn A. Constipation Withholding and Your Child. A Family Guide to Soiling and Wetting. London: Jessica Kingsley Publishers; 2006.

Patient information

Education and Resources for Improving Childhood Continence
    www.eric.org.uk
PromoCon
    www.disabledliving.co.uk/PromoCon

Case 72

Swollen joints

Dear Paediatrician,

Thank you for seeing this 8-year-old boy who has been limping for the last 2 months. He complains of pain in his knees and ankles and experiences joint stiffness in the morning. His parents report that his left knee looks swollen at times. Today the left knee felt warm to touch with a suggestion of an effusion. Thanks for assessing him.

Dr Shantini Patel

Case analysis

This referral suggests the likelihood of arthritis (joint inflammation). There is a distinction between joint swelling with or without pain. Arthritis is manifested as a swollen joint having at least two of the following conditions: limited range of motion, pain on movement, or warmth overlying the joint.

Differential diagnosis

Inflammatory arthritis e.g. juvenile idiopathic arthritis

An inflammatory arthritis, of which there are a number of types, is characterised by joint pain and/or swelling for more than 6 weeks, morning stiffness, a gelling phenomenon (stiffness after a period of rest, commonly first thing in the morning), constitutional upset (weight loss, poor eating, sleep disturbances), fever and rashes. There may be a positive family history. There are also associations with inflammatory bowel disease, psoriasis and connective tissue disorder as well as human leukocyte antigen HLA-B27. It is more common in girls. The diagnosis of juvenile idiopathic arthritis (JIA) is based on a history of joint inflammation for at least 6 weeks in the absence of any other cause or conditions. It represents a group of disorders, with a system of classification depending on presentation and symptomatology (Table 72.1). A systemic onset can present with fever every day for at least 2 weeks. Systemic onset is also usually associated with a salmon-pink, nonblanching, nonpuritic rash.

Trauma

Young children will jump onto and fall off things at height. An accidental injury is possible; however do not overlook the possibility of nonaccidental injury if there are significant injuries with little or no explanation, inconsistent stories, a worrying social set up or other supportive features. It would be unlikely for trauma not to resolve within a few days or so.

Table 72.1 Classification of juvenile idiopathic arthritis (JIA) in children

	Oligoarthritis*	Polyarthritis		Enthesitis-related (ER)	Psoriatic arthritis	Systemic-onset	Undifferentiated arthritis
		Rheumatoid factor negative	Rheumatoid factor positive				
Type	60% of JIA patients	20% of JIA is a polyarthritis		10–15% of patients	< 10% of patients	< 10% of patients	Arthritis which does not fit neatly into the other categories
		Majority of polyarthritis patients	about 10% of polyarthritis patients (< 5% of all JIA)				
Age	< 5 years	Onset any age; older onset → more similar to adult arthritis	Usually >10 years	Particularly >8 years (can be younger)	Usually 8–9 years	< 5 years	
Sex	< 8 years: F > M > 8 years: M > F	F > M	F>>M	M >> F	F > M	F = M	
Joints affected	< 5, most commonly one or both knees, ankle and wrist joints and sometimes elbows and small joints of hands and feet	Usually hands and feet; may also affect hips, knees, neck, elbows, shoulders or jaw	Quite severe form of disease which needs active medication to avoid joint damage	Inflamed entheses, mainly in hips, knees, ankles and sacroiliac joints	Usually small joints of hands or feet; can affect larger joints	Long-term development difficult to predict: joint symptoms may continue for years	
Associations	Chronic anterior uveitis (does not cause red or painful eye, but can cause reduced vision)	Onset can be sudden (simultaneously several joints become painful and swollen) or slow (steadily involve more joints over months)	Early treatment essential to prevent progression and long-term damage	Acute anterior uveitis 30–40% of ER JIA patients have on-going arthritis into adulthood, particularly if HLA-B27 positive (about 75% are positive). Often family history of AS or IBD because of HLA-B27 association	Painless uveitis Classic psoriatic rash may not develop until later. Psoriatic nail signs may be apparent Family history of psoriasis supports diagnosis	Presents with systemic illness, including fever, lethargy, rashes, loss of appetite and weight loss, and joint pain. Fever and rash usually settle. Very occasionally, myocarditis and pleural effusion	

AS, ankylosing spondylitis; F, female; IBD, inflammatory bowel disease; M, male.
* Called 'extended oligoarthritis' if extends to other joints.

Infection

Septic arthritis is unlikely to present to outpatients. But some viral (reactive) arthritidies may have already prompted a non-urgent referral for review.

Vasculitis

Inflammation of the small vessels in vasculitis can affect the joints, seen commonly in Henoch–Schönlein purpura.

Haematological

The presentation of a haematological condition such as a blood malignancy like leukaemia can present with a limp or swollen joint. A bleeding diasthesis can also cause swollen joints due to haemarthroses, haemophilia A being the most common.

Gastrointestinal conditions

Inflammatory bowel disease such as ulcerative colitis and Crohn's disease can be associated with arthritis in an individual with HLA-B27 histocomplex.

Rickets

Vitamin D deficiency in infants and children has an adverse effect on calcium metabolism resulting in rickets, as well as other manifestations such as convulsions, dental problems, general ill health, and poor growth. The main source of vitamin D is ultra-violet radiation from sunlight on the skin. There is a reduction of appropriate wavelength of light in the UK in winter months. Children with increased skin pigmentation have a reduced capacity to synthesise vitamin D in the skin. Recently, there has been a resurgence of rickets in British Asian children and recent immigrants to the UK and a decline in the routine use of vitamins over recent years. An affordable assay to vitamin D has led to more routine and less targeted measuring of serum vitamin D levels, and low vitamin D without abnormalities in other bone mineral parameters is being picked up.

Consultation essentials

History/examination

Assessment of the musculoskeletal system including joints will reveal any abnormality such as swollen joints, limited movement or deformity. A paediatric gait, arms, legs and spine examination (pGALS) will comprehensively assess the musculoskeletal system. Acutely swollen or tender joints at time of assessment is good evidence to back up the diagnosis.

Younger children may be reluctant to walk for short distances or seem to get tired quickly.

Tests/investigations

Blood tests

A rheumatoid factor will direct towards 'RF+' or 'RF−' arthritis/JIA. Similarly antinuclear antibodies (ANA) are autoantibiodies which can be positive, especially in children with oligoarthritis. It is also positive in systemic lupus erythematosis which can present with swollen joints. Children with positive ANA are more likely to have uveitis. ANA can be positive in 10% of the normal population. Inflammatory markers, especially erythrocyte sedimentation rate will be raised.

Radiographs and other imaging

X-rays of the affected joints should be done to assess joint space and the presence of an effusion radiologically. Ultrasound or MRI or joints can be helpful.

Diagnosis

This child has a swollen knee and his rheumatoid factor was negative, but ANA positive. He was referred to the paediatric rheumatology service for further assessment and management.

Management

Management includes medical, physical and psychosocial. The initial medical management is with nonsteroidal anti-inflammatory medications. Good doses of effective medications (such as naproxen) are prescribed. If the condition is more severe, disease-modifying drugs (such as methotrexate, corticosteroids, immune modulators and monoclonal antibodies) can be used. In significant joint inflammation, intra-articular injections may be required. Oral steroids can also be used. Since this is usually a chronic disease, family support and support for the young person in school is essential. School life may need to be modified if mobility is an issue. Physiotherapy and occupational therapy are important with attention to support activities of daily living. An early ophthalmology review should be arranged especially in younger children, who may have anterior uveitis without overt symptoms.

Follow up

Follow up will depend on the specific diagnosis. In the likelihood of a long-term condition, the child will need to be seen regularly by therapists and for medical assessment.

Discussion

As with any chronic condition, a co-ordinated approach with the local paediatric team is essential. Children on high risk medications, such as methotrexate will need regular blood tests. Arrangements for prescribing these medications need to be in place with close liaison between hospitals and health professionals.

Further reading

Petty RE, Southwood TR, Manners P, et al. International League of Associations for Rheumatology classification of juvenile idiopathic arthritis, 2nd edn. Edmonton, 2001. J Rheumatol 2004; 31:390–392.

Patient information

Arthritis research UK
    www.arthritisresearchuk.org

Case 73

Syncope

Dear Paediatrician,

I would value your opinion on Elizabeth as her family are becoming increasingly worried about her and have now been to see me three times.

Elizabeth is 13 years old. Over the last 6 months she has had four episodes of collapse. Elizabeth feels clammy and dizzy with some visual disturbance; she then falls to the ground and is unresponsive for up to 30 seconds. When she comes round she initially feels groggy but within about 15 minutes is back to normal. Last week Elizabeth collapsed at school and her teacher, who is qualified in first aid, said that she definitely had a seizure during the episode.

Elizabeth is normally fit and healthy and is doing very well at school. She is not on any regular medication.

Her cousin has epilepsy. Examination today was unremarkable. Her lying and standing blood pressures were 110/75 and 105/70 respectively.

I wonder if Elizabeth is developing epilepsy and feel that she requires further investigation.

Yours sincerely,

Dr Geraint Davidson

Case analysis

Elizabeth has had several episodes over a 6-month period but anxiety levels have likely been raised as a reliable observer has reported Elizabeth having a seizure. It is likely that this, plus the family history of epilepsy, has precipitated the referral. Initial thoughts from the history given are that these episodes are most likely vasovagal rather than epileptic in origin. The symptoms pre-collapse, the short duration and rapid recovery make epilepsy unlikely. The key issue in this case is to rule out any serious pathology and having done that, to reassure and offer mechanisms to reduce and manage the attacks.

Differential diagnosis

Vasovagal syncope

Syncope is a sudden and transient loss of consciousness, usually as a result of decreased cerebral blood flow causing anoxia. Syncopal episodes are usually of short duration (a few seconds), however on occasions they can last longer. Vasovagal syncope is by far the most common cause of syncope accounting for approximately 75% of cases, and is most common in adolescence. Episodes may be provoked by pain, stress, heat, prolonged standing or anxiety. A predisposition to postural hypotension may be present.

A prodrome of light-headedness, dizziness, cold sweat and pallor is common. There may also be visual or auditory disturbance just prior to the collapse. Collapse may be followed by twitching and jerking which can mimic an epileptic seizure. However these movements are due to the transient cerebral hypoxia rather than being epileptic in origin. Once laid down the patient will recover spontaneously and facial pallor will resolve. They may feel unwell and/or sleepy after the event. This is usually short lived but occasionally can mimic the excessive sleepiness associated with epileptic seizures.

Epilepsy

Epilepsy is much less common than syncope. There are an estimated 60 000 children under the age of 18 years with epilepsy in the UK. Some patients will get an aura before a seizure however this is different to the prodrome of vasovagal syncope. The aura can be varied and include unusual smells, a strange feeling in the head, a feeling of anxiety or visual disturbance. The visual aura of occipital lobe epilepsy usually involves colours and the patients will describe brightly coloured patterns. Patients are usually sleepy following a convulsive seizure and sleeping for an hour or more post-event would not be unusual.

A family history of epilepsy does increase the risk of epilepsy, however only 2–5% of children born to parents with epilepsy will develop the condition and the risk is even lower in second degree relatives.

Cardiac causes

Any syncope associated with exercise, shortness of breath or chest pain should raise the suspicion of a cardiac cause, as should a family history of sudden death. These causes are rare but must be checked for in the history and examination. Prolonged QT and hypertrophic cardiomyopathy are the silent killers.

Hypoglycaemia

It would be unusual to present at this age unless there was co-existing pathology such as anorexia. Collapse following a period of fast would suggest this diagnosis.

Psychogenic blackout

These occur most often in young adults but are seen in adolescence. The physiology is not yet fully understood but they are associated with stress or anxiety. Psychogenic blackouts can look just like syncope or an epileptic seizure but there are some subtle differences. Pallor and sweating are usually absent, they can occur when laid down, they often occur at the same time of day or in the same place and can be multiple or prolonged.

Consultation essentials

History/examination

As with many conditions a detailed history is the key, with emphasis on red flag symptoms. The history in this referral letter is highly suggestive of syncope. Events surrounding the collapse may point to triggers for the syncope, e.g. postural hypotension, warm environment, stress or fear. Any suggestion that these episodes are related to exercise should precipitate a detailed cardiac assessment. A child who has learning difficulties, is dysmorphic, or has a past history of birth trauma or brain injury should raise the question of epilepsy as the diagnosis.

Any abnormalities found on cardiac or neurological examination should precipitate further investigation.

Tests and investigations

Often the diagnosis is clear from the history. Supine and erect blood pressure measurements are often difficult to perform accurately and tilt-testing is impractical in all but the most resistant cases. If there is concern about a cardiac cause then an ECG seems reasonable. Otherwise an ECG is likely to provide little extra information, but may offer significant reassurance to the family. In a young girl post menarche a full blood count could be considered if anaemia is possible. Tilt testing may be used to confirm the diagnosis of vasovagal syncope but this is not usually required.

Electroencephalography (EEG) or further cardiac investigations are not required unless dictated by the history and examination.

Diagnosis

Elizabeth was diagnosed with vasovagal syncope.

Management

The management involves reassurance and advice on how to minimise further attacks and lifestyle advice such as avoiding prolonged periods of standing up, especially in hot environments. Advice should include lying down and raising the legs or sitting down and lowering the head at the first signs of an attack. There is minimal evidence that increasing salt and water intake improves symptoms but it should be tried in the first instance. In refractory cases medication such as fludrocortisone may be prescribed.

Follow-up

In simple vasovagal syncope follow up is not required unless the episodes are disabling due to frequency or severity. Most cases improve as the patient enters adulthood.

Discussion

Syncopal episodes are relatively common and, when associated with seizure-like activity, can be alarming. It is important to take an accurate history in order to make the diagnosis without over investigating. The most common age of onset of vasovagal syncope is around puberty when children experience a growth spurt.

Further reading

Armaganian L, Morillo CA. Treatment of vasovagal syncope: an update. Curr Treat Options Cardiovascular Med 2010:12(5).

Massin MM, Bourguignont A, Coremans C, et al. Syncope in paediatric patients presenting to an emergency department. J Paediatr 2004; 145(2):223–228.

Moodley M. Clinical approach to syncope in children. Semin Paedr Neurol 2013;20(1):12–17.

Patient information

The Syncope Trust And Reflex Anoxic Seizures
    www.stars.org.uk
Epilepsy Action
    www.epilepsy.org.uk

Case 74

Testicular problems

Dear Paediatrician,

Please see this 1-year-old boy who has had an absent left testicle since he was born. He has a normal right testicle but I am unable to feel the left. He was born at term and no one has documented that they have felt or seen the left testicle.

Yours sincerely,

Dr Megan Newcomb

Case analysis

The two central issues here are to find the left testicle and to bring it into the scrotum by the age of 9–12 months. Boys should be referred at 6 months of age if the testicle is not palpable. The past doctrine of completing surgery by age 2 years has been modified. There are essentially four options for the testicle:

i.   It is descended but retractile
ii. It is undescended
iii. It has maldescended (or is ectopic)
iv. It is absent

If it has been seen or felt before then it is likely that the testis is retractile, rather than undescended. It is important to find the testicle and bring it into the scrotum to improve fertility and reduce the risk of testicular cancer. In the majority of cases, the absent testis is noted at postnatal newborn examination (baby check) and parents are alerted then, with a referral to the general practitioner to reassess at the 6–8 weeks' check. It is well known that a percentage of testes will descend in the first 6 months of life and therefore referral for further assessment of an undescended or impalpable testis is by the general practitioner. 3–4% of boys will have an undescended testis at birth but only 1–2% by age of 1 year. Prematurity increases the risk of an undescended testis.

Differential diagnosis

Retractile testis

Most boys have very retractile testes. The testicle will disappear into the inguinal canal if stimulated, particularly on stroking the inner thigh. This is a reflex contraction of the cremaster muscle and known as the cremasteric reflex. This is a normal phenomenon.

Flat scrotum

The testes may be descended but a 'flat' scrotum, with minimal pouch, gives the appearance of undescended testes.

Consultation essentials

History

Was the boy born at term or prematurely? Were the testes present at the post-natal check? Have the parents ever seen or noticed both testes? Have the parents noted both testes to be down when the boy is bathed?

Examination

It is important to examine the child in a warm room. Quite often the testes will be visible when the nappy is first removed but will retract upwards almost immediately. Look at the size and shape of scrotum. If the scrotum is well developed it is likely that the testis is present in the inguinal canal. If the scrotum is very under-developed it is likely that the testis is intra-abdominal or absent, and likely not palpable. Examine the contra-lateral side if a testis seems large for the baby's age; this is often indicative that the contra-lateral side is absent or has undergone neonatal torsion.

When examining the inguinal canal sweep one hand down from above and firmly hold over the deep ring (mid-point of inguinal ligament), then with the other hand feel up from the scrotum and along the line of the inguinal canal. If you can feel anything, even if just sac material it is likely that the testis is in the groin. The most common place to find the testis is in the neck of the scrotum, just below the pubic tubercle where it gets stuck on decent during embryological development as it passes out of the superficial inguinal pouch. Sometimes a few squats (flexing a dextension of the hips and knees in succession) can aid a retractile testis to come down into the inguinal canal.

If the testis can be 'milked' into the scrotum and will stay there on release then it is a retractile testis and does not need an orchidopexy. If the testis needs tension to hold it in the scrotum then it needs an orchidopexy. Try not to confuse a testis that retracts due to the cremasteric reflex with one that is genuinely tight. Try to demonstrate both testis in the scrotum to the parents or how tight a testis is in needing tension to hold it in the scrotum.

Investigation

There is very little role for imaging. Testes are so retractile that ultrasound often causes testes to retract into the groin and then they are reported as undescended. MRI is time consuming and requires a general anaesthetic, and is therefore impractical. Laparoscopy is the investigation of choice.

Diagnosis

This child has an undescended, impalpable testicle and was managed accordingly, as detailed below.

Management

The clinical findings dictate the operation required. If a testis is palpable in the groin or ectopic then a standard groin approach orchidopexy is all that is required. The lower the testis the easier the operation, and the greater the success of the procedure. In cases of an impalpable testis then the management is more complicated and progressive.

The first stage is to examine the baby under anaesthetic; often an impalpable testis becomes palpable with a relaxed and compliant child. In this case, a standard groin approach orchidopexy is all that is required.

If the testis remains impalpable then the child should undergo a laparoscopy to look for an intra-abdominal testis and evidence of a vas deferens. If an intra-abdominal testis is found then the tethering testicular vessels are ligated, and the testis left in situ to allow the concurrent blood supply from artery to vas to develop. Then the testis is brought down at a second laparoscopic procedure in 6 months. If a remnant testis is found then it should be excised and the contralateral testis fixed in a subdartos pouch.

If a blind-ending vas is found then the contralateral testis should be fixed but it is assumed that there is no testis present. If the vas and vessels are found entering the deep ring then it is assumed that the testis is in the inguinal canal and the operation is converted to a groin approach with either an orchidopexy if a viable testis is found, or excision of a testicular remnant if that is all that is found.

The key point is that there must be closure on what has happened to the testis.

Follow up

The procedures are usually day case and follow up is required in 3–4 months. Follow up involves checking the position, size and consistency of the testis. The main risk of the operation is that the testis atrophies due to injury to the tethering blood vessels. If this occurs then the testis will wither away (usually painlessly) over a few months. The other major complication is that there is insufficient length and the testis remains high in the groin or even retracts up into the inguinal canal. Providing the testis is of adequate size and in a good position then no further follow up is requires. An atrophied testis does not need excision as no germ cells are left to become cancerous later on in life. An ascending testis requires further re-do surgery to attempt to bring it down to a palpable position.

Discussion

Fertility

Broadly speaking unilateral undescended testis has a small reduction in semen parameters but minimal effect on paternity which should be in excess of 80%. Bilateral undescended testes have a much worse outlook with only 25% being normospermic, 50% oligospermic and 25% azoospermic, and a paternity rate of 50%.

Cancer risk

There appear to be widely ranging estimates of cancer risk in undescended testes but the risk is of order of 3–7 × normal, i.e. about 1:100 compared to 1:500 for normal population. Orchidopexy does not completely normalise the risk and the contralateral testis also has a marginally greater risk of becoming cancerous. Orchidopexy crucially allows a cancer to be felt.

Tics

Dear Paediatrician,

Gordon is a 9-year-old boy who started on methylphenidate with some benefit just under 1 year ago but has recently developed unusual mannerisms. He grunts, has several facial twitches such as opening his mouth and pursing his lips, twitching his nostrils, blinking rapidly and rolling his eyes, and taking sudden intake of breath. When he is not grunting he tends to sigh or breathe rapidly. He does not stop what he is doing when he has these movements but he seems to be unaware that he is doing them and he cannot explain them. Originally, his behaviour had settled down in class on the medication but he is now a source of distraction with his noises. His teacher keeps telling him to be quiet and also not to make faces. Some children have been amused by the distraction whilst others have made fun of him. His mother says he twitches a lot at home in the evenings, especially when he is stressed.

Dr George Rogers

Case analysis

These episodes are likely to be tics; they are multiple in types, vary in morphology and intensity, occur involuntarily and are performed almost subconsciously. Gordon has both typical motor and vocal tics. Sniffing and grunting are common tics, hyperventilation is an unusual tic.

The tendency for the tics to be severe in the evening suggests he might be suppressing them at school but that they break through at home. There is a strong link between attention deficit hyperactivity disorder (ADHD) and tic disorders, but also tics are a known side effect of methylphenidate.

Differential diagnosis

Stereotypes and mannerisms (simple tics)

These are common and variable, the most frequent include, grimacing, throat clearing, shoulder shrugging and blinking. Body rocking, head banging or bobbing occur mainly in younger children. Classically tics evolve, so that they change. This distinguishes the movements from those with an underlying neurological pathology.

Management is with understanding and patience. Advice on tic management from Tourettes action (UK) can also be applied to children with simple tics.

(Gilles de la) Tourette's syndrome

This is a spectrum disorder with varying degrees of severity. Authorities differ as to where benign tics end and Tourette's syndrome begins. In the USA, Tourette's syndrome is viewed as a merging of tics, ADHD, obsessive-compulsive disorder and other behavioural difficulties (poor impulse control). UK authorities are more influenced by the severity of the tic, especially multiple motor and vocal tics lasting 1 year or more. Coprolalia is rare and certainly not a factor in diagnosing Tourette's syndrome.

Treatment includes assessing and treating any co-morbid conditions – especially anxiety, and educating schools so that children are not victimised. Some children will benefit from Child and Adolescent Mental Health Services (CAMHS) input to help with these issues. Children with severe Tourette's syndrome can benefit from tertiary referral to specialist clinics. Rarely drugs may be required. Common drugs used are haloperidol (the only one licensed for tics), clonidine, aripiprazole and risperidone.

Epilepsy

Juvenile myoclonic epilepsy can cause strange movements, but this is associated with violent jerks and there is not the same variety of movement. Episodes are usually less frequent.

Sydenham's chorea

This starts insidiously, often with myoclonic-like movements. Facial movements are prominent and the movements generalise and become continuous. Sydenham's chorea is classified as a paediatric autoimmune neuropsychiatric disorders associated with streptococcal infections (PANDAS) and it has been suggested tics might have a similar origin. Management includes long-term penicillin.

Metabolic disorders

These would usually present with more obvious neurological signs or symptoms. In this case, a metabolic cause was considered because of the episodes of heavy breathing, which the patient's mother recorded on a mobile phone, were not overt panting.

Wilson's disease

This autosomal recessive treatable disorder of copper metabolism presents usually after 8 years (but consider the diagnosis at any age) with neurological symptoms where facial grimacing is a classic feature. There could be speech impairment, also choreic and myoclonic movements. Kayser–Fleisher rings are visible on slit lamp examination. Features of liver failure are usually obvious. Treatment is with chelation therapy.

Tardive dyskinesia (late development of abnormal movements)

A movement disorder induced by neuroleptic drugs, especially the typical antipsychotics. The most common type is orofacial grimacing with stereotypic tongue protrusion, lip smacking or chewing. If this occurs the drugs should be stopped immediately. Unfortunately, the movements do not always resolve.

Consultation essentials

Clarify any suggestion of loss or clouding of consciousness during the tics which would imply an epileptic origin. An ability to continue activity uninterrupted is evidence against a diagnosis of epilepsy. The sheer variety of movement manifestations is also against that diagnosis. A history of recent sore throat would suggest possible streptococcal infection. A full drug history is clearly important. Enquire into aspects of behaviour and schooling.

History/examination

Tics might be observed in the clinic in which case one would be interested in the context, e.g. the child is busy with an activity. Very often tics are not apparent and it is useful to ask the parent to make a video-recording. Observing the tics can either confirm the diagnosis, or indicate what further specific examination is required.

Tests/investigations

Most authorities advise looking for and treating active streptococcal infection by performing a throat swab and anti-streptolysion O titre (ASOT) and commencing penicillin. Electroencephalography (EEG) would be important if epilepsy seemed likely. If there is any suspicion of Wilson's disease test serum copper, ceruloplasmin and liver function.

Diagnosis

In this case, the diagnosis is drug induced secondary tardive tics. It is not known why some children should react this way to stimulant medication. It is possible it has brought out a latent tendency. The tics themselves are not different from primary tics.

Management

As Gordon never liked the methylphenidate, this was stopped as soon as the tics developed, but the tics persisted. He was then started on atomoxetine for his ADHD. This produced little therapeutic response and the dose was limited due to its effect of drowsiness, and it was also discontinued. He similarly objected to its use. Gordon transferred to a special school for children with emotional and behavioural difficulty and he, and his tics, have settled down somewhat.

Follow up

This depends on several factors: the severity of the tics, the associated behavioural features and the decision to treat. Children on treatment will need monthly follow up, at least initially.

Discussion

Tics of any type can be extremely stigmatising, and this can lead to further problems. Unfortunately, until diagnosis, children may find themselves in trouble at school for tics, which are essentially involuntary. Tics are usually made worse by attracting attention, and calm down when they are ignored. They also tend to increase around the teenage years and become evident less towards the end of a child's teenage years. Tic suppression can be helpful, and allows children to limit the manifestation of tics at different times.

Further reading

Aicardi J. Diseases of the Nervous System in Childhood, Ist and 3rd edn. London: Mac Keith Press, 2009.
Robertson MM. The Gilles De La Tourette's syndrome: the current status. Arch Dis Child Educ Pract Ed 2012:9.
Chowdhury U, Heyman I. Tourette's syndrome in children, tic disorders are common and misunderstood. Br Med J 329 2004: 1356–1357. bmj.com
Jankovick J. Tourette's syndrome. N Engl J Med 2001; 345(16):1184–1192. www.nejm.org

Patient information

Tourettes action (UK)
www.tourettes-action.org.uk
Great Ormond Street Hospital
www.gosh.nhs.uk

Tongue tie

Dear Paediatrician,

The mother of this 4-week-old baby came to see me because of feeding difficulties and poor weight gain which the health visitor is attributing to a tongue tie. Mum remembers this was mentioned at the baby check and she was promised that she would be sent a referral to see a paediatrician, which hasn't materialised. She has researched tongue tie on the internet, and is concerned that it could cause later problems with speech and social adaptation. She would appreciate an appointment with a view to surgical intervention in the form of division of the tongue tie.

Yours sincerely,

Dr Jennifer Warburton

Case analysis

From the tone of the letter it seems likely that the family are coming to clinic with the clear purpose of having a frenotomy or frenuloplasty on the infant. An evaluation of the problem by a paediatrician to make a determination as to whether intervention is required may not be on their agenda. They may consider this appointment as part of the process to having surgery or may even be expecting that the procedure will be performed then and there.

If the child is genuinely failing to thrive then an immediate plan has to be made to combat this. It may include the use of high energy feeds and/or feeding via a nasogastric tube.

Differential diagnosis

Tongue tie meeting criteria for intervention

Ankyloglossia is the presence of an unusually short thick lingual frenulum. It can vary in severity from a mucous membrane band with just the inability to move the tip of the tongue beyond the lower incisor teeth, to a situation where the tongue is tethered to the floor of the mouth. The degree to which it affects feeding, speech, oral hygiene and its mechanical or social effects is variable. There is a difference of opinion amongst professionals as to how much of a problem this is, and how much of a solution can be provided by surgery. In studies, paediatricians do not perceive this as a major problem whilst lactation consultants, speech therapists and ENT surgeons perceive it as much more of an issue.

Other causes of feeding difficulty in early infancy

Although the health visitor has made a diagnosis of tongue tie, this is not confirmed. Other causes of poor feeding include:

Severe reflux/oral aversion

The baby may find feeding painful and feeding will be a struggle. In these cases always check for candida which is an easily treatable cause.

Suck-swallow in coordination

This can be a developmental issue. Coordinated sucking and swallowing should be present from about 34–36 weeks post conception. In some babies, it may be slower. If this baby is still around term, this could be a cause for poor feeding. Speech and language therapy might help, if there is no spontaneous improvement.

Cerebral palsy or neuromuscular problems

This covers a host of problems from hypotonia (and possibly hypothyroidism), to hypertonia (cerebral palsy). Management will depend on the diagnosis.

Cleft palate

A submucosal cleft can often only be diagnosed by looking, and is easily missed if the newborn exam has not incorporated this. If present it needs immediate referral to the specialist cleft palate team.

Micrognathia

This can be as part of Pierre-Robin sequence.

Macroglossia

Poor feeding and an abnormal tongue are often seen in macroglossia which can be idiopathic or syndromic.

Trisomy 21

Unfortunately, this is not always diagnosed at birth, and can be quite hard to diagnose in certain racial groups. It is often not diagnosed until the child is several months old. Usually, it would present with a protruding tongue.

Consultation essentials

History/examination

Establish any other reason for anxiety, e.g. family history of speech problems. Define nature of feeding difficulty – initial or sustained latch, sore nipples or mastitis in the mother, feed frequency and whether any breastfeeding advice has been offered and followed previously.

Specifically, assess if there is micrognathia. Observe the tongue focussing on whether it can protrude onto the lower lip margin and can touch the hard palate. Look at the appearance of frenulum, and see if there is any 'cupid' indentation of tongue on movement. Assess the palate by observation and look for any other local mouth problems, e.g. oral thrush.

Tests/investigations

Usually no tests are required.

Diagnosis

This child had significant tongue tie.

Management

He was referred to a paediatric surgeon who performed frenotomy in clinic to good effect.

Follow up

It is always sensible to have a further appointment, in case the intervention does not solve the problem. In this situation, a new hypothesis and plan needs to be made. If, however, the problem resolves the family can be advised to cancel the follow-up appointment.

Discussion

The management of tongue tie and particularly the role of frenotomy has always been controversial and in 1994 the National Institute for Health and Care Excellence interventional group assessed the evidence for this practice. Their guidance, recently updated, suggests that in some cases early frenotomy is indicated to help with the maintenance of breastfeeding. The evidence is less clear for speech problems where at best there may be some articulation issues which can easily be compensated for by the patient. It is well established that the frenulum naturally recedes during the process of a child's growth between 6 months and 6 years and adopting a wait-and-see approach, certainly in milder cases, is not unreasonable.

Further reading

National Institute for Health and Care Excellence (NICE). Division of ankyloglossia (tongue-tie) for breastfeeding. London: NICE, 1994.
www.nice.org.uk/IPG149

Patient information

NHS
www.nhs.uk
National Institute for Health and Care Excellence
www.nice.org.uk

Case 77

Tremor

Dear Paediatrician,

Thank you for seeing Albert who is now 9 years old and has very significant tremor and shaking. This can be extremely disabling, e.g. his writing is becoming difficult and he often spills his drinks. As this is clearly having a major impact on Albert and his family, I would appreciate your urgent help.

Yours sincerely,

Dr Catherine Bush

Case analysis

Although tremor is identified in the letter it is important to distinguish this from other movement disorders, such as myoclonus and dystonia. Tremor is a rhythmic, involuntary, oscillating movement, which has a frequency usually of 6–10 Hz. Whatever the cause of Albert's tremor, it is clearly having a major impact on his life. Ideally a cause and subsequent cure will be identified, but it maybe that the tremor is ameliorated rather than abolished; in which case he might need help dealing with its consequences.

Tremor can be divided into different types, and all tremors can be made worse by secondary causes, e.g. caffeine.

- Resting tremor occurs when the body is at complete rest and supported, e.g. tremor in the arms when they are resting on a table. The tremor amplitude usually decreases with activity. This tremor is uncommon in paediatrics, but may be seen in Wilson's disease, or in some drug-induced tremors. In adults it is common in Parkinson's disease or long-standing essential tremor
- Postural tremor occurs when trying to maintain a position against gravity, e.g. with an outstretched arm, the tremor amplitude usually increases with action
- Action or kinetic tremors occur during voluntary movement. Tremors may have postural and kinetic components. Causes of postural/kinetic tremors include:
  - Essential tremor (primarily postural)
  - Metabolic disorders (thyrotoxicosis, pheochromocytoma, hypoglycaemia)
  - Drug-induced parkinsonism (lithium, amiodarone, β-adrenergic agonists)
  - Toxins (alcohol withdrawal, heavy metals)
  - Neuropathic tremor (neuropathy)

Other forms of tremor are extremely rare in childhood. There are some specific tremors, such as writing tremor, and intention or terminal tremors, where there is a marked increase in amplitude at the end of a specific movement. Intention tremor can occur following cerebellar lesions and multiple sclerosis.

Differential diagnosis

Physiological tremor

Some degree of mild tremor is normal. If the tremor does not interfere at all with life, it may be labelled as physiological. Clearly, there will be some debate as to when physiological tremor becomes essential.

Essential tremor, benign essential tremor

Although this tremor has a benign pathology, the impact that it can have is often not so benign, and hence the benign label has been removed from its definition. Essential tremor (ET) occurs in about 5% of children, usually with a strong family history. Symptoms usually start in adolescence, and it is rare for ET to cause significant functional difficulties below the age of 10 years.

The tremor usually starts in the hands, but can progress. It is often both postural and kinetic, but may be one or the other, and tremor frequency increases slightly with age. It can cause significant difficulties, e.g. with drinking, eating and writing, texting or applying make-up. The tremor can be exacerbated by anxiety, which is problematic as tremor may itself generate anxiety. Similarly, fatigue or causes of secondary tremor can exacerbate the symptoms.

Management involves treating any secondary causes for tremor, and trying to manage the situation. Children with significant symptoms may need psychological support, and help at school, such as assistance to write their exam papers. Medication can be tried, although there is limited evidence of effectiveness. Propranolol is the most commonly used drug. There is some indication that the modern antiepileptic medications such as topiramate or gabapentin may be of benefit.

Orthostatic tremor

This is considered to be a variant of essential tremor. This type of tremor occurs in the legs immediately on standing and is relieved by sitting down. Orthostatic tremor is usually high frequency (14–18 Hz), and no other clinical signs or symptoms are present.

Psychogenic tremor

This usually has an acute onset, and is variable in amplitude and frequency, typically appearing in a much exaggerated form. It may shift around different parts of the body and usually stops when the young person is distracted. It is very uncommon, and should be straightforward to diagnose. Management is with psychological support.

Secondary tremor

Tremor can be caused or exacerbated by a number of factors.

Drug induced tremor

Numerous drugs may cause tremor including:
- Caffeine/alcohol/recreational drugs
- Opiate withdrawal
- β-adrenergic agonists, e.g. Salbutamol

- Anticonvulsants – sodium valproate, carbamazepine
- Endocrine drugs – thyroxine, hypoglycaemics, adrenocorticosteroids
- Tricyclic antidepressants, neuroleptics, lithium
- Others include cimetidine and monosodium glutamate

Metabolic disturbances

Metabolic abnormalities can cause or exacerbate tremor. In particular, hyperthyroidism, hypoglycaemia and even more rarely phaeochromocytoma or a Cushing's tumour.

Heavy metal poisoning

Heavy metal poisoning may cause tremor, but there would invariably be other symptoms.

Wilson's disease

Although this is extremely rare, many people worry about missing this. Invariably, children with Wilson's disease present with symptoms and signs of liver failure. Although tremor is a feature of Wilson's disease, it is almost unheard of for there not to be significant other, liver and neurological features. In Wilson's disease, there is a resting tremor, which can occur with movement as well. Diagnosis is confirmed by measuring copper and its metabolites and getting a slit lamp examination performed which should show the pathognomonic Kayser–Fleischer rings.

Brain injury

Tremor can follow acute brain injury. In an acute upper motor neurone lesion there may be fasciculation, but tremor may be a long-term side effect of spasticity. Similarly, dystonias may mimic or create tremors, and cerebellar lesions can also cause tremor. These are all rare events and will present with more than just tremor.

Juvenile myoclonic epilepsy

The myoclonus of juvenile myoclonic epilepsy (JME) may be reported as tremor. As episodes can occur at any time, the history often includes details such as spilling drinks or throwing food. However, there is no tremor with JME in between attacks.

Tic disorder

Some tics may present as tremor. In general tics will involve movement-like activity rather than simply shaking.

Consultation essentials

History

The history should include the age of onset of tremor, whether it has changed in any way and what factors make it better or worse. Causes of secondary tremor should be actively sought, and although there are drugs where tremor is a known side-effect, it may be an unknown side-effect of others. Therefore, any medication. the child is taking must be considered a potential culprit if there is a reasonable temporal link between starting it and the onset of tremor.

The presence of a family history, and the absence of any other symptoms makes essential tremor more likely.

Examination

Examination should clearly identify the nature of tremor. A resting tremor is invariably pathological, or psychological. A normal neurological examination makes a central nervous system disease, much less likely.

Tests/investigations

If the diagnosis is clearly essential tremor, then no further tests are required. As with many conditions, there are numerous potential investigations that may be undertaken.

Measuring thyroid function and copper and caeruloplasmin, may reveal diagnoses, which then respond to treatment. Other investigations will depend on clinical findings.

Imaging studies are rarely indicated, but frequently performed. Similarly, electrophysiology is unlikely to provide any useful information, unless there is diagnostic uncertainty.

Diagnosis

Albert clearly had features of essential tremor. There was a positive family history.

Management

Initially, no further action was required. However, over the years, his tremor became more marked, and significantly interfered with life, particularly at school. He commenced propranolol, but had to stop this due to side effects. He was commenced on a small dose of topiramate. Fortunately, his school was very understanding, although he did require some help from the school counsellor.

Follow up

Follow up depends on the severity of the symptoms. In Albert's case, he received follow up, essentially to monitor his response to medication.

Discussion

An understanding of causes of tremor can prevent over investigation. It is easy to focus too much on the cause of tremor, rather than its effects. In many cases of essential tremor, the tremor will become more troublesome in teenage years, and therefore the support, both medical and social that the child requires is likely to change over time.

Further reading

Crawford P, Zimmerman E. Differentiation and diagnosis of tremor. Am Fam Physician 2011; 83(6):697–702.
Tremor Disorders in Children: a guide for healthcare professionals
www.essentialtremor.org

Patient information

The International Essential Tremor Foundation
www.essentialtremor.org

Visual problems

Dear Paediatrician,

Please would you see this 3-month-old boy urgently. His parents are concerned that he doesn't seem to focus like his sister did at the same age. I was not able to see any obvious problem with his eyes. However, he doesn't have very good head control, and the family are not sure whether he is smiling or not.

He was born at full term and there were no problems with the pregnancy or delivery. He has had no illnesses. It took a week or so for him to establish breastfeeding but his weight gain has been satisfactory since.

Dr Richard May

Case analysis

The parents are worried. They are likely to be concerned that their child is blind. Because the list of possible causes could include serious problems and conditions with time-critical treatments, it is justifiable to see this child quickly, within a week or two at the most. The assessment could be with a developmental paediatrician or an ophthalmologist in a children's eye service.

Differential diagnosis

Eye problems

Cataract and other abnormalities of the eye, including extreme long sightedness may present like this. If the child cannot see well enough to fixate then he will not be able to follow gaze either.

Eye movement disorders

The child may be able to see but not move his eyes as the parents expect, and therefore they conclude he is not watching them. A squint or more serious neurological problem involving cranial nerves such as Mobius syndrome might be considered.

Brain problems

A cortical blindness may present with concerns about vision. Many children with brain injury have damage to the visual tracts and although they have normal eyes they behave as if they cannot see, because the visual information is not interpreted by the brain. These children usually have other evidence of brain injury such as signs of cerebral palsy and a history to explain their condition. These children may appear to be able to see better some days than others. Delayed visual maturation is a situation where the child also appears to have impaired vision in the presence of normal eyes. They are less likely to have a history of brain damage but often have other evidence of developmental delay. Their vision improves throughout the first few years of life, and MRI usually shows delayed myelinisation.

Other developmental problems

Consider cerebral palsy or a motor disorder restricting movement. If the parents are judging the child's visual ability on the presence of visual tracking, any condition which restricts the movement of the face and neck may be the cause.

Normal child with anxious parents

Sometimes the parents' concern is the single most important factor, and clinical assessment concludes that the child can fix and follow. While that does not preclude a more significant diagnosis, it can help to reassure while assessments are pending.

Consultation essentials

History

Take a birth and full developmental history to date. Ask about a family history of any visual problems. Detail the parents' concerns and what, if anything, the child looks at, including the distances where these objects appear to be seen. For example, does he fix at 50 cm but not at 2 m.

Examination

Check for a red reflex and pupillary responses.
Perform ophthalmoscopy: If there are any concerns, this may need to be performed by a specialist ophthalmologist. Assess fixation and tracking using a variety of sized and varyingly bright objects. If the child does not fix or track a face at 50 cm, or a bright red object at a similar distance, check to see whether he turns to diffuse light. Assess general muscle tone and for any other problems raised in the history.

Tests/investigations

The child may warrant a full ophthalmic assessment and consideration of visual-evoked response testing if there is no local reason for impaired vision. If there are additional neurological concerns then an MRI may be helpful. A strong family history may warrant further genetic investigation especially if associated with other physical or developmental abnormalities.

Diagnosis

The referral history for this child hints at other problems. Absence of definite smiling at this age is a concern, as is the poor head control. Lack of smiling is more likely to indicate developmental delay than visual impairment even if the impairment is severe. Assuming that neonatal checks were done thoroughly and the birth history is normal, the most likely reason for this baby's problem is delayed visual maturation (also known as cortical visual impairment) which can be associated with a variety of causes of developmental delay.

Management

The baby with delayed visual maturation requires a thorough neurological assessment, and referral to a paediatric ophthalmologist for assessment of visual pathways. If there are concerns about generally delayed development a full neurodevelopmental assessment would be planned for a later stage (typically around 2 years of age). If the child's vision is good enough at that time a Griffiths developmental assessment would be appropriate but if the child remains visually impaired a more specialised developmental assessment (Reynell – Zinkin scale) may be required.

Follow up

Physiotherapy may be indicated if the motor development is delayed. A programme of specific visual stimulation should be worked on by the parents and any other carers. This in principle would start by securing the child's visual attention (e.g. with a bright torch in a darkened room) and working on fixing and tracking in that setting, and then gradually working on focussing attention on smaller and duller objects at a greater distance. Children with significant visual impairment (even if thought to be temporary) should be referred to the specialist visual impairment teaching team, who will follow a developmental education programme, including visual stimulation and general learning.

Discussion

The prognosis for vision in children with delayed visual maturation is good, and their overall outcome depends on the underlying reason for the condition. They often continue to have mild or moderate learning problems.

Most cataracts should be detected at neonatal checks, but some are missed and some develop later. Therefore, a red reflex assessment or more definitive examination if available should be performed. Ophthalmoscopy to exclude other eye problems may also be needed if a cataract is confirmed.

Patient information

Royal National Institute of Blind People
    www.rnib.org.uk

Vulvovaginitis

Dear Paediatrician,

Please can you review Jenny who is 3 years old. She has had frequent episodes of vaginal discharge and irritation. In the most recent episode of discharge, a swab grew pseudomonas and she was treated with a week's course of ciprofloxacin. She is otherwise well and her mother wonders why she keeps getting infections. Please can you investigate her.

Dr Greg McElnay

Case analysis

The discharge is almost certainly caused by vulvovaginitis which is a common problem in young girls and is usually sorted with some simple measures as detailed below. The sensitive nature of dealing with a young girl's genitalia must be remembered but with the parent's/mother's support, assessment can be done carefully and without too much distress to child, doctor or parent.

Differential diagnosis

Vulvovaginitis

This is a common condition of lower urinary and genital tract of girls which manifests as irritation of, and discharge from, the vulva. Vaginal discharge is not uncommon in the first 3 months of life and then decreases through childhood to puberty. The reasons for the irritation are probably multifactorial encompassing a combination of the vulnerability of the prepubertal skin, local irritation due to hygiene, poor wiping and local infection or infestation. Sometimes there may be a physical issue such as fused labia. This will respond to topical oestrogen cream which mimics changes at puberty when labial separation would be expected as oestrogen levels rise. Sometimes surgical division is required. Repeated irritation of the skin in this area can contribute to fusion.

Lichen sclerosis

This is a skin condition of unknown aetiology, possibly autoimmune. It can present in a similar way to vulvovaginitis. It is characterised by atrophic, pale patches on the labia and may extend to the perineum. The patches may coalesce and be extensive in the genital area. There are often symptoms of local irritation and itch. When scratched, the skin is vulnerable to further inflammation and local minor bleeding. It can mistakenly be taken as a sign of sexual abuse. Often it will clear up on its own. Application of barrier greasy ointments may help. Topical mild steroid may be necessary for resistant cases.

Infection/bacterial vulvovaginitis

It may be difficult to resist swabbing a vaginal discharge in a young girl, especially when there is report of a foul smell to the discharge. Usually, this would be a vulval swab, rather than a vaginal swab (which is usually performed during an internal examination using a speculum, and is never performed in prepubescent children). Between the ages of 2 and 7 years vaginal discharge is common. This area is vulnerable because anatomically, the young girl has an exposed vaginal introitus once the maternal oestrogen effects have worn off. These create thick and well-developed labia majora in neonates. With low levels of oestrogen in prepubertal girls, the skin is thin and atrophic and vulnerable to infection. Similarly, a maternal oestrogen in neonates encourages presence of lactobacilli which cause acidic pH of the vaginal fluid. When oestrogens reduce, the lactobacilli reduce and the pH increases, reducing the resistance to infection. Isolated organisms include β-haemolytic *Streptococcus*, *Haemophilus influenzae* type B, *Klebsiella pneumoniae*, *Shigella flexneri*. Other bacteria such as *Streptococcus viridans*, proteus species and pseudomonas species are known to occur in healthy prepubertal girls but are not always considered to be pathogenic. Candida species has not been shown to be a major cause of infection in young girls with these symptoms.

Worms

The commonest infestation is threadworms (*Enterobius vermicularis*). They cause anal itching, particularly at night when they migrate out of the bowel and lay eggs in the perineal skin. This causes localised itching and symptoms are worse at night. Confirmation of the diagnosis is by the Sellotape test, applying the sticky tape to the anus at night and removing it in the morning. It is then examined under the microscope in the lab where ova may be seen. Treatment with mebendazole is usually sufficient. The whole family needs to be treated. Careful attention to hygiene and sharing towels can be helpful in preventing re-infection. The ova live under nails when perineal skin is scratched, and then ingested, to repeat the cycle.

Lower urinary tract infection

A lower urinary tract infection (UTI) is a possibility. Usually, a specimen will be sent for culture and the careful evaluation of a clean catch sample for leucocytes, nitrites, microscopy for white and red cells and culture will help identify a UTI. The distinction between a lower UTI (dysuria, frequency, lower abdominal discomfort, constipation) and upper UTI (fever, loin pain, generally unwell) is important.

Vaginal foreign body

A young girl with vaginal discharge and irritation could have a vaginal foreign body. Based on one small study, only about half the children will remember (or admit) inserting the object. Usual symptoms are vaginal bleeding and blood-stained or foul-smelling vaginal discharge. Often the foreign body can be seen, however removal (or examination) may need to be under general anaesthetic depending on the compliance of the child. Vaginal bleeding is also associated with a straddle injury, causing a vaginal or vulval laceration.

Gratification

Masterbation is not an uncommon behaviour in young girls. The repetitive rubbing or grinding can irritate the external genitalia and contribute to vulvovaginitis symptoms.

Behavioural modification with distraction techniques and positive reinforcement to avoid are effective strategies.

Sexual abuse

Child sexual abuse would not normally present in this way. A general question, 'I am sorry to have to ask this, but given the problem do you think that anybody could have been interfering with her' seems reasonable. In the absence of any disclosure or suggestive signs there is little indication to pursue this further. Vulval symptoms which are consistent with signs of trauma such as large, gaping hymeneal opening will necessitate discussion with the local safeguarding team and a formal examination by a designated doctor. Other signs and symptoms might include sexualised behaviour or soiling, and sexually transmitted infections.

Consultation essentials

History/examination

Question about duration and intermittent symptoms may suggest correlation with bathing or issues around hygiene. The amount, colour and odour of any discharge should be clarified. An assessment of their toileting habits would be helpful to know how frequently they micturate and open their bowels. This will also instigate discussion on their wiping, especially if they are self toileting.

A specific assessment of constipation would be important.

Discussing bathing or showering habits and the use of bubble bath, type of clothing, amount of drinks consumed through the day and any itching at night may also assist in aetiology.

Examination must include the rest of the skin (could be general skin disorder), abdomen (for palpable bladder and faecal loading) and external genitalia. Establish whether the child has a name for their genitalia and explain very carefully that you need to have a look. Parents are usually happy to facilitate this and many have managed this expectation before the consultation. Ask a nurse to chaperone. Ask the child to remove their underwear and lie on the couch with a sheet to cover them and keep their modesty. The girl should put her knees up in the midline and then drop them laterally to each side into the frog leg posture. This gives a view of the external genitalia for visual inspection. It may be helpful to look at the underwear to assess any discharge or soiling.

Tests/investigations

A swab might be appropriate in some situations. Urine sample might be indicated in dysuria and urinary symptoms.

Diagnosis

Jenny has vulvovaginitis. While pseudomonas on vulval swab of the discharge is less common than other organisms, it may not be pathogenic. It was treated and the symptoms seemed to improve. In reality, there may have been an element of constipation contributing as the whole episode coincided with her toilet training. There was slight redness of the labia and vulval skin on examination but no other abnormal features. A vulvovaginitis leaflet was given to her mother with an explanation of how to manage the condition. She was encouraged to increase Jenny's fluids and fibre in her diet. The symptoms settled and she was discharged back to the general practitioner at the follow-up appointment.

Management

An approach to this condition involves implementing the following strategies:
- Careful attention to wiping (down at the front and up at the back) after toileting. Children become more independent and with that independence comes the ineffective or vigorous wiping which can contribute to irritation
- Wearing 100% cotton underwear which will allow moisture to be absorbed, rather than polyester mixes which contribute to sweat production
- Loose-fitting clothing can help to 'air' – wear skirts rather than jeans or trousers
- Effective bladder emptying – encourage double voiding and ensure plenty of fluid intake
- Avoid constipation – fluids and fibre will help with this. Pay attention to wiping after passing stool
- Do not use bubble bath and do not wash hair in the bath. Or at least shower down after ensuring all soap suds are removed before patting the area dry
- Protecting the skin with a barrier cream and applying emollient can be helpful

Follow up

Follow up may be offered to review the symptoms and ensure there are no other problems. Sometime families need further support and encouragement to manage some of the strategies outlined in management.

Discussion

Working through the usual causes of vulvovaginitis can help rule in or out a specific trigger. Often parents will suggest they have tried some or all of those strategies. Very occasionally a resistant case may need formal dermatological input, or review by an adolescent gynaecologist who may be comfortable assessing young girls – often jointly with a paediatrician.

Further reading

Garden A. Vulvovaginitis and other common childhood gynaecological conditions. Arch Dis Child Educ Pract Ed 2011; 96:73–78.
Stricker T, Navratil F, Sennhauser FH. Vulvovaginitis in prepubertal girls. Arch Dis Child 2003; 88:324–326
Stricker T, Navratil F, Sennhauser FH. Vaginal foreign bodies. J. Paediatr. Child Health 2004; 40:205–207.

Patient information

The Royal Children's Hospital, Melbourne
    www.rch.org.au